SHORT TEXTBOOK OF PUBLIC HEALTH MEDICINE FOR THE TROPICS

SHORT TEXTBOOK OF PUBLIC HEALTH MEDICINE FOR THE TROPICS

4th edition

Adetokunbo O. Lucas

OFR MD DSc DPH DTM&H SMHyg FRCP FMCPH FFPH FRCOG
Adjunct Professor of International Health,
Harvard University, Cambridge, USA;
Visiting Professor, London School of Hygiene and
Tropical Medicine, University of London;
formerly Professor of Preventive and
Social Medicine, University of Ibadan

Herbert M. Gilles

UOH BSc MD MSc DSc FRCP FFPH FMCPH DTM&H DMedSc
Emeritus Professor, University of Liverpool;
Visiting Professor of Public Health, University of
Malta; formerly Professor of Tropical Medicine and
Dean, Liverpool School of Tropical Medicine,
Liverpool; formerly Professor of Preventive and
Social Medicine, University of Ibadan

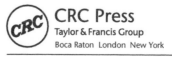

CRC Press
Taylor & Francis Group
Boca Raton London New York

CRC Press is an imprint of the
Taylor & Francis Group, an **informa** business

CRC Press
Taylor & Francis Group
6000 Broken Sound Parkway NW, Suite 300
Boca Raton, FL 33487-2742

© 2002 by AO Lucas and H M Gilles
CRC Press is an imprint of Taylor & Francis Group, an Informa business

No claim to original U.S. Government works

Printed and bound in Great Britain by CPI Group (UK) Ltd, Croydon, CR0 4YY
Version Date: 20151008

International Standard Book Number-13: 978-0-340-75988-2 (Pack - Book and Ebook) 978-0-340-81645-5 (Paperback)

Visit the Taylor & Francis Web site at
http://www.taylorandfrancis.com

and the CRC Press Web site at
http://www.crcpress.com

DEDICATION

To Kofo and Mejra

CONTENTS

CONTENTS

PREFACE

When the first edition of this book was published in 1973, it was designed to serve the needs of public health students in developing countries. Standard textbooks that were produced for use in developed countries in Europe and North America covered the basic principles of public health but the illustrative examples were drawn mainly from situations in advanced developed countries. Such textbooks did not adequately cover issues of concern to public health practitioners in developing countries of the tropics. This new edition retains the aims of previous editions of the textbooks but it also responds to important changes that have occurred in public health over the past three decades.

First, the process of epidemiological and demographic transition has altered the pattern of disease in developing countries. On the one hand, there has been steady progress in controlling the traditional health problems – childhood diseases and communicable diseases. On the other hand, chronic diseases such as cancers, cardiovascular diseases and diabetes are becoming increasingly prominent causes of morbidity and mortality. With the rising expectation of life, developing countries have to pay increasing attention to health problems of adults and the disabling disorders of the aged.

Second, important changes have also occurred in the scope and content of public health practice. Until recently, the role of public health was narrowly defined as being mainly concerned with programmes that were designed to promote health generally and to prevent specific diseases. The links of public health practitioners to the delivery of health care was largely confined to organizing community-based services as for example in maternal and child health programmes. Over the past few decades, public health work has expanded its scope to embrace broader issues with regard to policy making, planning and monitoring of health services including quality control, financing of health care, and equity throughout the entire health system.

The new edition has responded to these changes. Whilst retaining a strong emphasis on the control of communicable diseases, the section on chronic diseases has been significantly expanded. For example, there is a new section on the abuse of tobacco, a global problem that is having an increasing impact in developing countries. On the widening mandate of public health, the introductory chapter includes an analysis of the modern definition of public health and its functions. The authors have also thoroughly revised the chapter on the organization of health services and a guest author has produced a new chapter on health economics.

The textbook does not attempt to be a comprehensive reference manual on all aspects of public health; it provides illustrative models of the public health approach to identifying and solving health problems. Rather than offering stereotyped pre-packaged answers, the textbook provides the logical basis for analysing problems and devising appropriate solutions. For example, it provides guidelines for the national programmes for the control of HIV/AIDS and the principles involved in the control of occupational diseases which can be used as templates for devising programmes that are relevant and appropriate in the context of the local situation.

One new feature of the 4th edition is the inclusion of colour plates that illustrate some of the ecological situations in the tropics as well as photographs of vectors, tools for disease control and other pictures that facilitate the understanding of matters described in the text.

ACKNOWLEDGEMENTS

The authors acknowledge a grant from the Rockefeller Foundation in support of the preparation and printing of this edition thereby enabling the publisher to offer the book at a price more affordable to readers in developing countries.

We thank GlaxoSmithKline for their generous contribution towards the cost of the coloured plates.

We thank Harcourt Health Sciences for permission of the publisher Mosby to publish the following figures from W. Peters and H. M. Gilles (1995) *Atlas of Tropical Medicine and Parasitology*, 4th edition. Mosby, ISBN 0723 420696: 15, 16, 38, 83, 155, 171, 175, 300, 321, 386, 404, 408, 449, 479, 487, 539, 655, 702

We thank WHO for permission to publish many figures and plates, all of which are acknowledged in the respective captions.

CONTRIBUTORS

Ann Burgess
Freelance Nutrition Consultant
Craiglea Cottage
Glenisla
Blair Gowrie
PH11 8PS
Scotland

Steven S. Forsythe
The Futures Group International
ICSC 17th Street
NW Suite 1000
Washington DC 20036
USA

Niall Roche
Environmental Health Adviser
Concern Worldwide
Dublin
Ireland

CHAPTER ONE

CONCEPTS IN PUBLIC HEALTH AND PREVENTIVE MEDICINE

- The dimensions of public health
- Modern public health
- Key public health functions

- The tropical environment
- The ecological approach to public health
- References and further reading

When this textbook was first published in 1973, it was designed to fill a gap in the medical literature. It directed attention to the special problems of disease prevention in the tropics and it emphasized major health problems peculiar to the tropics with particular reference to parasitic infections and other communicable diseases that are prevalent in warm climates. However, it was not a textbook of parasitology or microbiology in that it provided epidemiological approaches to disease control. In effect it approached public health from the viewpoint of tropical countries.

Over the past few decades, the science and practice of public health has evolved and its mandate has been enlarged. Rather than being strictly confined to limited role in disease prevention, public health has progressively become a central feature of the health sector through its involvement in policy-making, management and evaluation at every level of the health services.

The evolution of the discipline has highlighted the confusing nomenclature that is used to describe public health and its component elements. The oldest term, hygiene, embodied the early knowledge about value of sanitation and personal cleanliness. The name still persists in the title of some old institutions (e.g. London School of Hygiene and Tropical Medicine). As knowledge grew, the term hygiene was felt to be too narrow and a broader term public health was used more widely. The term public health did not survive unchallenged as new terms were introduced to define special aspects of the discipline. Some used the term 'preventive medicine'; others preferred 'social medicine', 'community medicine', or 'community health'.

Winslow's classical definition suggests that the term 'public health' encompasses all the ideas contained in the newer names (Box 1.1).

In a modern interpretation of Winslow's definition, Beaglehole and Bonita (1997) identified the following essential elements of modern public health:

- collective responsibility;
- prime role of the state in protecting and promoting the public's health;
- partnership with the population served;
- emphasis on prevention;
- recognizing underlying socio-economic determinants of health and disease;

> **Box 1.1: Winslow's definition of public health**
>
> '... the science and art of preventing disease, prolonging life, and promoting physical health and efficiency, through organized community efforts, for the sanitation of the environment, the control of community infections, the education of the individual in the principles of personal hygiene, the organization of medical and nursing service for the early detection and preventive treatment of disease, and the development of the social machinery which will ensure to every individual in the community a standard of living adequate for the maintenance of health.'

- identifying and dealing with proximal risk factors;
- multidisciplinary basis for action.

Or succinctly, Acheson summarized public health as: *'the science and art of preventing disease, promoting health and prolonging life, through organized effort of society'*.

THE DIMENSIONS OF PUBLIC HEALTH

It would be useful to explore the concepts contained in the four terms that are commonly used to describe different aspects of public health (Fig. 1.1):

- preventive medicine;
- social medicine;
- community health;
- community medicine.

PREVENTIVE MEDICINE

Prevention is better than cure is one of the prime messages of public health. It differentiates public health from the clinical disciplines that are primarily involved with the care of the sick, whilst public health emphasizes the avoidance of illness. Prevention was initially construed narrowly in terms of protective measures like vaccination and improved nutrition that target only healthy people with the aim of preventing the onset of disease. This concept was extended to cover the early diagnosis and treatment of sick persons with the aim of preventing advanced diseases and in the case of communicable diseases, in preventing the spread within the community. A further extension of the definition covers the treatment of sick individuals aimed at reversing damage and restoring function. This concept led to the classification of prevention into three levels later to be differentiated into five stages (Table 1.1).

SOCIAL MEDICINE

'The poor die young'

The rise of social medicine coincided with increasing realization of the links between social status

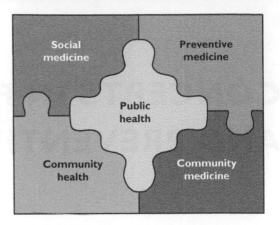

Figure 1.1: The dimensions of public health.

and the health of individuals and communities. Statistical analyses of mortality and morbidity data show strong correlation between the social stratification in society and the pattern of health and disease. At one end of the scale, the affluent educated privileged groups, including professional persons, senior managers, employers, enjoy significantly better health than the poor, deprived, illiterate and unemployed. Numerous studies in many countries confirm this association and point to the need for social interventions to complement biomedical tools in improving the health of the deprived sections of the community. The objective of social medicine is to identify the social determinants of health and disease in the community and to devise mechanisms for alleviating suffering and ill health through social policies and actions. Social medicine is based on certain fundamental assumptions:

- *Health as a birthright.* Everyone has the right to enjoy the highest possible level of health.
- *The responsibility of the state.* It is the duty of governments to ensure that the people have the basic elements that would enable families and individuals to maintain good health and that they have access to good quality health care.
- *Development and health are inter-related.* Good health promotes development, and development promotes health.
- *Education promotes health.* The strong association between health and level of education is particularly marked with regard to women's education. It affects their health status and behaviour as well as that of their children.
- *Social factors have a profound influence on health.* Culture, behaviour, social organization,

Table 1.1: Two classifications of preventive medicine

Three levels of prevention	Five stages of prevention
PRIMARY ■ *Target population*: entire population with special attention to healthy individuals ■ *Objective*: prevent onset of illness ■ *Methods*: education, immunization, nutrition, sanitation, etc.	1 *General health promotion* ■ *Target population*: entire population with special attention to healthy individuals ■ *Objective*: prevent onset of illness ■ *Methods*: education, nutrition, sanitation, life style changes, etc. 2 *Specific prophylaxis* ■ *Target population*: entire population with special attention to healthy individuals ■ *Objective*: prevent onset of specific diseases ■ *Methods*: education, immunization, nutritional supplement (vitamin A, iodine), chemoprophylaxis (e.g. against malaria)
SECONDARY ■ *Target population*: sick individuals ■ *Objective*: early diagnosis and treatment to prevent further damage to the individual and in cases of infectious diseases, spread to the community ■ *Methods*: screening of high risk groups e.g. Pap smears, sputum examination for TB; monitoring of vulnerable groups – children, pregnant women	3 *Early diagnosis and treatment* ■ *Target population*: sick individuals ■ *Objective*: early diagnosis and treatment to prevent further damage to the individual and in cases of infectious diseases, spread to the community ■ *Methods*: screening of high risk groups e.g. Pap smears, sputum examination for TB, blood test for HIV; monitoring of vulnerable groups – children, pregnant women
TERTIARY ■ *Target population*: sick patients ■ *Objective*: reduce damage from disease and restore function ■ *Method*: clinical care and rehabilitation	4 *Limiting damage* ■ *Target population*: sick patients ■ *Objective*: limit damage from disease ■ *Methods*: skilled clinical care and social support to limit physical and social damage from the disease 5 *Rehabilitation* ■ *Target population*: convalescent patients ■ *Objective*: restore function and capability ■ *Methods*: physical and social rehabilitation

allocation of family resources, healthcare seeking behaviour, etc.

■ *Health begins at home.* Many of the interventions required for promoting health in developing countries begin at home through changes in individual behaviour and lifestyle, in families and in households.

■ *Poverty* is a major underlying cause of ill health (Table 1.2).

The overall goal is to achieve equity in health. As noted in the Declaration at Alma Ata (p. 304):

'The existing gross inequality in the health status of the people particularly between developed and developing countries as well as within countries is politically, socially and economically unacceptable and is, therefore, of common concern to all countries'.

Alma Ata Declaration, WHO (1978)

Health and human behaviour

Human behaviour is an important dimension of social medicine. The link between health and human behaviour is a major area of interest in public health with medical anthropologists and sociologists providing specific professional expertise. The link between lifestyle and health is gaining more attention as chronic diseases increasingly dominate the epidemiological pattern. The risk factors associated with cancers, cardiovascular diseases, diabetes and other chronic diseases relate

Table 1.2: Comparing some health indicators of the poor versus the non-poor in selected countries. Source: WHO (1999)

| Country | Percentage of population in absolute poverty* | Probability of dying per 1000 | | | | Prevalence of tuberculosis | |
| | | Between birth and age 5 years, females | | Between ages 15 and 59 years, females | | | |
		Non-poor	Poor:non-poor ratio	Non-poor	Poor:non-poor ratio	Non-poor	Poor:non-poor ratio
Chile	15	7	8.3	34	12.3	7	8.0
China	22	28	6.6	35	11.0	13	3.8
Ecuador	8	45	4.9	107	4.4	25	1.8
India	53	40	4.3	84	3.7	28	2.5
Kenya	50	41	3.8	131	3.8	20	2.6
Malaysia	6	10	15.0	99	5.1	13	3.2

*Poverty is defined as income per capita less than or equal to $1 per day in dollars adjusted for purchasing power.

to such lifestyle choices as the use of tobacco and alcohol, diet, nutrition and exercise. The pandemic of HIV/AIDS has highlighted the health importance of sexual behaviour, making sex literally a matter of life and death: life in its reproductive function and death in its association with the risk of acquiring deadly diseases.

Access to and utilization of health services

Behavioural scientists are also interested in health-care seeking behaviour of individuals and families ranging from the self-treatment at home, to consultations with traditional or orthodox medical practitioners.

Information about beliefs, attitudes and behaviour provides the rational basis for developing programmes of health education for individuals and communities. Social medicine emphasizes the relationship between social factors and health status. It draws attention to the need for a multidisciplinary approach to health with deep involvement of social and behavioural scientists, economists, ethicists and political scientists.

COMMUNITY HEALTH

Community health deals with the services that aim at protecting the health of the community. The interventions vary from environmental sanitation including vector control to personal health care, immunization, health education and such like. It includes an important diagnostic element – 'community diagnosis' – aimed at surveying and monitoring community health needs and assessing the impact of interventions.

COMMUNITY MEDICINE

This usually refers to services that are provided at the community level and is now often encompassed in the new term primary care. Community physicians, nurses and other health-care personnel are involved in providing care at clinics, health centres and in people's homes.

MODERN PUBLIC HEALTH

The modern concept of public health includes all these elements – preventive medicine, social medicine, community medicine, community health. Important features of modern public health include the following characteristic features. It is:

- multidisciplinary;
- multisectoral;
- evidence-based;
- equity-oriented.

MULTIDISCIPLINARY

Although medical practitioners constitute a vital segment of the public health practitioners, the contributions from other health-related disciplines are absolutely essential for achieving the goals of public health. Thus, the public health team would include, as required, doctors, nurses, midwives, dentists and pharmacists; anthropologists, economists and other social scientists; philosophers, ethicists and other experts on moral sciences, as well as educationists, communications experts and managers. It is noteworthy that at the peak of its achievements, the late James Grant, a lawyer by profession, led UNICEF. Leadership in public health has to be earned from demonstrated ability and performance and not granted as a matter of course to the individual with a medical degree.

MULTISECTORAL

The health sector has two distinct roles. It is primarily responsible for planning and delivering health services. It also has an important leadership function in mobilizing intersectoral action. It should work with other ministries: with public works on water and sanitation; with education on the health of school children and health promotion; with transport on the control of road traffic accidents; and with agriculture on food security, nutrition, use of pesticides and the control of zoonotic infections.

EVIDENCE-BASED

Modern public health demands that decisions should be science-based and knowledge-based. As far as possible, policy-making should be made only after objective analysis of relevant information. Where information is lacking, there is a clear indication for gathering data and carrying out research to inform decision-making. It is often stated that researchers should present their results in a way that decision-makers can apply their findings. By the same token, policy-makers have the responsibility to ensure that their decisions are based on the best available scientific evidence. Both researchers and policy-makers with their common interest in promoting the health of the population need to work closely together in generating and using sound evidence as the basis of decision-making.

EQUITY-ORIENTED

Public health programmes must be designed to promote equity as the ultimate goal of all health action. The aim is to ensure for each member of society the highest possible level of health. Public health programmes should actively monitor equity and make necessary corrections. Public health practitioners must adopt a strong advocacy role in persuading decision-makers and influential members of society that, in the long run, equity in health is to everyone's advantage as a means of securing sustainable development and strengthening the social contract among citizens from a wide variety of backgrounds and between them and their governments. It should be made clear that solidarity with the poor is not merely an act of charity but a mechanism for promoting the welfare of all peoples (p. 284).

KEY PUBLIC HEALTH FUNCTIONS

Public health services perform a wide range of functions, which can be classified as four key elements (Fig. 1.2):

- assessing and monitoring of the health of the population;
- planning, implementing and evaluating public health programmes;
- identifying and dealing with environmental hazards;
- communicating with people and organizations to promote public health.

ASSESSING AND MONITORING OF THE HEALTH OF THE POPULATION

The objective is to identify and deal with health problems of the population. The activities range from the investigation of an acute epidemic outbreak to longer-term definition of the priority health problems and their determinants. The

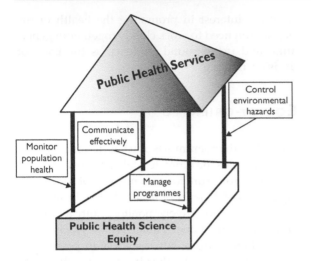

Key public health functions:
* Founded on a solid base of science to provide evidence-based decision-making
* Equity as the explicit goal
* Four pillars of support to the health services: monitoring population health, protecting against environmental hazards, designing and managing public health progammes and communicating effectively in support of public health.

Figure 1.2: Graphic representation of the role of public health.

public health approach also includes a ranking of problems in terms of their contribution to the burden of disease and their amenability to control through cost-effective interventions. The information gathered provides a sound basis for making decisions about the best approach for dealing with an acute emergency such as an outbreak of an epidemic disease like cholera; it also provides the basis for broader and longer-term decisions about policy, priorities and programmes (see Chapter 2).

PLANNING, IMPLEMENTING AND EVALUATING PUBLIC HEALTH PROGRAMMES

Public health practitioners are also concerned with the design and management of public health programmes at district, regional and national levels. Their role is dominant at the primary health-care level but they are also involved in decisions that affect services for the referral and specialist services (see Chapter 10).

IDENTIFYING AND DEALING WITH ENVIRONMENTAL HAZARDS

Protection of the population against environmental hazards including accidents is a prime function of public health. This is a well-recognized traditional role of public health with regard to the provision of safe water, the disposal of wastes, control of vectors and modern hazards from toxic wastes and radioactive chemicals (see Chapter 13).

COMMUNICATING WITH PEOPLE AND ORGANIZATIONS TO PROMOTE PUBLIC HEALTH

Effective communication is an important tool that public health workers use to bring about change in the behaviour of individuals and communities as well as in advising organizations within and outside the public sector (see Chapter 13).

THE TROPICAL ENVIRONMENT

The total environment of human beings includes all the living and non-living elements in their surroundings. It consists of three major components: physical, biological and social. The relationships of human beings to their environment is reciprocal in that the environment has a profound influence on them and they in turn make extensive alterations to the environment to meet their needs and desires (Fig. 1.3).

PHYSICAL ENVIRONMENT

This refers to the non-living part of the environment – air, soil, water, minerals – and climatic factors such as temperature and humidity. The physical environment is extremely variable in the tropics covering deserts, savannahs, upland jungle, cold dry or humid plateaux, marshlands, high mountain steppes or tropical rainforest.

Climatic factors such as temperature and humidity have a direct effect on humans, their comfort and their physical performance. The physical environment also exerts an indirect effect by determining the distribution of organisms in the biological

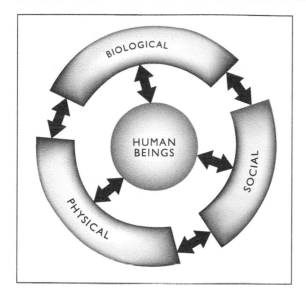

Figure 1.3: The interaction between human beings and their environment.

environment: plants and animals which provide food, clothing and shelter; animals which compete with humans for food; and parasites and their vectors which produce and transmit disease.

Humans alter the natural characteristics of the physical environment sometimes on a small scale but often on a very large scale: from clearing a small patch of bush, building a hut and digging a small canal to irrigate a vegetable garden to the building of large cities, draining of swamps, irrigating arid zones, damming rivers and creating large artificial lakes. Many such changes have proved beneficial but some aspects of these changes have created new hazards.

On the global scale, there is increasing concern that human activities are steadily leading to a significant rise in the earth's temperature with forecasts of dire results.

BIOLOGICAL ENVIRONMENT

All the living things in an area – plants, animals and micro-organisms – constitute the biological environment. They are dependent on each other and ultimately, on their physical environment. Thus, nitrogen-fixing organisms convert atmospheric nitrogen into the nitrates that are essential for plant life. Plants trap energy from the sun by photosynthesis. A mammal may obtain its nourishment by feeding on plants (herbivore) or on other animals (carnivore) or both (omnivore). Under natural conditions, there is a balanced relationship between the growth and the size of the population of a particular species, on the one hand, and its sources of food and prevalence of competitors and predators, on the other hand.

Humans deliberately manipulate the biological environment by cultivating useful plants to provide food, clothing and shelter, and raising farm animals for their meat, milk, leather, wool and other useful products. They hunt and kill wild animals, and destroy insects which transmit disease or which compete with them for food.

In many parts of the tropics, insects, snails and other vectors of disease abound and thrive. This is partly because the natural environment favours their survival but also because, in some of these areas, relatively little has been done to control these agents.

SOCIAL ENVIRONMENT

This is the part of the environment that is entirely made by humans. In essence, it represents the situation of human beings as members of society: family groups, village or urban communities, culture including beliefs and attitudes, the organization of society – politics and government, laws and the judicial system, the educational system, transport and communication, and social services including health care.

HEALTH AND DEVELOPMENT

The close link between health and development in other sectors is clearly recognizable. There is a clear correlation between economic, industrial and other indices of development and the health status of populations and communities. At one end of the spectrum are the industrialized, affluent developed countries and at the other end are the least developed countries that still rely largely on traditional agricultural practices and simple crafts. The term 'developing countries' is used to describe countries that have not as yet achieved a high level of industrial and economic development. Characteristic features of developing countries include relatively low income, low literacy rates, low access to electricity and other modern sources of energy, and high mortality rates among vulnerable groups (children, pregnant women). These factors interact: illiteracy is associated with poverty; poverty predisposes to ill health; and ill health aggravates poverty. The World Bank summarized the key indicators of the development gap:

- of the world's 6 billion people, 1.2 billion live on less than $1 a day;
- about 10 million children under the age of 5 years died in 1999, most from preventable diseases;
- more than 113 million primary school age children do not attend school – more of them girls than boys;
- more than 500 000 women die each year during pregnancy and childbirth from complications that could have been easily treated or prevented if the women had access to appropriate care;
- more than 14 million adolescents give birth each year.

The World Bank, the International Monetary Fund, the members of the Development Assistance Committee of the OECD, and many other agencies have adopted International Development Goals which set targets for reductions in poverty, improvements in health and education, and protection of the environment (Box 1.2).

There is much variation in the extent of technical development in the various countries in the tropics. Some of these countries are now highly developed whilst others are still in the early stages. Some of the developing countries show certain common features: limited central organization of services, scattered populations living in small self-contained units, low level of economic development, limited educational facilities, and inadequate control of common agents of disease. Some of these communities are still held tightly in the vicious circle of ignorance, poverty and disease (Fig. 1.4).

Two maps illustrate the diversity in income, life expectancy and fertility rates (Plates 1 and 2).

Many areas in the tropics are in transition. Rapid economic development and the growth of modern industries are causing mass migrations from rural to urban areas. Faster means of transportation, progress in education, the control and eradication of major endemic diseases, and other developments are effectively breaking the chains of disease, poverty and ignorance. At the same time new problems are emerging, including those resulting from the social and psychological stresses imposed by these bewildering changes and their destructive effects on traditional family life and communal relationships.

In these transitional societies there have been marked changes in the patterns of disease. Non-communicable diseases and conditions are now

---

Box 1.2: International development goals

Source: World Bank, World Development Indicators (2001)

- Halve the proportion of people living in extreme poverty between 1990 and 2015.
- Enroll all children in primary school by 2015.
- Empower women by eliminating gender disparities in primary and secondary education by 2005.
- Reduce infant and child mortality rates by two-thirds between 1990 and 2015.
- Reduce maternal mortality ratios by three-quarters between 1990 and 2015.
- Provide access to all who need reproductive health services by 2015.
- Implement national strategies for sustainable development by 2005 so as to reverse the loss of environmental resources by 2015.

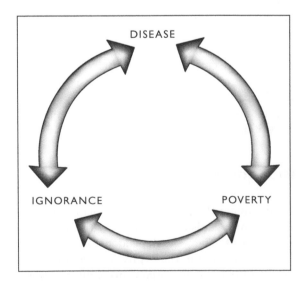

Figure 1.4: The cycle of ignorance, poverty and disease.

replacing communicable diseases which were formerly the predominant causes of disability, disease and death. Malnutrition in the form of the deficiency of specific nutrients is being succeeded by problems resulting from over-indulgence, thus obesity is replacing marasmus as the predominant nutritional problem. Alcoholism and drug abuse are emerging as manifestations of social stresses and tensions.

THE ECOLOGICAL APPROACH TO PUBLIC HEALTH

In public health, it is useful to consider the reciprocal relationship between humans and their total environment. In the search for the causes of disease, it is not sufficient merely to identify the specific agent of a disease, such as a virus or a parasite, but it is desirable to identify the influence of environmental factors on the interaction between humans and the specific agent. For example, the typhoid bacillus (*Salmonella typhi*) is known to be the causative agent of disease but the occurrence of outbreaks of typhoid is determined by various environmental factors: water supply, methods of sewage disposal, prevalence of typhoid carriers, personal habits of the people (cleanliness), use of raw water, attitude to and use of medical services, including vaccination. Similarly, a specific nutritional deficiency, such as ariboflavinosis, should not be viewed merely as a discrete metabolic defect but it should be seen in the context of the food habits of the community including food taboos, the level of education and income of the population and the local agriculture.

From this ecological approach, one can derive a rational basis for the control of disease within the population. Typhoid control should go beyond the treatment of the individual patient, to include immunization of susceptible groups, protection of water supplies, safe disposal of waste and improvement of personal hygiene. Malnutrition is managed not only by giving pills containing concentrated nutrients but also by giving suitable advice about diet and promoting the cultivation of nutritional foods both commercially by farmers and privately in home gardens; in more complex situations management may extend to promotion of welfare services such as unemployment benefits and food supplements for the needy. *The health*

worker should seek suitable opportunities for improving the health of the people through action on the environment. It is important that these lessons should be repeatedly emphasized.

The individual and the family can do much about the cleanliness of the home and its immediate surroundings, thereby reducing the occurrence of a number of infectious diseases. Domestic accidents, especially in such high-risk areas as the kitchen and the bathroom, can be prevented by careful attention to the environment in the home. The individual needs to recognize *how* the environment in the home affects the health of the family, *why* each person must act to improve the situation and *what* the individual and the family can do to deal with the problem.

The community should be approached as a whole to deal with the widespread problems that affect many families, and also for help with those problems which require action beyond the means of individual families. For example, certain environmental situations may require organization at the community level and must be designed in the context of the culture of the local community:

- collection and storage of water to ensure that each family has an adequate supply of safe water;
- disposal of human and other wastes;
- control of other environmental hazards (see Chapter 12).

In most developing countries, modern development projects and urbanization are introducing new risks (Plates 3–5). It is therefore necessary to ensure that these new initiatives should be carefully examined at the community level with regard to their appropriate siting and safe management, with minimal risk to the environment.

At the national and international level, large-scale projects such as the creation of artificial lakes, irrigation projects and mining of minerals including oil, require careful assessment of their environmental impact. The adverse effects can best be minimized by careful planning so that as far as possible protective measures can be incorporated into the design of these projects.

Some developed countries facing problems of disposing of toxic chemicals and radioactive waste have resorted to dumping them in developing countries. The serious concerns raised by these events should lead to tighter international controls.

Developing countries are also involved in dealing with environmental issues which are of global dimensions: the denudation of the tropical forest and its probable adverse effects on climate; the use of chlorofluorocarbons (CFCs) that destroy the ozone layer; and the extensive use of fossil fuel and consequent increase in greenhouse gases identified as the main cause of global warming.

REFERENCES AND FURTHER READING

Beaglehole R. & Bonita R. (1997) *Public Health at the Crossroads*. Cambridge University Press, Cambridge.

Evans T., Whitehead M., Diderichsen F. *et al.* (Eds) (2001) *Challenging Inequities in Health: From Ethics to Action*. Oxford University Press, New York.

Gwatkin D.R. (2000) Critical reflection: Health inequalities and the health of the poor: What do we know? What can we do? *Bull. WHO* 78, No. 1, 3–18.

Marmot M. (2001) Economic and social determinants of disease. *Bull. WHO* 79: 906–1004.

Marmot M. & Wilkinson R.G. (Eds) (1999) *Social Determinants of Health*. Oxford University Press, Oxford.

WHO (1976) *Health Hazards from New Environmental Pollutants*. Technical Report Series No. 586. WHO, Geneva.

WHO (1985) *Environmental Pollution in Relation to Development*. Technical Report Series No. 718. WHO, Geneva.

WHO (1992) *Our Planet, Our Health*. WHO Commission on Health and Environment, Geneva.

WHO (1994) *Environmental Health in Urban Development*. Technical Report Series No. 807. WHO, Geneva.

WHO (1999) *The World Health Report 1999 Making a Difference*. World Health Organization, Geneva.

WHO (2001) *Macroeconomics and Health: Investing in Health for Economic Development*. Report of the Commission on Macroeconomics and Health, December.

ADDENDUM ADDED AT REPRINT

MILLENNIUM DEVELOPMENT GOALS

At the Millennium Conference in New York in 2000, all 191 United Nations Member States have pledged by 2015 to:

1   Eradicate extreme poverty and hunger:
   ■ Reduce by half the proportion of people living on less than a dollar a day;
   ■ Reduce by half the proportion of people who suffer from hunger.
2   Achieve universal primary education:
   ■ Ensure that all boys and girls complete a full course of primary schooling.
3   Promote gender equality and empower women:
   ■ Eliminate gender disparity in primary and secondary education preferably by 2005, and at all levels by 2015.
4   Reduce child mortality:
   ■ Reduce by two-thirds the mortality rate among children under five.
5   Improve maternal health:
   ■ Reduce by three-quarters the maternal mortality ratio.
6   Combat HIV/AIDS, malaria and other diseases:
   ■ Halt and begin to reverse the spread of HIV/AIDS;
   ■ Halt and begin to reverse the incidence of malaria and other major diseases.
7   Ensure environmental sustainability:
   ■ Integrate the principles of sustainable development into country policies and programmes; reverse loss of environmental resources;
   ■ Reduce by half the proportion of people without sustainable access to safe drinking water;
   ■ Achieve significant improvement in the lives of at least 100 million slum-dwellers, by 2020.
8   Develop a global partnership for development:
   ■ Develop further an open trading and financial system that is rule-based, predictable and non-discriminatory. Includes a commitment to good governance, development and poverty reduction – nationally and internationally;
   ■ Address the least developed countries' special needs. This includes tariff- and quota-free access for their exports; enhanced debt relief for heavily indebted poor countries; cancellation of official bilateral debt; and more generous official development assistance for countries committed to poverty reduction;
   ■ Address the special needs of landlocked and small island developing States;
   ■ Deal comprehensively with developing countries' debt problems through national and international measures to make debt sustainable in the long term;
   ■ In cooperation with the developing countries, develop decent and productive work for youth;
   ■ In cooperation with pharmaceutical companies, provide access to affordable essential drugs in developing countries;
   ■ In cooperation with the private sector, make available the benefits of new technologies – especially information and communications technologies.

For more information on the Millennium Development Goals, see the following web sites: www.un.org/millenniumgoals; www.undg.org/login.cfm.

CHAPTER TWO

HEALTH STATISTICS: INFORMATION FOR HEALTH

- Types of data
- Collection of data
- Notification of diseases
- Analysis of data

- Modern information technology
- Geographical Information System (GIS)
- Presentation of data
- References and further reading

The assessment of the health of the individual is made on clinical grounds by medical history, physical examination, laboratory tests and other special investigations. Theoretically, one could assess the health of a whole community by conducting repeatedly a detailed clinical examination of each individual. In practice, the health status of the population is assessed less directly by the collection, analysis and interpretation of data about important events that serve as indicators of the health of the community – deaths (mortality data), sickness (morbidity data) and data about the utilization of medical services. The lack of reliable data in developing countries is an important obstacle to the effective management of health care and other social services. It is necessary to develop and improve information systems which decision makers and health-care givers can use for planning, implementing and evaluating services.

TYPES OF DATA

VITAL STATISTICS

These are records of vital events – births, deaths, marriages and divorces – obtained by registration (see p. 14). The data are used for generating birth and mortality rates for whole populations or subgroups.

MORBIDITY STATISTICS

Data on the occurrence and severity of sickness in a community may be obtained from a number of sources within the medical services (see Table 2.1). They are both more difficult to collect and to interpret than the data of vital statistics (see p. 19 and Fig. 2.2) but allow a more detailed analysis of health status and services.

HEALTH SERVICE STATISTICS

Two types of data can be derived from the operation of the health services:

- resources data;
- institutional records.

RESOURCES

For the efficient management of health services, it is useful to collect and analyse data about the resources available for the delivery of health care. The inventory should include data on all health institutions, both government and private (hospitals, health centres, dispensaries, medical clinics) and details of the numbers of various types of health personnel (doctors, nurses, midwives, etc.). The distribution of these resources in relation to the population should also be noted. This would show, for example, how far people in each community have to travel to reach the nearest institution which can provide them with various types of care. For example, how far is the nearest antenatal clinic, the referral centre at which caesarean section can be performed or blood transfusion given?

INSTITUTIONAL RECORDS

Records generated by health facilities can provide much useful information about the demand for and utilization of health services and about the extent to which various target groups within the population are being served. For example, what proportion of eligible children have been immunized? How many pregnant women received antenatal care and gave birth under the supervision of trained personnel? Such information can be used to plan, monitor and modify the health services. By relating the performance of the institutions to their resources, one can monitor efficiency and guide health policy. For a discussion of the use of statistics in monitoring the performance of health services, see Chapter 10.

DATA FROM OTHER SECTORS

Apart from data derived from the health services, information relevant to health can be obtained from other sectors of government:

- education (literacy rates, especially in girls and women);
- public works (housing, water supply, sanitation);
- agriculture (food production and distribution);
- economic planning and development (poverty, economic indicators).

COLLECTION OF DATA

A variety of mechanisms are used for the collection of the data which form the basis of health statistics

(Table 2.1). In order that health statistics from various communities can be compared, standardization of these methods is essential nationally and desirable internationally.

CENSUS OF THE POPULATION

This is required to provide the essential population base for calculating various rates. The census usually includes not only a total count of the population but also a record of the age and sex distribution, and some other personal data.

POPULATION PYRAMID

The age and sex structure of the population is often displayed in the form of a histogram showing the percentage distribution of each sex at 5-year age intervals. In the past, the shape of this diagram was roughly pyramidal in all parts of the world: the base, representing the youngest age group, tapering to a narrow peak in the oldest age group. In developing countries, the shape of the pyramid is determined by the high birth rate and high child death rate in these communities (Fig. 2.1a): with a broad base and a rapid tapering off in the older age groups. In more developed countries, the population pyramid shows more gradual decline, indicating the relatively older population with a low death rate in childhood (Fig. 2.1b).

NATIONAL CENSUSES

In most countries, national censuses are held periodically, usually every 10 years. In addition to the standard demographic information about age and sex, the census may also be used to gather additional information that can be used for planning in health and other sectors.

LOCAL CENSUSES

The public health worker may need to conduct a census on a small scale in a local area where national census data are unobtainable or not sufficiently

Table 2.1: Sources of different types of health statistics

Source	Examples	Type of data
Census	Local, national	Total count; age, sex distribution
Epidemiological surveys		
Questionnaires	Sickness surveys	Sickness absence from work/school
Physical examination	Nutritional survey	Anthropometric measurements
	Goitre survey	Physical examination
Special investigations	Serological surveys	Prevalence of HIV infection
	Tuberculosis survey	Tuberculin sensitivity established
Medical institutions		
Outpatient clinics	Health centre	Clinical records – pattern of diseases
Special clinics	Specific groups: e.g. maternal and child welfare	Attendance records Health profile of women and children
	Specific disease clinic: e.g. tuberculosis, sexually transmitted diseases	Clinical and epidemiological features
Inpatient services	General hospitals Specialist hospitals	Clinical records, laboratory results, autopsy data
Data collected for other purposes		
Routine medical examination	School entrants	Nutritional status, immunization rates
	Pre-employment/army recruits	Profile of health status of young adults
	Insurance	Baseline data, prevalence of risk factors
Sickness absence records	Schools, industry	Early warning of epidemics

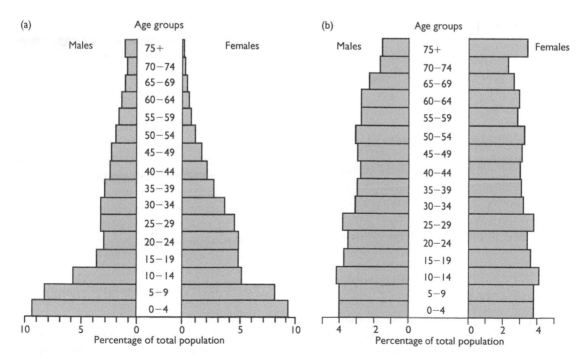

Figure 2.1: Population pyramids showing the distribution of males and females amongst different age groups (a) in a developing country, (b) in an industrialized country.

accurate for a proposed epidemiological survey. For some studies, the census is conducted on the basis of the number of persons who are actually present on the census date in the defined area; this *de facto* population may include temporary residents and visitors but may exclude permanent residents who happen to be away. For other studies, especially where a longitudinal survey is planned, the census enumerates all persons who are normally resident in an area; that is, this *de jure* population would exclude temporary residents and visitors but include permanent residents who are temporarily away.

REGISTRATION OF BIRTHS AND DEATHS

The registration of births and deaths is compulsory in the developed countries but only in some of the developing countries. Births and deaths are two important events which can be clearly recognised by lay persons and as such the data can be collected and recorded by trained literate persons. In addition to recording the fact of death, it is useful to establish the cause of death. The certification of the cause of death is done at various levels of sophistication, ranging from simple diagnoses that can be made by health auxiliaries to more difficult diagnoses that can only be obtained from elaborate investigations of the patients by highly trained personnel and post-mortem examination by competent pathologists.

Methods to improve registration

In many developing countries it is difficult to obtain a complete registration of births and deaths. Even where the local laws make such registrations compulsory, the enforcement of these regulations is difficult and unpopular. Various devices have been tried to improve the quality of the data.

REGISTRATION CENTRES

These should be conveniently sited so that each person has reasonable access to the registration centre in his or her district. The registration centre should be adapted to the local social structure, using such persons as village heads, heads of compounds, religious scribes, or institutions that are appropriate in the particular area.

REWARDS AND PENALTIES

In some countries the population is induced to register births by attaching rewards to the possession of birth certificates. For example, the government free primary school may be available only to children whose births have been registered. Unduly harsh penalties against defaulters are not to be recommended because such actions may antagonize the public and alienate them from other public health programmes and personnel. The system should emphasize positive inducements ('carrots') rather than sanctions ('whips').

Education

Regardless of the method of registration adopted, the success of the scheme will depend on being able to get appropriate and sufficient information to the general public about the programme. They must know why the procedure is considered necessary and what benefits it may bring to both the individual and the community.

NOTIFICATION OF DISEASES

NATIONAL NOTIFICATION

In every country there is a list of certain diseases, cases of which must be reported to the appropriate health authority. It includes communicable diseases, but in addition there are specific regulations about the reporting of certain industrial diseases. The notification of acute epidemic diseases is designed to provide the health authorities with information at an early stage so that they can take urgent action to control outbreaks of these infections. For example, the early notification of a case of typhoid would enable the health authorities to confine the epidemic to the smallest possible area in the shortest possible time. The notification of chronic and non-epidemic infections provides information which can be used in the long-term planning of health services and also in the assessment and monitoring of control programmes.

THE VALIDITY OF NOTIFICATIONS

Various factors may limit the usefulness of notifications in the control of disease. These problems, and their possible solutions, are summarized in Table 2.2.

Concealment of cases

Fear of forcible confinement in an isolation hospital, or of ostracism by the community (in diseases that carry a social stigma, e.g. leprosy, HIV/AIDS, other sexually transmitted diseases) may result in concealment of disease. This may be avoided by *education* to explain how notification can help both the individual and the community. *Feedback* of the compiled data allows those who contributed to see how this information is being used (see Table 2.2).

Errors of diagnosis

In well-equipped hospitals and health centres, laboratory and other diagnostic services facilitate clinical diagnosis: haematology, microbiology, histopathology, radiology, etc. These facilities are usually more limited in small peripheral institutions such as the primary health-care clinics in remote rural areas. In such situations, and sometimes in poorly equipped hospitals in developing countries, health personnel have limited access to laboratory services and have to rely on their clinical skills.

Under these conditions, diagnosis may be missed, particularly in cases that are atypical, mild or subclinical. In certain diseases, a high proportion of those infected do not feel or appear ill but may transmit infection (i.e. they act as carriers). Over-diagnosis may also occur. The quality and

comparability of the diagnoses obtained in such situations may be improved by:

- providing good laboratory services – with particular emphasis on simple techniques which the staff can use effectively and on equipment which can be maintained locally;
- training health personnel to improve their clinical and laboratory skills;
- establishing standard diagnostic criteria – including the use of simple algorithms.

Incomplete reporting

Correctly diagnosed cases may remain unreported due to ignorance or negligence on the part of the health worker. Simple forms assist case reporting. Where levels of literacy are low, health officials have used colour-coded cards carrying the address of the health office; the local informant can alert the health authorities about new cases of the reportable illnesses simply by dropping a card of the right colour in the post box. The village head can notify a case merely by posting a card of the appropriate colour.

INTERNATIONAL NOTIFICATION

A few diseases are subject to notification on the basis of international agreement. These internationally notifiable diseases, known also as 'quarantinable' or 'convention' diseases, are governed by International Sanitary Regulations. Formerly, six diseases were included (smallpox, plague, cholera, yellow fever, louse-borne typhus and louse-borne relapsing fever). Diseases currently notifiable to the World Health Organization are:

- plague;
- cholera;
- yellow fever.

Where health services are poorly developed, many cases of notifiable diseases are not recognized and are not reported. Thus, the official records include an incomplete and uncertain proportion of the cases that have occurred. In some instances, national authorities are reluctant to publicize outbreaks of communicable diseases for fear that such information could affect their tourist industry or have other damaging effects on the image of the country. The World Health Organization is therefore putting emphasis on strengthening the

Table 2.2: Factors limiting the usefulness of notification and how to overcome them

Problems	Solutions
Concealment of cases	Education Feedback
Errors of diagnosis: ■ Missed diagnosis ■ Over-diagnosis	Improved diagnosis: ■ Laboratory services ■ Training ■ Standard diagnostic criteria
Incomplete reporting	Simple forms Better supervision

capabilities of developing countries to carry out effective surveillance of major communicable diseases, and on its co-ordinating role in collecting information about infections which tend to spread from country to country (e.g. influenza, HIV infection). Some national authorities who suppress public health information that they find embarrassing sometimes frustrate these mechanisms for international exchange of information. Thus, notifications of diseases such as cholera and dengue are delayed or censored. For a long time, many African countries denied the occurrence of HIV/AIDS or grossly understated the number of cases in their countries. This led to long delays in instituting effective preventive measures.

DATA FROM MEDICAL INSTITUTIONS

Hospitals, health centres, clinical laboratories and other medical institutions provide easily accessible sources of health statistics (see Table 2.1), but such institutional data must be used and interpreted most cautiously.

Limitations

The pattern of disease, as seen in hospitals and in other medical institutions, is distorted by many factors of selection which operate from the patient's home to the point of being seen and the condition diagnosed in an institution (Fig. 2.2). The patient's action depends on awareness of being sick and knowledge that relief is available at a particular institution. The person then makes a choice of treatment from the available alternatives:

- self-treatment with traditional or modern drugs;
- treatment by traditional healers;
- treatment by quacks or other unqualified persons;
- modern medical treatment by a private medical practitioner or at the dispensary, health centre or hospital.

Factors in the institutions that can influence the pattern of disease include:

- the types of services offered by the institution;
- accessibility of the institution including such factors as the distance from home and the fees charged;

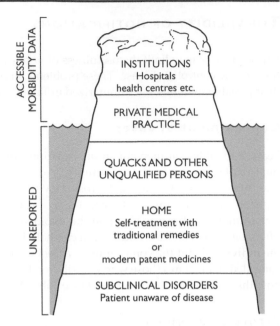

Figure 2.2: The iceberg phenomenon of morbidity assessment. Data from institutions such as hospitals represent an unknown proportion, and in some cases a very small proportion, of the cases in the community. Institutional cases are often no more than the tip of the iceberg; the nature and extent of the larger mass beneath the surface can only be discovered by well-designed epidemiological studies.

- the special interests and reputation of the personnel.

Thus, for example, the establishment of a bacteriological laboratory in a hospital might lead to an increase in the frequency with which certain diseases such as typhoid are diagnosed. The appointment of a specialist obstetrician in a hospital may lead to a concentration of difficult obstetric problems as a result of referrals from other doctors and self-selection by patients who have heard of the specialist's reputation. A free clinic may attract large numbers of patients, including relatively large numbers of the poor, whereas mainly the rich will use an expensive private clinic and those who have financial provision through insurance.

In addition to these selection effects, another defect of institutional data is that although the numerator (i.e. number of cases) is known, the denominator (i.e. the population at risk) is not easy to define. Comparisons from community to community on the basis of institutional data are difficult and fraught with the danger that erroneous conclusions may be based on the distorted pattern of hospital data.

In spite of these limitations and dangers, the information derived from medical institutions can usefully supplement data from other sources (see Table 2.1).

ANALYSIS OF DATA

RATES

Health statistics may be presented as absolute numbers but they are often expressed as rates (i.e. the number of events are related to the population involved) and, in order to simplify comparisons, rates are usually expressed in relation to an arbitrary total (e.g. 1000, 100 000 or 1 000 000).

$$\text{Rate} = \frac{\left[\begin{array}{c}\text{No. of persons affected or} \\ \text{number of events}\end{array}\right]}{\text{Population at risk}} \times 1000$$

Crude rates

Rates which are calculated with the total population in an area as the denominator are known as crude rates (Table 2.3). Crude rates from different populations cannot be easily compared, especially where there are striking differences in the age and sex structure of the population. Thus, the crude death rate may be relatively high in a population which has a high proportion of elderly persons compared with the rate in a younger population. If the death rate is to be used as an indicator of the health status of a population, adjustment of the crude rate is required. Standardizing the crude rate for age, sex or other peculiarities of the population may do this. The adjustment is made to a standard population.

Specific rates

Alternatively, rates may be calculated using data from specific segments of the population. These rates, using the particular population at risk as the denominator, are called specific rates (Table 2.3). For example:

Age/sex specific death rate

$$= \frac{\left[\begin{array}{c}\text{No. of deaths in people of} \\ \text{a specified age/sex}\end{array}\right]}{\left[\begin{array}{c}\text{No. of people in the specified} \\ \text{age/sex group}\end{array}\right]} \times 1000$$

The age-specific death rate in a total population may be analysed separately for each sex in 1-year age groups, or more conveniently, in 5-year or 10-year age groups.

VITAL STATISTICS: MORTALITY RATES

The various rates calculated from vital statistics may be used either to reflect the health status of a community as a whole, or to study the health problems and needs of specific groups. For example, rates of maternal death, stillbirth and perinatal mortality are of value in the analysis of obstetric problems and obstetric services.

The overall health of the community may be assessed using standardized death rates, although in practice, the mortality rates of the most susceptible age groups have proved to be more sensitive indicators.

INFANT MORTALITY RATE

The infant mortality rate is widely accepted as one of the most useful single measures of the health status of the community.

The infant mortality rate may be very high in communities where health and social services are poorly developed. Experience has shown that it can respond dramatically to relatively simple measures. Thus, with the establishment of maternal and child health services, the infant mortality rate may fall from being very high (200–300/1000 live births) to a moderate level (50–100/1000 live births).

In the most advanced nations the rate is low (below 20/1000 live births). Even in these developed communities, the infant mortality rate shows striking differences in the different socioeconomic groups: it may be as low as 10 deaths/1000 live births in the upper socioeconomic group whilst it is 40 deaths/1000 live births in the lower socioeconomic group of the same country.

Table 2.3: Some commonly used mortality rates in public health

Rate	Calculation (× 1000)
Crude rates	
Crude birth rate	$= \dfrac{\text{No. of live births in a year}}{\text{Mid-year population}}$
Crude death rate	$= \dfrac{\text{No. of deaths in a year}}{\text{Mid-year population}}$
Natural increase rate	$= \dfrac{\text{No. of live births minus no. of deaths in a year}}{\text{Mid-year population}}$
Specific rates	
Pregnancy and puerperium	
Fertility rate	$= \dfrac{\text{Total no. of births in a year}}{\text{No. of women aged 15–49 years}}$
Maternal mortality ratio	$= \dfrac{\left[\begin{array}{c}\text{Annual no. of maternal deaths due to pregnancy, childbirth} \\ \text{and puerperal conditions}\end{array}\right]}{\text{Total no. of births in a year}}$
Stillbirth rate	$= \dfrac{\text{Annual no. of foetal deaths after 28 weeks' gestation}}{\text{Total no. of births in a year}}$
Perinatal mortality rate	$= \dfrac{\text{Annual no. of stillbirths and deaths in the first 7 days}}{\text{Total no. of births in a year}}$
Infants and children	
Neonatal mortality rate	$= \dfrac{\text{Annual no. of deaths in the first 28 days}}{\text{No. of live births in a year}}$
Postneonatal mortality rate	$= \dfrac{\text{Annual no. of deaths between 28 days and 1 year}}{\text{No. of live births in a year}}$
Infant mortality rate	$= \dfrac{\text{Annual no. of deaths in the first year}}{\text{No. of live births in a year}}$
Child death rate	$= \dfrac{\text{Annual no. of deaths between 1 and 4 years}}{\text{No. of live births in a year}}$
Under five mortality rate	$= \dfrac{\text{Annual no. of deaths under 5 years}}{\text{No. of live births in a year}}$

NEONATAL AND POSTNEONATAL MORTALITY

The infant mortality rate is usually subdivided into two segments: the neonatal and the post-neonatal death rates (Table 2.3).

The neonatal death rate is related to problems arising during:

- pregnancy (congenital abnormalities, low birth-weight);
- delivery (birth injuries, asphyxia);
- after delivery (tetanus, other infections).

Thus, neonatal mortality rate is related to maternal and obstetric factors. The postneonatal mortality rate on the other hand is related to a variety of environmental factors and especially to the level of child care.

Improvement in maternal and child health services brings about a fall in both the neonatal and the postneonatal death rates, but the fall occurs more dramatically in the latter rate. Thus, at high infant mortality rates (200 deaths/1000 live births), most of the deaths occur in the postneonatal period but at very low levels (20 deaths/1000 live births), a high proportion of the deaths are neonatal and are mainly due to such problems as congenital abnormalities and immaturity.

UNDER FIVE MORTALITY RATE

In developed countries, the first year of life represents the period of highest risk in childhood and the death rate is very low in older children. In many tropical developing countries, although the first year does represent the period of highest risk, a high mortality rate persists in the older children. Thus, the infant mortality rate taken by itself underestimates the loss of child life. The under five mortality rate (U5MR), defined as the annual number of deaths of children under 5 years of age/1000 live births, is used to complete the picture.

The U5MR is low (below 20/1000) in developed countries, but shows a wide range in developing countries. Some developing countries – Chile, Costa Rica, Cuba – have achieved low U5MRs comparable with the rates in developed countries. However, the rates are above 150/1000 in a number of developing countries, especially in Africa.

The United Nations Children's Fund (UNICEF) advocates the use of U5MR as 'the single most important indicator of the state of the world's children'. UNICEF made this choice because it found that:

> U5MR reflects the nutritional health and the health knowledge of mothers; the level of immunization and ORT[1] use; the availability of maternal and child health services (including prenatal care); income and food availability in the family; the availability of clean water and safe sanitation; and the overall safety of the child's environment.

LIFE TABLES

By applying age-specific death rates to a cohort of persons, one can generate a life table which shows

the probability of survival at different ages. A life table from birth – *life expectancy at birth* – shows the average longevity of the population. In developed countries, life expectancy at birth is over 70 years but it is under 50 years in some developing countries.

MORBIDITY STATISTICS

In addition to vital statistics, data about the occurrence of sickness within the community can provide more detailed assessment of the health of the community.

Collecting morbidity data

Morbidity data are more difficult to collect and interpret than the records of births and deaths (see Table 2.2).

- Lay persons can easily recognize and record births and deaths. Success in the collection of morbidity statistics depends on the extent to which individuals recognize departures from health and also on the availability of facilities for the diagnosis of illnesses. Thus, the quality of morbidity statistics depends on the extent of coverage and the degree of sophistication of the medical services.
- Whereas each vital event of birth and death can occur only on one occasion in the lifetime of any person, sickness may occur repeatedly in the same person. In addition one person may suffer from several disease processes concomitantly.

Table 2.4 gives examples of sources of morbidity data.

Morbidity rates

In describing the pattern of sickness in a community, various morbidity rates are calculated (Table 2.4). These fall into four major groups.

INCIDENCE RATES

These describe the frequency of occurrence of new cases of a disease or spells of illness. The incidence rate may be defined in terms of numbers of persons who start an episode of sickness in a particular

---

[1]ORT, oral rehydration therapy.

Table 2.4: Morbidity rates

Rate		Calculation (× 1000)
Incidence rate (persons)	=	$\dfrac{\text{No. of persons starting an episode of illness in a defined period}}{\text{Average no. of persons exposed to risk during the period}}$
Incidence rate (episodes)	=	$\dfrac{\text{No. of episodes of illness starting during the defined period}}{\text{Average no. of persons exposed to risk during the period}}$
Prevalence rate	=	$\dfrac{\text{No. of persons who are sick at a given time}}{\text{Average no. of persons exposed to risk}}$
Fatality rate	=	$\dfrac{\text{No. of deaths ascribed to a specified disease}}{\text{No. of reported cases of the specified disease}}$
Average duration of illness	=	$\dfrac{\text{Sum of duration of illness of cases in the sample}}{\text{No. of cases in the sample}}$

period, or alternatively, in terms of the number of episodes during that period.

PREVALENCE RATE

The prevalence rate of illness can be defined as the number of persons who are currently sick at a specific point in time.

FATALITY RATE

This is the number of deaths in relation to the number of new cases of a particular disease. It is, in part, a measure of the severity of the disease, efficacy of therapy and the state of host immunity.

DURATION OF ILLNESS

The average duration of illness can be calculated per completed spell of illness, per sick person, or per person. For example, in an outbreak of guinea worm infection, record the duration in weeks of disability for each case (defined arbitrarily as the period when the infection prevented attendance at work, school or usual occupation). Find the average duration of disability per case by dividing the sum by the number of affected persons.

NEW STATISTICAL APPROACHES IN HEALTH

Policy-makers are using new statistical tools to provide an objective basis for their decisions:

- measurement of the burden of disease;
- estimates of the cost-effectiveness of interventions;
- analysis of national health accounts.

Burden of disease

New methods of measuring the burden of disease are increasingly being used to make objective decisions for setting priorities in the health sector. These new indicators attempt to summarize the impact of specific health problems in terms of disease, disability and premature death. In Ghana, Morrow and his colleagues developed a summary that was based on the calculation of the number of useful days of life lost from premature death (mortality) and from disability (morbidity) (Ghana Health Assessment Project Team, 1981). A new measure, disability-adjusted life years (DALYs), an advance on the Ghana model, similarly combines losses from death and disability, but also makes allowance for:

- a discount rate, so that future years of healthy life are valued at progressively lower levels;
- age weights, so that years lost at different ages are given different values.

Quite understandably, there are relatively good-quality data from the developed countries and the more advanced developing countries, but in the least developed countries data are scanty, and some of the estimates of the global burden of disease were derived from extrapolations. The results showed that in developing countries communicable diseases and perinatal problems accounted for the largest part of the burden of diseases, whereas in the industrial countries chronic diseases were the predominant causes of loss of DALYs (Plate 6).

The DALY is proving a useful tool, for ranking diseases and conditions and to estimate the cost-effectiveness of interventions by comparing the cost of averting a DALY. More work is required to refine and simplify it. Refinements of the DALY have been developed to emphasize specific aspects of the burden of disease. For example, disability-adjusted life expectancy (DALE) measures the number of years lived without disability.

Estimation of cost-effectiveness

Policy-makers use cost-effectiveness analyses to compare different interventions for the same condition. Such analyses provide the basis for selecting the interventions that give the largest gain in DALYs per unit cost, and how to modify interventions and make them more cost-effective. The most cost-effective interventions like vitamin A supplementation or measles vaccination require US$1–10 per DALY gained; but more expensive interventions like the treatment of leukaemia may require US$1000–10 000 per DALY gained.

National health accounts

This is a new valuable tool for monitoring the flow of financial resources for health. The analysis of national health accounts provides a comprehensive overview of health expenditures, both public and private. It extends the analysis of health financing beyond spending within the public sector to include private spending through insurance, corporate arrangements and employee schemes, and out-of-pocket spending. It combines data on health spending from all sources – public and private, corporate and personal – into comprehensive health accounts. The results affect the choices made within the public sector and influence the public role in providing guidelines to the private sector and communities on the most cost-effective uses of their personal expenditures. It also provides useful guidance for promoting equity by identifying those in greatest need as specific targets for public funds.

National health accounts are usually presented in the form of a matrix. The columns of the matrix list all sources of health spending: public (taxation and national social insurance) and private sources, including employment-based schemes, privately financed insurance, and out-of-pocket expenditure. The rows of the matrix show the distribution of expenditure for personal health care, public health and environmental sanitation services, and administration.

In more detailed analyses, the items in the columns and rows are subdivided, thereby providing more detailed information about the sources and patterns of spending. The analyses can show variations by time, by geography, by population subgroups, or by any other policy-relevant variables. The data from African countries show that a relatively heavy proportion of health expenditure is derived from private sources and out-of-pocket spending.

STATISTICAL CLASSIFICATION OF DISEASE

The use of standard classification of diseases and injuries has greatly aided the statistical analysis of morbidity and mortality data. Through the United Nations and the World Health Organization, an internationally recommended classification has been evolved, which is periodically revised. Although this classification may be extended or modified to suit local and national conditions, the essential structure for international comparisons must be preserved.

The cause of death can be defined as 'the morbid condition or disease process, abnormality, injury or poisoning leading directly or indirectly to death. Symptoms or modes of dying such as heart failure, asthenia, etc. are not considered to be the cause of death for statistical purposes'. These causes of death are classified broadly under seventeen main sections (Table 2.5).

In the rural areas of the tropics where facilities are limited and autopsies infrequent (e.g. in many provincial hospitals), the use of individual headings gives an impression of precision to diagnoses which is often not justified. The use of cause groups (e.g. diarrhoeal disease) in these circumstances permits a more valid estimate of the size of the problem, focuses on the necessity for corrective action and makes it easier to detect change over a period of time.

Table 2.5: Classification of diseases. Based on the International Classification of Diseases, 10th Revision, WHO.

I	Infective and parasitic diseases
II	Neoplasms
III	Allergic, endocrine, metabolic and nutritional diseases
IV	Diseases of the blood and blood-forming organs
V	Mental, psychoneurotic and personality disorders
VI	Diseases of the nervous system and sense organs
VII	Diseases of the circulatory system
VIII	Diseases of the respiratory system
IX	Diseases of the digestive system
X	Diseases of the genito-urinary system
XI	Complications of pregnancy, childbirth and the puerperium
XII	Diseases of the skin and cellular tissue
XIII	Diseases of the bones and organs of movement
XIV	Congenital malformations
XV	Certain diseases of early infancy
XVI	Symptoms, signs and ill-defined conditions
XVII	Accidents, poisoning and violence*

*Alternative classifications of items in group XVII are: E XVII (external cause) and N XVII (natural cause). The E and N classifications are independent and either or both can be used.

CERTIFICATION OF THE CAUSE OF DEATH

This is usually provided by the physician who was in attendance on a sick patient during his or her last illness. The certificate is made out on a form which is usually based on the international form of medical certificate of cause of death. This form is in two parts (Fig. 2.3).

In many developing countries, only a small proportion of deaths occur under the supervision of trained doctors. In the other cases, a certificate of death may be provided by other categories of staff including health auxiliaries. Attempts have been made to evolve for the use of such staff simple classifications of causes of death, based mainly on symptoms and broad descriptions. Such methods of recording crude causes of death can be of great value if the data are interpreted with care. These statistics should, however, be tabulated separately from certifications from qualified physicians.

MODERN INFORMATION TECHNOLOGY

Major advances in information technology make new effective tools available to public health

CAUSE OF DEATH		Approximate interval between onset and death
I Disease or condition directly leading to death	(a) _____ due to (or as a consequence of)	
Antecedent causes Morbid conditions, if any, giving rise to the above cause, stating the underlying condition last	(b) _____ due to (or as a consequence of) (c) _____	
II Other significant conditions contributing to the death, but not related to the disease or condition causing it	_____	

I This does not mean the mode of dying, e.g. heart failure, asthenia, etc. It means the disease, injury, or complication which caused death.

Figure 2.3: International form of the medical certificate for the cause of death. Details vary from country to country but usually include the items in this example.

practitioners. These new developments including computers and the internet offer many different applications that are increasingly accessible in developing countries.

COMPUTERS IN HEALTH SERVICES

Computers are being used for storing and analysing data in public health programmes, epidemiological surveys and community-based research projects. Technical advances in recent years have made available compact, affordable computers that are simple to operate ('user friendly'). New, small, laptop models are more powerful than some large mainframe computers of a few decades ago which cost 10 times as much. Hand-held equipment is being used in the field for the direct entry of data which is subsequently transferred to larger machines for storage, analysis and mathematical modelling. Used imaginatively, computer technology is a powerful management tool for monitoring and evaluating health programmes and special projects.

The new technology should be introduced cautiously. Before selecting hardware and software, there should be a careful analysis of needs, capabilities of staff, reliability of power supplies and facilities for servicing equipment. There should be provision for the training of staff so that they can follow established procedures in a disciplined manner.

THE INTERNET

The internet is a global network that makes it possible for an individual to have access to information that is stored in computers all over the world. The specific interest is in the World Wide Web (WWW) which allows access to material that is stored at various web sites. The typical storage mechanism is a web page that includes graphics and texts; important features of such home pages are the links to related sites. Home pages on the WWW use the hypertext markup language (HTML).

Public health workers are exploring many innovative applications of modern information technology. In essence, the various systems provide facilities for holding, transferring and retrieving information. These mechanisms are helping to overcome the isolation of health workers in developing countries by giving them access to information and opportunities for interaction with their peers throughout the world.

Public health workers can use the internet to:

1 Access information provided by major organisations:
   - United Nations agencies – World Health Organization, UNICEF, FAO;
   - major health initiatives (Mectizan Donation Programme, International Trachoma Initiative, Children's Vaccine Programme, International AIDS Vaccine Initiative, etc.);
   - private foundations (Ford, Melinda and Bill Gates, Rockefeller foundations and the Wellcome Trust);
   - academic institutions – (most universities and large academic institutions e.g. London School of Hygiene and Tropical Medicine, Institute of Tropical Medicine, Amsterdam);
   - scientific databases – MEDLINE, Cochrane database (Box 2.1);
   - scientific publications – e.g. *Lancet*, *British Medical Journal*, *International Journal of Epidemiology* – abstracts and/or full texts available free or on payment of fee;
   - news agencies – CNN, British Broadcasting Corporation, major newspapers in developed and developing countries.
2 Communications:
   - electronic mail – send and receive messages;
   - list servers – this provides a group of people with facility for on-going communications with each other. Enrolling on a list server of a particular group may provide the individual with regular information on a particular topic of interest.
   - electronic networks – communication linkage among persons sharing a common interest for exchanging information and ideas.

GEOGRAPHICAL INFORMATION SYSTEM (GIS)

Geographical Information System is a newly developed tool for combining geographical and other variables in a database for display as maps and other graphical or textual format. Advances in satellite and computer technologies have facilitated the acquisition, storage and analysis of data in electronic form. Public health applications of GIS

Box 2.1: The Cochrane database

Abstracted from the Cochrane website: http://www.cochrane.org/cochrane/.

In 1979, Archie Cochrane, a British physician, criticized the medical profession for not having established a system for producing up-to-date summaries of the results of reliable research about the effects of health care. He recognized that people who want to make more informed decisions about health care do not have ready access to reliable reviews of the available evidence. In 1979, he wrote:

> *It is surely a great criticism of our profession that we have not organised a critical summary, by specialty or sub-specialty, adapted periodically, of all relevant randomized controlled trials.*

The Cochrane Collaboration was founded in 1993 to respond to Cochrane's challenge. Cochrane reviews (the principal output of the Collaboration) are published electronically in successive issues of *The Cochrane Database of Systematic Reviews*. Preparation and maintenance of Cochrane reviews is the responsibility of international collaborative review groups. The members of these groups – researchers, health-care professionals, consumers, and others – share an interest in generating reliable, up-to-date evidence relevant to the prevention, treatment and rehabilitation of particular health problems or groups of problems. How can stroke and its effects be prevented and treated? What drugs should be used to prevent and treat malaria, tuberculosis and other important infectious diseases? What strategies are effective in preventing brain and spinal cord injury and its consequences, and what rehabilitative measures can help those with residual disabilities?

---

have evolved over the past three decades. For example, by combining physical information with climatic data, epidemiologists are now producing GIS maps showing the distribution of risks of transmission of malaria, schistosomiasis and other vector-borne diseases. GIS maps can also be applied to the study of health services by relating epidemiological, demographic transportation and other variables with the aim of designing the most cost-effective organization of services.

PRESENTATION OF DATA

The aim of presenting data is to produce a precise and accurate demonstration of the information, summarized to simplify and highlighted to draw attention to the most important features. This may be achieved both numerically and graphically. Computer-based tools are available for data entry, analysis and presentation (Box 2.2).

NUMERICAL PRESENTATION

At its simplest, numerical presentation may be no more than an arrangement of the figures in order of magnitude, so that the range of the data from the smallest to the largest is clearly displayed.

Box 2.2: Statistical and epidemiological packages

EPI-INFO, a statistical and epidemiological package, is widely used with over 100 000 users globally. It is particularly popular with health departments. Originally written for the DOS operating system, the current version, EPI-INFO 2000 is based on Windows operating system. The US-based Center for Diseases Control, Atlanta, which produced the package and updates it, has placed the product in the public domain; it can be acquired by downloading it free from their website or installed from a CD-ROM. It provides user-friendly processes for data entry and backup as well as flexible analytical tools and numerical and graphical presentations. EPIMAP, a companion tool, is used for drawing maps to show disease distribution and other health data.

SUMMARY STATISTICS

Simple statistical calculations can indicate salient features of the data. For example, a series of values can be summarized by calculating statistics such as:

- Mean, median or mode. Each is a single value which is representative of the series of figures, (i.e. an average).
- Range or standard deviation. These are measures of dispersion which show the degree of variability within the series of values.

TABULATION

For tabular presentation, data are sorted, arranged, condensed and set out in such a way as to bring out the essential points. Often the raw data are classified, compressed and grouped into a frequency distribution. For example, rather than showing the individual ages of persons, data may be classified into 5-year or 10-year age-groups, with a record of the number of persons in each group. For effective presentation, a few simple rules must be observed:

- *Title*. This should clearly describe the material contained within the text. Three elements commonly featured in the title are: (i) What? – the material contained in the table; (ii) Where? – location of the study; and (iii) When? – time of the study.
- *Labelling*. Each column and each row should be clearly labelled and the units of measurement stated. If a rate is used, the base of measurement and the number of observations must be stated.
- *Totals*. The totals for columns and rows should be shown where appropriate.
- *Footnotes*. Abbreviations and symbols should be explained in footnotes except when they are well known and universally familiar (e.g. £, $, etc.).

GRAPHIC REPRESENTATION

Statistical data can be summarized and displayed in the form of graphs, geometric figures or pictures. The aim of the graphic representation is to provide a simple, visual aid such that the reader will rapidly appreciate the important features of the data.

BAR CHART

A bar, the length of which is proportional to the absolute or relative frequency of events, represents each item in the group. It is particularly useful in representing discrete variables (Fig. 2.4).

HISTOGRAM

A histogram is a special type of bar chart used to display numerical variables. The variable of interest is shown on one axis as a continuous scale split into

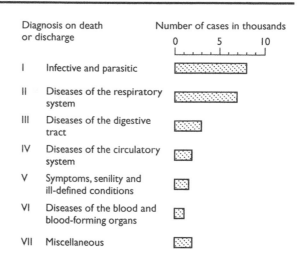

Figure 2.4: Bar chart analysis of the cases admitted to Laciport Hospital in 1989.

classes. Adjoining bars are drawn, their areas representing the frequency of events. If the class intervals are constant, the frequency may be given on the other axis (Fig. 2.5). The age and sex distribution of a population may be displayed in the form of a histogram to produce a population pyramid (see Fig. 2.1).

PIE CHART

This consists of a circle, which is divided into sectors, with the area of each sector proportional to the value of each variable (Fig. 2.6).

GRAPHS

The simplest graph shows two variables: one on the horizontal axis and the other on the vertical axis (Fig. 2.7).

THE USE OF HEALTH STATISTICS

There is a tendency to over-emphasize the collection of statistics and to pay insufficient attention to their use. Much information collected at great cost remains unused in the archives of health departments. A few examples illustrate how statistics can be used in a dynamic way to identify and deal with problems affecting the health of the community.

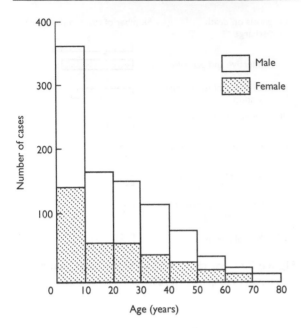

Figure 2.5: Histogram showing the age and sex distribution of cases of tetanus, Laciport Hospital 1986–89 inclusive.

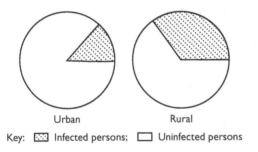

Key: ▓ Infected persons; ☐ Uninfected persons

Figure 2.6: Pie chart showing the prevalence of hookworm infection in Laciport State in 1989.

Local uses

The delivery of health care at the primary level generates much raw data. At the health post, the dispensary, the maternal and child welfare clinic and the general practitioner's clinic, data can be collected and used in a simple but effective manner. For example, the pattern of diseases seen at the clinic can be summarized using simple classification in broad diagnostic groups. In this way the proportion of attendances due to common problems – diarrhoeal diseases, acute respiratory infections, minor injuries – can be monitored. A sudden change can call attention to an epidemic, and trends over time can also be observed.

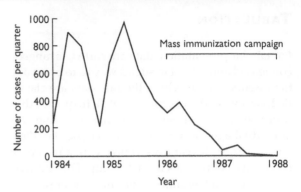

Figure 2.7: Graph of the numbers of cases of poliomyelitis notified in Laciport State from 1984–88.

At a health centre, for example, each service unit should collect and display statistics on high priority problems. The section of the clinic, which treats sick patients, could, for example, show cases of acute diarrhoea in a simple graph so that comparisons can be made day by day, week by week, and month by month. These statistics may alert the staff of the institution to sudden changes in the number of cases of a particular disease and it could provide some assessment of the performance of the services. The child welfare clinic should display the number of children they have immunized to show both the uptake over time (by comparing vaccination and birth rates) and the proportion completing the course (by indicating the numbers entering and finishing the programme).

No specific list can be prescribed for all centres but each centre should select a few priority problems for careful scrutiny. These data can form the basis of discussions among the staff and with the community for the strategy to deal with specific problems.

District and national collation and planning

In addition to the collection of data for local use, the primary health-care unit should also pay attention to the need to contribute accurate data for use at the district and national level.

DISTRICT LEVEL

The district health team should use the data derived from peripheral units to obtain an indication of the pattern of diseases and operation of the health services. Trends that may not be apparent in one local unit may become obvious on compilation of data from several villages or communities. For example, an outbreak of diarrhoeal disease may be confined to a small area involving one or two villages, but an increase in the number of cases over a wider area may call attention to a more serious problem.

The district officer should also select data that would give information about the health problems within the district and the operation of the health services should be examined. What proportion of children are being immunized community by community? What proportion of pregnant women receive antenatal care and how many deliver their babies under skilled supervision? Scrutiny of such information would enable the district officer to assess the performance of the health teams, and to gauge the community response.

NATIONAL LEVEL

At the national level, the statistical unit serving the Ministry of Health can be a most valuable resource for decision-making. Data that are carefully collected, evaluated and interpreted should form the basis of defining the priorities for health care, for allocating resources and for monitoring progress. Such national data can be analysed to show distribution by geography, and other relevant variables. National health data can also be compared with data from other countries especially with countries that have a similar ecological setting.

MANAGEMENT INFORMATION SYSTEMS

'Information for action'

Rather than deal with health information as discrete pieces of data, it is best to develop a Management Information System (MIS). The objective of the MIS is to generate information that decision-makers and managers can use to support health programmes. The aim is to collect, analyse data and interpret findings as the basis for making decisions,

monitoring trends and evaluating programmes. A good MIS depends on:

- careful identification of the users and their needs;
- the specific information that they require;
- a data collection system using appropriate tools;
- an analytic process for interpreting the data; and
- a mechanism for disseminating information to those who need to know.

The MIS may combine the routine reporting system with epidemiological surveillance and special surveys.

REFERENCES AND FURTHER READING

Berman P.A. (1997) National health accounts in developing countries: appropriate methods and recent applications. *Health Economics* 6(1): 11–30.

Ghana Health Assessment Project Team (1981) A quantitative method of assessing the health impact of different diseases in less developed countries. *International Journal of Epidemiology* 10(1): 73–80.

Hyder A.A., Rotllant G. & Morrow R.H. (1998) Measuring the burden of disease: healthy life-years. *American Journal of Public Health* 88(2): 196–202.

Murray C.J. (1994) Quantifying the burden of disease: the technical basis for disability-adjusted life years. *Bulletin World Health Organization* 72: 429–445.

Murray C.J.L. & Lopez A.D. (Eds) (1996) *The global burden of disease: a comprehensive assessment of mortality and disability from diseases, injuries, and risk factors in 1990 and projected to 2020.* Cambridge, Harvard School of Public Health on behalf of the World Health Organization and The World Bank (Global Burden of Disease and Injury Series, Vol. 1).

UNICEF (1989) *The State of the World's Children.* Oxford University Press, Oxford.

WHO (1977) *New Approaches to Health Statistics.* Technical Report Series No. 599. WHO, Geneva.

WHO (1987) Evaluation of the strategy for health for all by the year 2000. In: *Seventh Report on the World Health Situation. Volume 1: Global Review.* WHO, Geneva.

WHO (1994) *Information Support for New Public Health Action at District Level.* Technical Report Series No. 845. WHO, Geneva.

CHAPTER THREE

EPIDEMIOLOGY

- Disease distribution
- Epidemiological methods
- Epidemiological data
- The uses of epidemiology
- General introduction
- Infectious diseases and development
- Epidemiology of communicable diseases

- Control of communicable diseases
- The use of drugs in the control of infections
- Antimicrobial resistance
- Surveillance of disease
- Epidemiology of non-infectious diseases
- References and further reading

Originally, the term 'epidemiology' meant 'the study of epidemics', but the techniques that were originally used in the study and control of epidemics have also been usefully applied in the study of other types of diseases including non-communicable diseases and accidents. In its modern usage, the term epidemiology refers to the study of the distribution of disease in human populations, against the background of their total environment. It includes a study of the patterns of disease as well as a search for the determinants of disease. It exploits the technologies from other disciplines – microbiology, parasitology, social sciences, etc. in analysing the frequency, distribution and determinants of health and disease in populations. New advances in genetics and molecular biology have stimulated the development of *molecular epidemiology*; it investigates the contributions of genetic and environmental risk factors that are identified at the molecular level in the aetiology and distribution of health and disease in groups and populations.

The modern definition of epidemiology includes three important elements:

- *All diseases included*. The term is no longer restricted to the study of infections but it includes cancer, malnutrition, road accidents, mental illness and other non-communicable diseases. Epidemiological techniques are also being applied to the study of the operation of health services.

- *Populations*. Whereas clinical medicine is concerned with the features of disease in the individual, epidemiology deals with the distribution of disease in populations, communities or groups.
- *Ecological approach*. The frequency and distribution of disease are examined against the background of various circumstances in man's total environment – physical, biological and social. This is an ecological approach: the occurrence of disease is examined in terms of the interrelationship between human beings and their total environment.

Table 3.1 lists examples of applications of epidemiology in various types of diseases.

DISEASE DISTRIBUTION

Three major questions are usually asked in epidemiology:

- *Who*? What is the distribution of the disease in terms of persons?
- *Where*? What is the distribution of the disease in terms of place?
- *When*? What is the distribution of the disease in terms of time?

Answers to these questions provide clues to the factors which determine the occurrence of the disease.

Table 3.1: Brief summaries illustrating the contributions of epidemiology to public health

Topic	Brief summary
Infectious diseases*	
Smallpox	Edward Jenner, in late 18th century, noted that milkmaids were apparently spared during epidemics of smallpox and he reasoned that prior infection with cowpox had protected them. This led to the use of cowpox and provided the foundation for modern concepts of immunization
Cholera	John Snow in the 1830s showed a strong link between the risk of cholera and the source of water supply. An epidemic subsided after the removal of the handle from the pump of a suspect well
Puerperal sepsis	Ignatius Semmelweiss, a Hungarian obstetrician, analysed data which showed association between childbed fever and dirty hands of doctors who attended the births. He also showed that the risk of the disease could be reduced if attendants washed their hands with chloride of lime
Nutritional disorders	
Scurvy	Classical studies by James Lind, late 18th century, showed scurvy could be treated and prevented by small doses of lemon juice. This finding antedated the discovery of vitamins by over a century
Tropical neuropathy	Osuntokun in Nigeria adduced clinical, epidemiological and biochemical evidence linking a tropical ataxic neuropathy with cyanide intoxication of dietary origin – a staple diet of cassava root, which contains cyanogens
Vitamin A	Vitamin A deficiency was associated with night blindness and xerophthalmia. Studies by Somers showed marked fall in child mortality in children who were given vitamin A supplement
Cancers	
Cigarette smoking	In the 1950s the role of cigarette smoking in the aetiology of cancer of the lung was shown through case-control studies in the USA (Wynder and colleagues) and in Britain (Doll and Hill). This association was confirmed in cohort studies
Childhood cancers	Studies analysed risk factors for childhood cancers. One prominent finding was a strong association between abdominal X-rays of pregnant women and leukaemia in children
Other conditions	
Heart disease	Community-based longitudinal study in Framingham, Massachusetts, USA showed the association of ischaemic heart disease with hypertension, level of serum cholesterol and other risk factors
Congenital abnormalities	Gregg, an Australian ophthalmologist, observed a high frequency of congenital cataract and other abnormalities in babies born to mothers who had German measles in early pregnancy
Road traffic accidents	A case control study of drivers who died from road traffic accidents in New York showed higher frequency of raised blood alcohol in fatal cases as compared with controls

*Epidemiological studies in these classical cases generated useful knowledge that led to practical control measures before modern knowledge of bacteria and other infective agents.

EPIDEMIOLOGICAL METHODS

The basic tool of epidemiology is the rate – it relates the number of cases to the population at risk. In order to compare populations of different sizes easily, the rate is usually expressed as the number of events in an arbitrary total, for example 1000 or 100 000.

Two main types of rates are calculated.

INCIDENCE RATE

This indicates the occurrence of new cases within a stated period:

$$\text{Incidence rate} = \frac{\begin{bmatrix} \text{No. of new cases in a} \\ \text{stated period} \end{bmatrix}}{\text{Population at risk}} \times 1000$$

PREVALENCE RATE (POINT PREVALENCE RATE)

This is the number of cases that are present within the population at a particular point in time:

$$\text{Prevalence rate} = \frac{\begin{bmatrix} \text{No. of current cases at} \\ \text{a specified time} \end{bmatrix}}{\text{Population at risk}} \times 1000$$

INCIDENCE, PREVALENCE AND DURATION

There is obviously some relationship between the rate at which new cases occur and the number of cases present at any particular point in time. The third factor to be considered is the *duration* of the illness.

The prevalence rate would rise if:

- the incidence of illness increases but the average duration remains unchanged;
- the incidence rate remains unchanged but the average duration of the illness increases.

Thus, the prevalence rate is dependent on the combination of these two factors, incidence rate and duration of illness. Under certain conditions where no marked changes are occurring in these factors, there is a simple mathematical relationship:

$$\text{Prevalence rate} = \text{Incidence rate} \\ \times \text{Average duration}$$

This relationship changes if the incidence rate is rapidly changing, as in an acute epidemic; if the disease is episodic; or if the average duration of the illness is changing, perhaps in response to treatment.

EPIDEMIOLOGICAL STUDY DESIGN

There are three main types of epidemiological studies: descriptive, analytical and experimental.

Descriptive epidemiology

This is the first phase of epidemiological studies in which the distribution of disease is described in terms of the three major variables: people, place and time. The various characteristics needed to qualify the questions: 'Who is affected? In what place? And at what time?' are listed in Table 3.2.

The answers to these questions together with knowledge of the clinical and pathological features of the disease and information about the population and its environment, assist in developing hypotheses about the determinants of the disease. These hypotheses can be tested by analytical studies.

Analytical epidemiology

Two types of study are employed (Fig. 3.1).

CASE-CONTROL STUDIES

For case-control studies (also known as retrospective studies or case-history studies), a group of affected persons is compared with a suitably matched control group of non-affected persons. For example, in a study designed to test the hypothesis that

Table 3.2: Some of the variables used to describe the distribution of disease in descriptive epidemiology

People	Age, sex, marital status
	Race, ethnic group, religion
	Occupation, education, socioeconomic status
	Personal habits – use of alcohol and tobacco
Place	Climatic zones
	Country, region, state, district
	Urban or rural
	Local community, city wards
	Precise location in an institution
Time	Year, season, day
	Secular trends, periodic changes
	Seasonal variations and other cyclical fluctuations

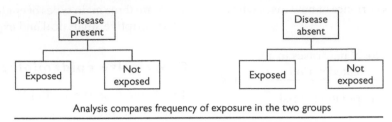

CASE-CONTROL STUDY

Subjects selected on the basis of disease

Disease present		Disease absent	
Exposed	Not exposed	Exposed	Not exposed

Analysis compares frequency of exposure in the two groups

COHORT STUDY

Subjects selected on the basis of exposure

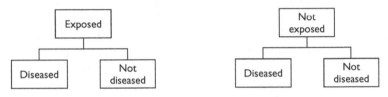

Exposed		Not exposed	
Diseased	Not diseased	Diseased	Not diseased

Analysis compares incidence of disease in the two groups

Figure 3.1: Comparing the design of case-control study with that of cohort study.

Table 3.3: The relationship between the results of a screening test and the true disease status of subjects

		True disease status		
		Present (+)	**Absent (−)**	
Test result	Positive (+)	True positives (TP)	False positives (FP)	Total positive tests (TP + FP)
	Negative (−)	False negatives (FN)	True negatives (TN)	Total negative tests (FN + TN)
		Total disease present (TP + FN)	Total disease absent (FP + TN)	

cigarette smoking is an important factor in causing lung cancer, a number of patients with this disease (cases) were questioned about their smoking habits. Similar questions were asked of a group of patients who had cancer at other sites (controls). This enquiry showed significant differences in the smoking habits of cases compared with controls. It was a case-history study in that the subjects were selected on the basis of being *affected* or *non-affected* persons.

COHORT STUDIES

For cohort studies, a group of persons who are exposed to the suspected aetiological agent are

compared with matched control subjects who have not been similarly exposed. For example, in a further study on cancer of the lung, a large group of persons were questioned about their smoking habits. During the follow-up period, the incidence rate of cancer of the lung among the smokers (exposed) was compared with the rate among non-smokers (non-exposed). In this cohort study, the subjects were selected on the basis of *exposure* or *non-exposure* (Tables 3.3–3.6).

CASE-CONTROL VERSUS COHORT DESIGN

Compared with cohort studies, case-control studies have the advantage of being relatively quick, easy

Table 3.4: Analysis of the results of screening tests

		True disease status		
		Present (+)	**Absent (−)**	
Test result	Positive (+)	True positives (TP)	False positives (FP)	Predictive value (+) TP/(TP + FP)
	Negative (−)	False negatives (FN)	True negatives (TN)	Predictive value (−) TN/(FN + TN)
		Sensitivity TP/(TP + FN)	Specificity TN/(FP + TN)	

Sensitivity: indicates the extent to which the test identifies diseased persons; out of all persons in whom the disease is present (TP + FN), what proportion are correctly identified by the test, TP/(TP + FN).
Specificity: indicates to what extent the test identifies healthy persons; out of all the persons in whom the test is negative (FP + TN) what proportion are truly free of the disease, TN/(FP + TN).
Predictive value positive (PVP): what proportion of persons testing positive actually have the disease.
Predictive value negative (PVN): what proportion of persons testing negative are truly free of the disease.

Table 3.5: Analysis of case-control studies

	Exposure		
	Exposed (+)	**Not exposed (−)**	**Incidence**
Disease (+)	A	B	A/(A + B)
No disease (−)	C	D	C/(C + D)

Table 3.6: Analysis of cohort study

	Disease		
	Present (+)	**Absent (−)**	**Incidence**
Exposed (+)	A	B	A/(A + B)
Not exposed (−)	C	D	C/(C + D)

$$\text{Relative risk} = \frac{\text{Risk in exposed}}{\text{Risk in non-exposed}} = \frac{a/(a + b)}{c/(c + d)}$$

$$\text{Attributable risk} = \frac{(\text{Incidence in exposed group}) - (\text{Incidence in non-exposed group})}{\text{Incidence in exposed group}}$$

$$= \frac{a/(a + b) - c/(c + d)}{c/(c + d)}$$

and relatively inexpensive. A significant number of cases can be assembled for the case-history study and a variety of hypotheses can be rapidly screened. The more promising theories can be further examined by the more laborious, time-consuming and expensive cohort studies. The latter have the advantage of giving a more direct estimation of the risk from exposure to each factor.

Experimental epidemiology

This involves studies in which one group which is deliberately subjected to an experience is compared with a control group which has not had a similar experience. Field trials of vaccines and of chemo-prophylactic agents are examples of experimental epidemiology. In such trials, one group receives the vaccine or drug, whilst the control group is given a placebo; alternatively, a new vaccine or drug may be compared with a well-established agent of known potency. Apart from trials of pro-phylactic and therapeutic agents, there are not many opportunities for experimental epidemi-ology in humans; studies that are theoretically pos-sible may not be feasible or ethical.

EPIDEMIOLOGICAL DATA

As in clinical medicine, epidemiological data may be obtained in the form of answers to questions, physical examination of persons and results of laboratory and special investigations. In assessing the value of a particular method the following qualities should be considered:

1 *Sensitivity* – the ability of the test to detect the condition when it is present (true positive). A highly sensitive test will be positive whenever the condition is present; a less sensitive test will be positive in a proportion of cases, but will give a *false negative* result in others.
2 *Specificity* – the ability of the test to differentiate cases in which the condition is present from those in which it is absent. A highly specific test will be negative whenever the disease is absent (*true negative*); a less specific test will give some *false positives*. Table 3.4 shows how the speci-ficity and sensitivity of a screening test may be calculated.
3 *Repeatability* – the extent to which the same result is obtained when the test is repeated on the same subject or material. The variation which occurs on repeating the test may be due to the following:
   - variation in the item being measured, for exam-ple changes in heart rate, blood pressure and other physiological variables during exercise;
   - limitation in the accuracy of the instrument of measurement.

OBSERVER VARIATION

Observer variation (also known as observer error or bias) may occur between repeated measurements by the same observer (*intra-observer variation*) or there may be differences between the findings of two or more observers when they measure or clas-sify the same object (*inter-observer variation*).

Observer variation can be minimized by:

- *Standardizing the procedures* for obtaining the measurements and classifications, for example for an anthropometric survey, the procedure for measuring height should be clearly specified: the subject is barefooted, standing erect against the measuring pole, keeping head in a position such that the subject looks straight ahead.
- *Defining the criteria* in clear objective terms to differentiate case from non-case.
- *Training observers* in the methods to be adopted to ensure uniform standard techniques.
- *Providing standard reference material* such as photographs or standard X-ray films for direct comparison.
- *Taking 'blind' measurements* and making the classi-fications without knowledge of the status of the patient, whether the individual is a 'case' or a 'control' subject. In the *double-blind* technique, subjects are randomly allocated to treatment and control groups; neither the subjects nor the observers know to which group each subject is assigned. Thus, there is 'blind' assignment of sub-jects as well as 'blind' assessments of the results.

It is generally accepted that a 'randomized double-blind' design is highly favoured as a means of reducing bias.

THE USES OF EPIDEMIOLOGY

Epidemiology is a powerful tool of proven value in public health practice. The epidemiological approach should be more extensively used in defining and solving health problems in develop-ing countries. The key role of epidemiological sur-veillance in the control of disease is discussed on page 44. Specialist epidemiologists have an import-ant role in planning and managing the epidemi-ological services at district and national level, for designing and executing major epidemiological studies, for tackling difficult problems and for training personnel. However, other health personnel who are not specialized in this discipline can and should use epidemiological methods in their work.

At the primary health care unit epidemiological methods should be used to determine the most common causes of death, disease and disability; to find out which persons are at highest risk; and to identify the determinant factors. Epidemiological methods should also be used to solve specific health problems. If, for example, data show that acute diarrhoeal diseases are among the commonest causes of death in a rural district, the most appropriate interventions can best be designed on the basis of epidemiological analyses of the problem. What is the distribution of the cases according to age, sex, geographical area and season? Among the cases, what is the case fatality rate in different age-groups? The data obtained at the health clinic or other institution may not be sufficient to provide answers to these questions. A simple house to house survey will provide some of the missing data and additional information about sources of water supply, cooking practices, food storage and other relevant matters. Such surveys could draw attention to polluted water supplies, unhygienic practices in the home and the need to promote the use of simple oral rehydration for young children who have acute diarrhoea. These studies do not call for elaborate protocols or for sophisticated statistical analyses and yet the findings can be very valuable in guiding and evaluating public health measures.

EMERGING AND RE-EMERGING INFECTIOUS DISEASES (PLATE 7)

In many of the countries of the developed world, infectious diseases – of childhood in particular – have been generally conquered. This, however, is far from being the case in developing countries, where they are responsible for 45% of all deaths (Plate 8). The leading killers are acute respiratory infections, HIV/AIDS, diarrhoeal diseases, tuberculosis, malaria and measles (Plate 9). The background is a combination of factors: poverty and hence their relatively new description 'poverty diseases'; poor sanitation; uncontrolled urbanization; mass population movements; population growth, poor access to essential inexpensive drugs, lack of political will and lack of community demand for action.

In addition, some of these typical diseases cause severe disability and hence economic loss (Plate 10); some chronic infections (e.g. hepatitis B and C) cause hepatoma while the interaction of malnutrition and infection has long been established.

A window of opportunity, however, does exist and success stories have been recorded even in low income countries (e.g. Guinea) where within 4 years of launching its TB control programme using the WHO DOTS strategy (directly observed treatment strategy), the case detection rate doubled and nearly 80% of patients were cured.

Polio and guinea worm disease are on the verge of being eliminated.

Despite the development over the years by WHO of low-cost strategies to combat many of the killer infectious diseases, many countries are still not using them and not deploying them enough to make an impact on morbidity or mortality (Plate 11).

INFECTIOUS DISEASES AND DEVELOPMENT

Changes in land and water use, deforestation, agricultural development, dams and irrigation schemes can have major positive or negative impact on the pattern of disease (Plate 12). Large outbreaks of communicable diseases periodically occur worldwide (Plate 13).

EPIDEMIOLOGY OF COMMUNICABLE DISEASES (PLATE 14)

THE COMPONENTS OF COMMUNICABLE DISEASE

Communicable diseases are characterized by the existence of a living infectious agent which is transmissible. Apart from the infectious agent, two other factors, the host and the environment, affect the epidemiology of the infection. The relationship between these three components may be illustrated using the following analogy:

Agent:	The seed
Host:	The soil
Route of transmission:	The climate

INFECTIOUS AGENTS

These may be viruses, rickettsiae, bacteria, protozoa, fungi or helminths. The biological properties of the agent may play a major role in its epidemiology.

In order to survive an infectious agent must be able to do the following:

- multiply;
- emerge from the host;
- reach a new host;
- infect the new host.

Knowledge of the mechanisms that the organism uses at each of these four stages may help in identifying the most vulnerable stage at which to direct control measures. The ability of the infective agent to survive in the environment is an important factor in the epidemiology of the infection. The term, *reservoir of infection*, is used to describe the specific ecological niche upon which it depends for its survival. The reservoir may be human, animal or non-living material; for some infective agents, the reservoir may include several elements. The infective agent lives and multiplies in the reservoir from which it is transmitted to other habitats but cannot survive indefinitely at these other sites. For example, from its human reservoir, *Salmonella typhi* the cause of typhoid fever, can contaminate water supplies, milk and other food products and can infect susceptible hosts. Since the bacilli cannot survive indefinitely in these habitats, these other sites do not represent the reservoir of typhoid infection but may serve as a *source of infection*.

HUMAN RESERVOIR

This includes a number of important pathogens that are specifically adapted to man – the infective agents of measles, AIDS, typhoid, meningococcal meningitis, gonorrhoea and syphilis. The human reservoir includes both ill persons and healthy carriers. In some cases (e.g. salmonellosis) humans share the reservoir with other animals.

Carriers

A carrier is a person who harbours the infective agent without showing signs of disease but is capable of transmitting the agent to other persons. Different types of carriers are described depending on when they excrete the organism in relation to the illness:

- A *healthy carrier* remains well throughout the infection.
- An *incubatory* or *precocious carrier* excretes the pathogens during the incubation period, before the onset of symptoms (e.g. HIV/AIDS) or before the characteristic features of the disease (e.g. the measles rash or glandular swelling in mumps) are manifested.
- A *convalescent carrier* continues to harbour the infective agent after recovering from the illness. The carrier may excrete the agent for only a short period; or may become a *chronic carrier*, excreting the organism continuously or intermittently over a period of years.

WHY CARRIERS ARE IMPORTANT IN THE EPIDEMIOLOGY OF SOME INFECTIONS

Carriers play an important role in the epidemiology of certain infections (poliomyelitis, meningococcal meningitis, typhoid and amoebiasis):

- There may be *large numbers of carriers* far outnumbering the sick patients.
- Since neither the *healthy carriers* nor their contacts are aware of the infection, they may not take precautions to avoid transmission of the infection, e.g. using condoms to avoid sexually transmitted infection. Thus, whilst the sick patient's contacts may be restricted to close family members, friends and visitors, the carrier can continue with normal daily routine, moving freely from place to place, and making contacts with uninfected persons over a wide area.
- *Chronic carriers* may serve as a source of infection over a very long period and as a means of

repeatedly reintroducing the disease into an area which is otherwise free of infection.

ANIMAL RESERVOIR

Some infective agents that affect humans have their reservoir in animals. The term *zoonosis* is applied to those infectious diseases of vertebrate animals which are transmissible to man under natural conditions:

- where humans use the animal for food, e.g. taeniasis;
- where there is a vector transmitting the infection from animals to humans, e.g. plague (flea), viral encephalitis (mosquito);
- where the animal bites human beings, e.g. rabies;
- where the animal contaminates human environment including food, e.g. salmonellosis.

Health workers should collaborate closely with veterinary authorities in identifying and dealing with these zoonoses.

NON-LIVING RESERVOIR

Many of these agents are saprophytes living in soil and are fully adapted to living free in nature. The vegetative forms are usually equipped to withstand marked changes in environmental temperature and humidity. In addition, some develop resistant forms such as spores which can withstand adverse environmental conditions, for example clostridial organisms – the infective agents of tetanus (*Clostridium tetani*), gas gangrene (*C. welchii*) and botulism (*C. botulinum*).

THE SOURCE OF INFECTION

This term refers to the immediate source of infection; that is, the person or object from which the infectious agent passes to a host. This source of infection may or may not be a portion of the reservoir. For example, human beings are the reservoir of shigella infection; a cook who is a carrier may infect food that is served at a party; that item of food, rather than the reservoir is the source of infection in that particular outbreak.

ROUTE OF TRANSMISSION

This refers to the mechanism by which an infectious agent is transferred from one person to another or from the reservoir to a new host. Transmission may occur by:

- *Contact*, either directly, person to person, or indirectly through contaminated objects (fomites). Contact infections are more likely to occur where there is overcrowding, since this increases the likelihood of contact with infected persons. Hence they tend to be more marked in urban than in rural areas, and they are associated with overcrowding in households. Some highly contagious infections spread through casual contact – the type of contact that occurs in day to day activities at home, work or school. Other infections may require close, intimate contact for transmission (e.g. sexually transmitted disease usually requires intimate contact with exchange of body fluids for infection to occur).
- *Penetration of skin*, directly by the organism itself (e.g. hookworm larvae, schistosomiasis), by the bite of a vector (e.g. malaria, plague) or through wounds (e.g. tetanus).
- *Inhalation of air-borne infections*. Poor ventilation, over-crowding in sleeping quarters and in public places are important factors in the epidemiology of air-borne infections.
- *Ingestion*, from contaminated hands, food or water.
- *Transplacental infection*. Some infective agents cross the placenta to infect the foetus in the womb, producing congenital infections (e.g. HIV, syphilis, toxoplasmosis).

For some infective agents, infection occurs through more than one route of transmission. For example, plague is transmitted by flea bite (bubonic plague) but in some cases, direct person to person transmission occurs through the respiratory route (pneumonic plague).

HOST FACTORS

The occurrence and outcome of infection are in part determined by host factors. The term immunity is used to describe the ability of the host to resist infection. Apart from determining the occurrence of infection, the host's immune responses also modify the nature of the pathological reaction to infection. Allergic reactions in response to infection may significantly contribute to the clinical and pathological reactions. Resistance to infection is determined by non-specific and by specific factors.

Non-specific resistance

This depends on the protective covering of skin which resists penetration by most infective agents, and the mucous membranes, some of which include ciliated epithelium which mechanically scavenges particulate matter. Certain secretions – mucus, tears and gastric secretions – contain lysozymes which have antibacterial activity; in addition, the acid content of gastric secretion also has some anti-microbial action.

Reflex responses such as coughing and sneezing also assist in keeping susceptible parts of the respiratory tract free of foreign matter.

If penetration has occurred, the organisms may be eliminated through the actions of macrophages and other cells or through the effects of non-specific serological factors.

Specific immunity

Specific immunity may be due to genetic or acquired factors.

GENETIC FACTORS

Certain organisms that infect other animals do not infect humans, and vice versa. This species specificity is, however, not always absolute and there are some infective agents which regularly pass from animals to human beings (zoonoses).

There are also variations in the susceptibility of various races and ethnic groups, for example some people of African origin tend to have a high level of resistance to vivax malaria infection.

Specific genetic factors have been associated with resistance to infection, for example persons who have haemoglobin S are more resistant to infection with *Plasmodium falciparum* than those with normal haemoglobin AA (see p. 250).

ACQUIRED FACTORS

Acquired immunity may be active or passive. In active immunity the host manufactures antibodies

and develops other protective mechanisms including cellular immunity, in response to an antigenic stimulus. In passive immunity, the host receives preformed antibodies.

Active immunity may be naturally acquired following clinical or subclinical infection; or it may be induced artificially by administering living or killed organisms or their products.

The new-born baby acquires passive immunity by the transplacental transmission of antibodies; in this way the newborn babies of immune mothers are protected against such infections as measles, malaria and tetanus in the first few months of life. Passive immunity is artificially induced by the administration of antibodies from the sera of immune human beings (homologous) or animals (heterologous). Protection from passive immunity tends to be of short duration, especially when heterologous serum is used.

FACTORS AFFECTING HOST IMMUNITY

The resistance of the host to infection is affected by such factors as age, sex, pregnancy, nutrition, trauma and fatigue (see below). Certain infections (e.g. HIV, the aetiological agent of AIDS), some systemic diseases (e.g. diabetes mellitus, nephrotic syndrome) and immunosuppressive therapy may also undermine the resistance of the host.

Age

For some infections, persons at both extremes of age tend to be most severely affected (i.e. children and the elderly). Some infections predominate in childhood: this usually occurs in situations in which most children become infected and thereby acquire lifelong immunity. Other infections predominate in adults: this may be determined by exposure, for example industrial (anthrax) or sexual (gonorrhoea). Age may also influence the clinical pathological form of an infection, for example miliary tuberculosis is more likely in children whilst cavitating lung lesions are more likely in adults.

Sex

Some infective diseases show marked differences in their sex incidence; this is apart from infections which specifically affect the genital and other sex organs. Infections such as poliomyelitis and diphtheria often show a preponderance in females.

Pregnancy

Pregnancy increases susceptibility to certain infections: these occur more frequently, show more severe manifestations and have a worse prognosis than in non-pregnant women of a similar age group, for example viral infections such as poliomyelitis; bacterial infections such as pneumococcal infection; and protozoal infection such as malaria and amoebiasis. However, there does not appear to be a uniform depression of resistance to all infections. Certain infections, for example typhoid and meningococcal infection, do not occur more frequently nor show greater clinical severity in pregnant women.

Nutrition

Good nutrition is generally accepted as an important measure in enhancing resistance to infection. Severe specific deficiency of vitamin A renders the cornea and the skin more liable to infection. In addition to such specific effects it has been noted that poorly nourished children are more liable to succumb to gastro-enteritis and measles. Conclusive evidence has accumulated showing that significant reduction in mortality occurs when vitamin A supplementation is administered to children in poorly nourished communities.

Trauma and fatigue

Stress in the form of trauma and fatigue may render the host more susceptible to infections. One classical example is the effect of trauma and fatigue on poliomyelitis. The paralytic form of the disease may be precipitated by violent exercise during the prodromal period or by trauma in the form of injections of adjuvanted vaccine; paralysis tends to be most severe in the limb into which the vaccine was injected or which was subjected to most fatigue.

Herd immunity

The level of immunity in the community as a whole is termed 'herd immunity'. When herd immunity is low, introduction of the infection is likely to lead to severe epidemics. For example, the introduction of measles into an island population which had no previous experience of the infection resulted in massive epidemics. On the other hand, when herd immunity is high, the introduction of infection may not lead to a propagated spread. A disease may be brought under complete control when a high proportion of the population has been immunized; even though a small proportion remains non-immune the transmission of infection may virtually cease. The current programme for the global elimination of poliomyelitis includes the strategy of mass immunization on national immunization days (NID). The NID approach gives a big boost to herd immunity and helps to eliminate the wild poliovirus from the community.

CONTROL OF COMMUNICABLE DISEASES

ESTABLISHING A PROGRAMME

A programme for the control of a communicable disease should be based on a detailed knowledge of the epidemiology of the infection and on effective public health organization to plan, execute and evaluate the project. The epidemiological information should include knowledge of the local distribution of the infection, the major foci and the overall effect of the infection on the population.

The programme must include some mechanism for:

- recognizing the infection and the confirmation of the diagnosis;
- notifying the disease to the appropriate authority;
- finding the source of infection;
- assessing the extent of the outbreak by finding other cases and exposed persons.

RECOGNITION OF THE INFECTION

For the early recognition of communicable diseases, it is necessary that physicians and medical auxiliaries should be able to recognize the clinical manifestations of the major infective diseases in the area. This is particularly important in the case of acute epidemic diseases such as cholera, where prompt action is required to prevent the disastrous spread of infection. The health personnel at the most peripheral unit should be able to recognize epidemic outbreaks and take appropriate action. Laboratory services should be used to support clinical diagnosis. Ideally there should be a public health laboratory system which can process specimens from patients and from the environment.

NOTIFICATION OF DISEASES

A notifiable disease is one the occurrence of which must be reported to the appropriate health authority. The group includes the major epidemic diseases and other communicable diseases about which the health authorities require information. Some diseases are also notifiable internationally (see p. 372).

IDENTIFICATION OF THE SOURCE OF INFECTION

Epidemiological investigations are directed to finding the source of infection. This involves analysis of the information about the time sequence of the occurrence of cases and the history of the movements of the patients.

INCUBATION PERIOD

Knowledge of the incubation period of the infection (the interval between infection and onset of symptoms) is of great value in interpreting the data (Fig. 3.2). For example, in tracing the likely source of a case of gonorrhoea the patient should list all sexual contacts in the preceding 5 days before the onset of symptoms. Similarly, in a case of syphilis, the suspects would include all sexual partners in the 3-month period preceding the appearance of the chancre. Figure 3.3 gives the range of values for the incubation periods of some common infectious diseases.

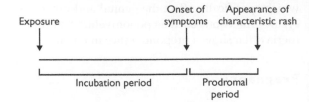

Figure 3.2: The dynamics of infection. The incubation period, defined as the time from infection of the host to the first appearance of symptoms, is in practice taken from time of first exposure, which is easier to determine. The prodromal period is the interval between the onset of symptoms and appearance of clinical manifestations, for example in measles infection, the symptoms of fever and coryza will occur within 10 days of exposure (incubation period) with the characteristic rash appearing about 4 days later (prodromal period).

Knowledge of the incubation period is also helpful in identifying whether an outbreak has resulted from a simple common exposure (a point source epidemic) or from multiple sources. Propagation of an epidemic from a single source will give rise to cases which will all be present within the incubation period of the infection. The occurrence of cases later than the maximum known length of the incubation period indicates propagation of the epidemic from more than one source.

Certain infections can be prevented by immunization of the host during the incubation period:

- *Passive immunization* with immunoglobulin can prevent or modify an attack of measles in a child who has been in contact with the infection.
- *Active immunization* early in the incubation period can protect those exposed to the risk of infection – as for possible exposure to rabies.

ASSESSMENT OF THE EXTENT OF THE OUTBREAK

This involves finding other infected persons in addition to those who have been notified, and identifying others who also have been exposed to the risk of infection – the contacts of known patients and others who have been exposed to a common source such as a polluted stream.

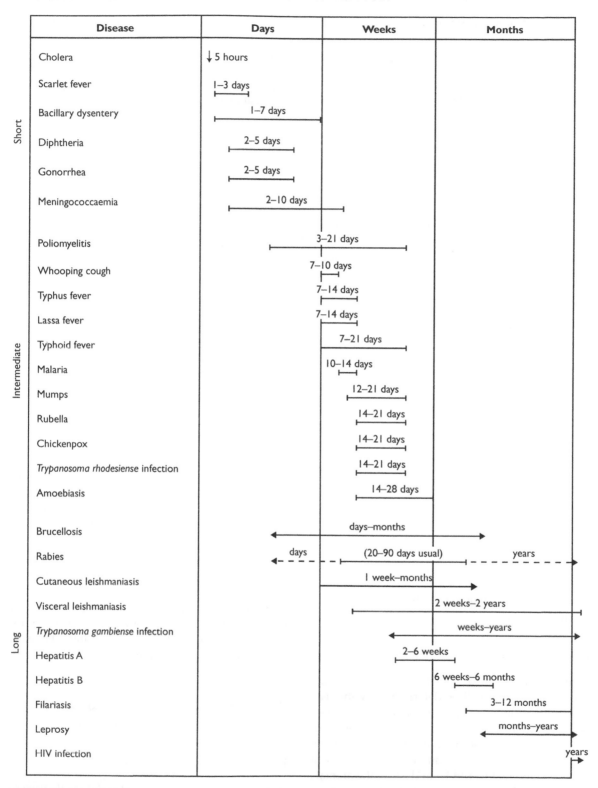

Figure 3.3: The range of values for the incubation periods of some common infectious diseases.
Source: Geddes (1988).

METHODS OF CONTROL

There are three main methods of controlling a communicable disease:

- eliminate reservoir of infection;
- interrupt the pathway of transmission;
- protect the susceptible hosts.

Elimination of the reservoir

HUMAN RESERVOIR

Where the reservoir is in human beings, the objective would be to find and treat all infected persons, both patients and carriers, thereby eliminating sources of infection. For some infections, segregation of infected persons through isolation or quarantine of those at risk may be required.

Isolation of patients

Isolation of patients is indicated for infections which have the following epidemiological features:

- high morbidity and mortality;
- high infectivity;
- no significant extrahuman reservoir;
- infectious cases easily recognizable;
- chronic carriers are not a significant part of the reservoir.

Quarantine

This refers to the limitation of movement of persons who have been exposed to infection. The restriction continues for a period of time equal to the longest duration of the incubation period usual for the disease.

THE ZOONOSES

Where the reservoir of infection is in animals, the appropriate action will be determined by the usefulness of the animals, how intimately they are associated with human beings and the feasibility of protecting susceptible animals. Where, as in the case of the plague rat, the animal is regarded as a pest, the objective would be to destroy the animals and exclude them from human habitations. Where, as in the case of rabies in an urban area, pet dogs are susceptible, the approach would be to protect them with rabies vaccine whilst destroying stray dogs. Animals that are used as food should be examined and the infected ones eliminated. This examination may take place in life, for example tuberculin testing of cattle, or it may take place after slaughter during meat inspection.

NON-LIVING RESERVOIR

Where the reservoir is in soil, elimination of the reservoir is not feasible but it may be possible to limit man's exposure to the affected area, for example in some areas, infection with *Histoplasma capsulatum* occurs in persons who go into bat-infected caves. Such exposure can be avoided.

Interruption of transmission

This mostly involves improvement of environmental sanitation and personal hygiene. The control of vectors also depends largely on alterations in the environment and, in addition, the use of pesticidal agents.

Protection of the susceptible host

This may be achieved by active or passive immunization. Protection may also be obtained by the use of antimicrobial drugs, for example chemoprophylaxis is used for the prevention of malaria, meningococcal meningitis and bacillary dysentery.

Mass campaigns are sometimes indicated for dealing with acute epidemics or as a method of controlling or eradicating endemic diseases. Any vaccine or drug used for a mass campaign must be effective, safe, cheap and simple to apply. Following the emergency operation of a mass campaign, the programme should be integrated into the basic health services of the community.

ARTIFICIAL IMMUNIZATION IN THE CONTROL OF INFECTION

Passive immunization

Preformed antibodies are used mainly in the protection of individuals who are at risk of exposure to a specific infection or as treatment for sick patients.

For example, travellers to places where infective hepatitis (hepatitis A virus) is highly endemic may be protected by inoculation with immunoglobulin. Passive immunization is also recommended for protecting individuals who are unusually susceptible to infections, for example varicella–zoster immune globulin is indicated in a child under immunosuppressive therapy who is exposed to chickenpox.

Active immunization

Since Edward Jenner demonstrated the value of cowpox in protecting against smallpox, active immunization has evolved to become a powerful tool in public health. In developing countries, vaccination has proved to be a cost-effective approach to disease control requiring relatively simple technology. Vaccination is usually the preferred intervention in those diseases for which effective vaccines are available. Traditionally, vaccines may contain one of the following:

- attenuated live organisms (e.g. measles, poliomyelitis);
- killed organisms (e.g. pertussis, typhoid, cholera);
- toxins–denatured toxins (e.g. tetanus, diphtheria);
- genetically engineered vaccines including the use of live carriers.

In order to be effective vaccines, the altered live organisms or their products must retain their ability to induce a protective immune response.

STRATEGIES FOR USING ACTIVE IMMUNIZATION

Routine childhood immunization

Routine immunization of children against diphtheria, pertussis, tetanus, measles, poliomyelitis and tuberculosis is an important tool for the control of these infections and for the promotion of child health (see Chapter 11). Many developing countries have had difficulty in ensuring that children receive the prescribed course of immunizations. WHO and UNICEF have jointly sponsored ventures aimed at improving the immunization programmes in developing countries. The WHO Expanded Programme for Immunization (EPI)

assists health authorities to design, implement and evaluate their immunization programmes, train their health personnel and acquire vaccines and other essential supplies. UNICEF has included immunization as an important component of its Child Survival Programme (p. 326).

These organizations are also involved in research aimed at solving the problems encountered in running the immunization programmes. For example, live vaccines must be refrigerated to maintain their potency otherwise they would deteriorate. WHO has tackled the problem of ensuring a continuous 'cold chain' from the point of manufacture of the live vaccine to its delivery to children in the most remote rural areas of hot tropical countries. A new initiative, the Global Alliance for Vaccine Initiatives (GAVI) has expanded the base of support for global immunizations by bringing together other stakeholders including the private sector.

Epidemic control

Vaccines are also used to control outbreaks of diseases, for example yellow fever (see Table 12.4).

The global eradication of smallpox and the elimination of poliomyelitis, first in the western hemisphere, now being extended to other regions, are outstanding examples of the successful application of immunization in disease control, elimination and eradication.

NEW VACCINES

Recent advances in immunology, molecular biology and genetic engineering have stimulated new approaches to the development of vaccines. Scientists are now able to identify more precisely the process by which immunity is acquired; to identify the antigenic components which induce protective immunity; and to produce relevant biological materials through the cloning of genes or the synthesis of peptides. These developments hold out the prospect of replacing the crude products of traditional vaccines with well-defined antigens. There is also the hope that effective vaccines can be developed against malaria and other parasitic infections. These biomedical advances have made possible a new generation of vaccines with increased efficacy, safety profile and affordability.

THE USE OF DRUGS IN THE CONTROL OF INFECTIONS

Apart from the treatment of individual patients, antimicrobial agents are used as part of the strategy for controlling infectious diseases. The drug may:

- protect the uninfected individual;
- arrest the progression of disease and reverse pathological damage;
- eliminate infection and thereby prevent further transmission of disease.

These qualities are exploited in the use of drugs for:

- *chemotherapy* – the treatment of sick individuals (although the term is also applied more broadly to cover other uses of drugs, including prophylaxis);
- *chemoprophylaxis* – the protection of persons who are exposed to the risk of infection, e.g. malaria;
- *chemosuppression* – the prevention of severe clinical manifestations and complications in infected persons.

STRATEGIES

Drugs have been used successfully as the main strategy for the control of some endemic diseases. Strategies for large-scale use of drugs in disease control include the following variants:

Mass chemotherapy

This strategy entails the treatment of all persons in the community, whether infected at the time of the survey or not. If a single examination of faeces, blood or urine shows that a high infection rate, say 50% or over, serial examinations will reveal that transmission is very high and that at some time or another, most of the community will acquire the infection. In such situations, it is more cost-effective to treat everyone without establishing the presence of infection in each subject. Mass chemotherapy with penicillin was used extensively in the yaws campaign and is currently used for the control of onchocerciasis (p. 231).

Selective population chemotherapy

This involves treatment of all persons that are found to be infected at initial and subsequent surveys, for example control of intestinal parasite infections, schistosomiasis control programmes, malaria eradication programmes.

Targeted chemotherapy

This involves treating only those individuals harbouring heavy infections and/or high risk groups, for example treatment of persons aged 5–20 years for *S. haematobium* infection.

In highly endemic areas and in the absence of an integrated approach to disease control (involving sanitation, health education and community participation) prevalence rates of infection tend to return to pretreatment levels within a relatively short time, usually a year. However, the intensity of infection remains low for a longer if variable period. Simulation models suggest that for some parasitic infections, targeted chemotherapy is most effective for the control of morbidity as opposed to the control of transmission. These various strategies for large-scale use of drugs are being applied in the control of several infectious diseases notably trachoma, schistosomiasis, malaria and onchocerciasis (see pp. 123, 206 and 231 respectively).

DRUG SPECIFICATIONS

Given the circumstances under which they will be administered, the ideal drugs for use in developing countries should meet the following specifications:

1 *Efficacy*. The drug should be effective against all strains of the pathogen; the occurrence or emergence of resistant strains would limit the usefulness of the drug.
2 *Safety*. The drug can be used safely by health personnel who have limited skills; it can be safely administered to persons who would not remain under continuous medical supervision; there should be a wide margin between the effective and the toxic dose; and there should be no dangerous side-effects.
3 *Simple regimens*. The dosage regimen should be simple and preferably administered by mouth; single dose treatments should be available.

4 *Acceptable*. The drug should be well tolerated by persons of the target age group and should have no unpleasant side-effects.
5 *Affordable*. The cost of the drug should permit its use within the limited budgets of developing countries.

Few drugs have all these qualities but the specifications serve as a checklist for assessing the value of any drug that is proposed for large-scale use. When such widespread drug therapy is administered in public health programmes it must be realized that resistant strains may emerge and that some individuals will show undesirable side-effects.

ANTIMICROBIAL RESISTANCE (PLATE 15)

Antimicrobial resistance has now become a serious public health concern. Thus, resistance to the first-line drugs for tuberculosis ranges from 2 to 40%; up to 90% of cases of *Salmonella dysenterae* are resistant to cotrimoxazole and naladixic acid; multiresistant *Salmonella typhi* is widespread in endemic countries; chloroquine-resistant malaria is global (except in Central America) while in South East Asia there has been a progressive decline in response to several antimalarial drugs (Plate 16).

The development of resistance is multifactorial namely: (i) overuse and misuse if antimicrobials by doctors and health personnel; (ii) poor compliance; (iii) self-medication; (iv) counterfeit drugs; (v) poor control of antimicrobials in hospitals; (vi) poor standards of hygiene – personal and environmental in hospitals; (vii) use of antibiotics in animal husbandry, horticulture and aquaculture; and (viii) international travel and trade.

SURVEILLANCE OF DISEASE

Surveillance of disease means the exercise of continuous scrutiny and watchfulness over the distribution and spread of infections and the related factors, with sufficient accuracy and completeness to provide the basis for effective control. This modern concept includes three main features:

- the systematic collection of all relevant data (Table 3.7);

Table 3.7: Examples of sources of epidemiological data in the surveillance of disease

- Registration of deaths
- Notification of disease and reporting of epidemics
- Laboratory investigations
- Data from routine screening, e.g. blood donors
- Investigation of individual cases and epidemics
- Epidemiological surveys
- Data from clinics, health centres, hospitals and other service institutions
- Distribution of the animal reservoir and the vector
- Production, distribution and care of vaccines, sera and drugs
- Demographic and environmental data
- Non-medical statistics, e.g. consumption of specific foods

- the orderly consolidation and evaluation of these data;
- the prompt dissemination of the results to those who need to know, particularly those who are in a position to take action.

The surveillance of communicable diseases has two main objectives. The first objective is the recognition of acute problems that demand immediate action. For example, the recognition of an outbreak of a major epidemic infection such as cholera or the fresh introduction of it into a previously uninfected area, must be recognized promptly so that infection may be confined to the smallest possible area in the shortest possible time. Second, surveillance is used to provide a broad assessment of specific problems in order to discern long-term trends and epidemiological patterns, to guide and monitor interventions, and finally to assess their impact. Thus, surveillance provides the scientific basis for ascertaining the major public health problems in an area, thereby serving as a guide for planning, implementation and assessment of programmes for the control of communicable disease.

The techniques of surveillance are now being applied to the control of non-infectious disease (see below):

- environmental hazards associated with atmospheric pollution, ionizing radiation and road traffic accidents;
- diseases such as cancer, atheroma and other degenerative diseases;

- social problems such as drug addiction, juvenile delinquency and commercial sex work.

EPIDEMIOLOGY OF NON-INFECTIOUS DISEASES

Epidemiological methods have been widely applied in the study of non-infectious diseases. Such studies have yielded many fruitful results, especially in providing the basis for taking effective preventive action long before the specific aetiological agent is identified or the mechanism of the pathogenesis of the disease are understood. For example, in the 18th century Lind demonstrated that the occurrence of scurvy was associated with lack of fresh fruit in the diet of sailors. He was able to take effective action in preventing scurvy by the use of lime juice more than 150 years before the recognition of vitamin C as the specific factor involved.

Epidemiological studies have made important contributions to knowledge of the aetiology of various diseases including the following examples:

- *nutritional disorders* (scurvy, beriberi, pellagra, dental caries, goitre);
- *cancer* (skin, lungs, penis, cervix uteri, breast, bladder, leukaemia);
- *congenital abnormalities* (Down's syndrome, thalidomide poisoning);
- *intoxications* (chronic beryllium poisoning, alcoholic cirrhosis);
- *mental illness* (postpartum psychosis, neuroses, suicide);
- *accidents* (home, road and industrial accidents) (Plates 17 and 18)
- *degenerative diseases* (tropical neuropathy, coronary artery disease, hypertension, arthritis).

THE COMPONENTS IN THE AETIOLOGY OF NON-INFECTIOUS DISEASE

For the study of infectious diseases, it is convenient to use the simple model of 'agent', 'mode of transmission' and 'host'. This model needs to be modified in dealing with non-infectious diseases. First, instead of a specific aetiological agent, the non-infectious disease may result from multiple factors. Second, since there is no infective agent being transmitted, it is more appropriate to replace this with 'environmental or behavioural factors'. Third, host factors cannot be analysed in terms of active or passive immunity but rather in terms of various host factors – genetic, social, behavioural, psychological, etc. – which modify the risk of developing these various diseases.

RISK FACTORS

The concept of risk factors is increasingly used in the study of non-communicable disease. For example, many factors are associated with the occurrence of ischaemic heart disease including diet, exercise, and the use of cigarettes. From the public health point of view it is desirable to be able to assign different weights to each of these factors. How much does cigarette smoking contribute to the risk of the occurrence of ischaemic heart disease? Conversely, how much change in the rate can be expected if a group alters its smoking habits? Similarly, the same question can be asked with regard to diet and exercise. Furthermore, there is the possibility that the effects of individual factors are not merely additive but may interact. It is possible to obtain numerical estimates of the risk factors by the use of statistical methods including multiple regression and partial correlations.

Apart from the study of the aetiology of non-communicable diseases, the concept of risk factors has been applied to other health phenomena. In obstetric practice, for example, the outcome of pregnancy is influenced by maternal factors, environmental factors and in the health care given to the mother and the new-born baby. Thus, the perinatal mortality rate is associated with such factors as the age of the mother, the number of previous pregnancies, her past obstetric history, her stature (especially her height and the size and shape of her pelvis), and her state of health (especially the presence of diseases such as hypertension, diabetes and anaemia).

In some cases the risk factors relate directly to aetiological factors (cigarette smoking and cancer of the lung) but in other cases the risk factor identified may be a convenient, easily identified and measured indicator of an underlying aetiological factor.

For example, the level of education of the mother can be identified as a risk factor in relation to the health status of the infant. The effect of the mother's education is indirect. It would have been more direct to measure maternal practices with regard to child care (specific indicators of care can be devised and validated). In many communities, however, the level of maternal education serves as an index of important environmental, social and economic factors which affect the health of the child.

In spite of these apparent differences, the basic epidemiological approach is identical: the epidemiological investigation of non-communicable disease involves a study of the distribution of the disease (descriptive), a search for the determinants of the distribution (analytical), and deliberate experiments designed to test hypotheses (experimental). The basic strategy is to discover populations or groups in which the disease is relatively rare: these groups can then be compared and contrasted in the hope of discovering the probable causes of the disease. The effects of making alterations in these supposed factors can be examined by controlled trials.

REFERENCES AND FURTHER READING

Buck C., Llopis A., Nájera E. & Terris M. (1988) *The Challenge of Epidemiology: Issues and Selected Readings.* Pan American Health Organization, Washington, DC.

Geddes A.M. (1988) *Medicine International Infections.* Part 1, p. 8.

Last J.M. (Ed.) (1988) *A Dictionary of Epidemiology,* 3rd edn. Oxford Medical Publications, New York.

Vaughan J.P. & Morrow R.H. (Eds) (1989) *Manual of Epidemiology for District Health Managers.* WHO, Geneva.

WHO (1975) *The Veterinary Contribution to Public Health Practice.* Technical Report Series No. 573. WHO, Geneva.

WHO (1979) *Parasitic Zoonoses.* Technical Report Series No. 637. WHO, Geneva.

WHO (1997) *Anti-TB Drug Resistance in the World.* Report on Malarial Control Programme and Drug Resistance in Thailand, Sirichaisintop and Banchongaksorn, 1997, WPRO.

WHO (2000) *Communicable Diseases 2000.* WHO/CDS/2000.1. WHO, Geneva.

Wilson M.E. (1991) *A World Guide to Infections: Diseases, Distribution, Diagnosis.* Oxford University Press, Oxford.

CHAPTER FOUR

COMMUNICABLE DISEASES: INFECTIONS THROUGH THE GASTRO-INTESTINAL TRACT

- Infective agents
- Control of the infections acquired through the gastro-intestinal tract
- Diarrhoeal diseases
- Viral infections

- Bacterial infections
- Protozoal infections
- Helminthic infections
- References and further reading

INFECTIVE AGENTS

A number of important pathogens gain entry through the gastro-intestinal tract. Some of these cause diarrhoeal diseases (e.g. *Salmonella* and *Shigella* spp.) whilst others pass through the intestinal tract to cause disease in other organs (e.g. poliomyelitis, viral hepatitis). The pathogens include viruses, bacteria, protozoa and helminths. Box 4.1 lists all the infections described in this chapter.

PHYSICAL AND BIOLOGICAL CHARACTERISTICS

In considering the epidemiology of these infections, it is useful to note some of the physical and biological properties of each infective agent. The organisms vary in their ability to withstand physical conditions such as high or low temperatures and drying, and they also differ in their susceptibility to chemical agents, including chlorine. The vegetative form of *Entamoeba histolytica* is rapidly destroyed in the stomach but the cyst form survives digestion by gastric juices. Differences in the sizes of the organisms are also of epidemiological importance. Thus, simple filtration through a clay filter will eliminate most of the large organisms – bacteria, protozoa, and the eggs or larvae of helminths – from polluted water, but the filtrate will contain the smaller organisms such as viruses.

TRANSMISSION

Viruses, bacteria and cysts of protozoa are directly infectious to man as they are passed in the faeces, but in the case of helminths, the egg may become infectious only after maturation in the soil (e.g. *Ascaris*) or after passing through an intermediate host (e.g. *Taenia saginata*). The most important pattern of transmission is the passage of infective material from human faeces into the mouth of a new host and this is known as 'faeco-oral' or 'intestino-oral' transmission. It should be noted, however, that not all the pathogens which infect through the mouth are excreted in the faeces; for example guinea worm infection (see p. 81) is acquired by mouth but the larvae escape through the skin. On the other hand, the ova of hookworm (see p. 137) are passed in faeces but the route of infection is most

Box 4.1: List of infections

Viral infections
Gastro-enteritis/meningitis (coxsackie, echo, reo, rotaviruses)
Poliomyelitis (poliovirus)
Viral hepatitis* (hepatitis A and E viruses)

Bacterial infections
Enteric fevers (*Salmonella typhi, S. paratyphi*)
Gastro-enteritis (*Escherichia coli, Campylobacter* spp.)
Bacillary dysentary (*Shigella* spp.)
Cholera (*Vibrio cholera*)
Brucellosis (*Brucella* spp.)
Food poisoning (*Salmonella typhimurium, Staphylococcus aureus, Clostridium welchii*)

Protozoal infections
Amoebiasis (*Entamoeba histolytica*)
Giardiasis (*Giardia lamblia*)
Balantidiasis (*Balantidium coli*)
Toxoplasmosis (*Toxoplasma gondii*)
Cryptosporidiosis (*Cryptosporidium*)

Helminthic infections
Nematodes (roundworms)
Ascariasis (*Ascaris lumbricoides*)
Toxocariasis (*Toxocara canis, T. cati*)
Trichuriasis (*Trichuris trichiura*)
Enterobiasis (*Enterobius vermicularis*)
Dracontiasis/guinea worm (*Dracunculus medinensis*)
Trichinosis (*Trichinella spiralis*)
Angiostrongyliasis (*Angiostrongylus cantonensis*)
Gnathostomiasis (*Gnathostoma* spp.)

Cestodes (tapeworms)
Taeniasis (*Taeniae* spp.)
Diphyllobothriasis (*Diphyllobothrium latum*)
Hymenolepiasis (*Hymenolepis* spp.)
Hydatid disease (*Echinococcus* spp.)

Trematodes (flukes)
Paragonimiasis (*Paragonimus* spp.)
Clonorchiasis (*Clonorchis sinensis*)
Opisthorchiasis (*Opisthorchis* spp.)
Fascioliasis (*Fasciola hepatica*)
Fasciolopsiasis (*Fasciolopsis buski*)
Heterophyiasis (*Heterophyes heterophyes*)
Metagonimiasis (*Metagonimus yokogawi*)

*Other types of hepatitis not acquired through the gastro-intestinal tract are also dealt with here.

frequently by direct penetration of the skin by the infective larvae.

The faeco-oral route

The direct ingestion of gross amounts of faeces is uncommon, except in young children and mentally disturbed persons. Faeco-oral transmission occurs mostly through inapparent faecal contamination of food, water and hands – the three main items that regularly make contact with the mouth (Fig. 4.1). It should be noted that minute quantities of faeces can carry the infective dose of various pathogens. Thus, dangerously polluted water may appear sparkling clear, contaminated food may be free of objectionable odour or taste, and apparently clean hands may carry and transmit disease.

As shown in Figure 4.1, food occupies a central and important position. Not only can it be contaminated directly by faeces but it can also be contaminated indirectly through polluted water, dirty hands, contaminated soil and filth flies. Water may be polluted directly by faeces but also indirectly from the polluted soil on the riverbank. There are many opportunities for the contamination of hands: the person may contaminate hands on cleaning after defaecation or in touching or handling contaminated objects, including soil. Contamination of the soil with faeces plays an essential role in the transmission of certain helminths which must undergo a period of maturation before becoming infectious (e.g. *Ascaris*).

Filth flies, in particular the common housefly, spread faecal material and play a role in the transmission of gastro-intestinal infections. The housefly mechanically transfers faecal pollution by:

- carrying faeces on its hairy limbs;

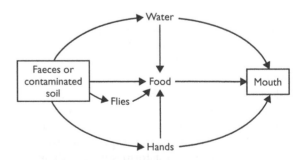

Figure 4.1: Pathways of faceo-oral transmission.

- regurgitating the contents of its stomach on to solid food as a means of liquefying it ('vomit drop');
- defecating on the food: its faeces may contain surviving organisms derived from human faeces.

Although flies are physically capable of transmitting these infections, it is not easy to determine how important they are in particular epidemiological situations and it is likely that their significance has been exaggerated in relation to the other mechanisms of transmission.

Epidemic patterns in relation to the mode of transmission

Some of the infections that are acquired through the gastro-intestinal tract characteristically occur in epidemic form, for example typhoid. The pattern of an epidemic is affected by the route of transmission. A water-borne epidemic is typically explosive: it may affect people over a wide area who have no other traceable connection but the use of the same water supply. Food-borne outbreaks may be more localized, affecting persons from the same household or boarding institution, those who feed communally at a hotel, restaurant, aeroplane or staff canteen, or those who have taken part in a festive dinner or picnic.

HOST FACTORS

Certain non-specific factors in the host pay some part in preventing infection through the gastro-intestinal tract. The high acid content and the antibacterial lysozyme in the stomach, and the digestive juices in the upper part of the intestinal tract destroy potentially infective organisms but do not constitute an impenetrable barrier to infection.

More significant is the specific immunity which can be derived from previous infections or from artificial immunization. Immunity is in part related to specific antibodies in the sera of those previously infected or artificially immunized. It has also been demonstrated that the intestinal mucosa may acquire resistance to certain pathogens such as cholera or poliomyelitis: this local resistance is mediated through a fraction of immunoglobins (IgA) which are secreted by the mucosa.

CONTROL OF THE INFECTIONS ACQUIRED THROUGH THE GASTRO-INTESTINAL TRACT

The most effective method of controlling these diseases can best be determined from a knowledge of the epidemiology of the infection with particular reference to the local community. Control can operate on each of the three components of infection:

1 The infective agent:
   - sanitary disposal of faeces;
   - elimination of human and animal reservoirs.
2 The route of transmission:
   - provision of safe water supply;
   - protection of food from contamination;
   - control of flies;
   - improvement of personal hygiene.
3 The host:
   - specific immunization;
   - chemoprophylaxis;
   - specific treatment.

The measures directed at infective agents and their transmission relate to the improvement of environmental sanitation and are mostly not specific to any particular infection.

Action can be taken at the level of the individual, the family, and the community. Control at community level may be investigating specific outbreaks, for example at school or parties, instituting surveillance charts in the dispensary or primary health unit, or through health education.

DIARRHOEAL DISEASES

Diarrhoeal diseases, as a group, remain a major cause of death in developing countries, especially in preschool children. Children under 3 years of age may experience as many as 10 episodes of diarrhoea per year. The main agents are:

- Enteroviruses, e.g. rotavirus;
- *Escherichia coli*
   (a) Enterotoxigenic *E. coli* (ETEC)
   (b) Localized-adherent *E. coli* (LA-EC)
   (c) Diffuse-adherent *E. coli* (DA-EC)
   (d) Enteroinvasive *E.coli* (EIEC)
   (e) Enterohaemorrhagic *E. coli* (EHEC);

- *Campylobacter* spp.;
- *Shigella*;
- *Vibrio cholerae* 01 and 0139;
- *Salmonella* (non-typhoid);
- *Entamoeba histolytica*;
- *Giardia lamblia*;
- *Cryptosporidium*.

See sections below on each of these agents and on gastro-enteritis for further details.

ACUTE DIARRHOEA

Most episodes of diarrhoea last less than 7 days and can be effectively treated with oral rehydration, combined with an appropriate diet. Limited evidence suggests that vitamin A deficiency predisposes to increased risk of diarrhoeal illness and to increased risk of death in preschool children.

Children with diarrhoea but no dehydration should receive extra fluids at home – as much as the child will take in small sips. If the child is being breast-fed, more frequent and longer breast-feeding is advocated; supplemented with oral rehydration solution (ORS) or clean water. For non-exclusively breast-fed children give ORS, rice water, or clean water. If some dehydration is present – restlessness, instability, thirsty – take child to nearest clinic if possible.

If the child is severely dehydrated – lethargy, swollen eyes, drinking poorly – take child to nearest hospital.

A reduced osmolarity rehydration solution has been found to reduce stool output and vomiting and results in fewer failures requiring the use of intravenous fluids compared with the standard WHO solution (see page 65).

PERSISTENT DIARRHOEA

Persistence of an acute diarrhoeal episode for at least 14 days occurs in 3–20% of cases. This leads to significantly increased mortality: 14% of persistent cases are fatal compared with 1% of acute cases. Risk factors in the development of persistent diarrhoea include:

- age;
- nutritional status;
- immunological status;
- previous infections;

- concomitant enteropathogenic bacteria (e.g. enteroadherent *E. coli*; enteropathogenic *E. coli* and cryptosporidia).

The main goal in the clinical management of persistent diarrhoea is to maintain the child's hydration and nutritional status while the intestinal damage is being investigated and treated.

CONTROL

Programmes for the reduction of morbidity and mortality include:

- oral rehydration therapy – highly effective in preventing death from dehydration in acute episodes;
- promotion of breast-feeding (exclusively for 4 months: continue for 2 years);
- improving weaning practices (soft mashed cereals, pulses: small serving of vegetable oil);
- improving water supply and sanitation (safe water: use of latrines: safe disposal of stools);
- promoting personal and domestic hygiene (handwashing: prevent contamination of food);
- immunization (measles);
- specific chemotherapy for invasive bowel infections or presence of *Helicobacter pylori*;
- zinc supplementation.

Not all interventions are appropriate everywhere. Each country must decide which package of measures is likely to be most feasible and cost-effective. Rota viruses and cholera immunization must await the results of field trials of the new vaccines.

VIRAL INFECTIONS

The most common viral infections transmitted through the gastro-intestinal tract are:

- rotaviruses;
- poliomyelitis;
- viral hepatitis A.

ENTEROVIRAL DISEASES

The enteroviruses, in addition to poliovirus, mainly include the coxsackie, echo (enteric cytopathogenic human orphan), reo, norwalk and rotaviruses.

These viruses were first isolated from the faeces of patients during poliomyelitis investigations. Healthy persons may excrete enteroviruses for short periods, and in areas where standards of environmental sanitation are low, subclinical infection is prevalent among infants and young children. *It should be noted that the enteroviruses may interfere with oral poliomyelitis vaccination campaigns in the tropics.*

Coxsackie viruses are classified into two groups, A and B, and although frequently isolated from healthy persons they may cause a variety of human illnesses (e.g. herpangina, summer grippe, vesticular stomatitis, virus meningitis, etc.). The presence of coxsackie group B virus can interfere with poliomyelitis virus multiplication, while a mixed coxsackie group A and poliomyelitis virus infection might result in a more severe paralysis.

Echo viruses are also excreted by healthy persons, particularly children, but may cause illnesses such as diarrhoea and meningitis.

Reoviruses were first isolated from the faeces of healthy children but have also been found in children with diarrhoea and steatorrhoeic enteritis.

ROTAVIRUSES

Occurrence:	Worldwide
Organisms:	Rotaviruses groups A and B
Reservoir:	Humans
Transmission:	Faeco-oral, person to person, water
Control:	High level of personal sanitary practices
	Improved environmental hygiene

Rotaviruses are the most common cause of diarrhoea worldwide, accounting for 134 million episodes yearly. Virtually all children have been infected by the age of 4 years.

The incubation period is short – 24–48 hours – with vomiting, fever and a watery diarrhoea the presenting clinical features.

Epidemiology

Most infections are caused by group A viruses, although group B have caused widespread outbreaks in China. The reservoir of infection is humans and transmission occurs by the faeco-oral route due to poor standards of personal and environmental hygiene. Virus shedding continues for about 8 days. The peak age-specific prevalence is in children between 6 and 24 months.

Diagnosis

Rotaviruses are identified in the stool by ELISA, electron microscopy, or passive particle agglutination techniques.

Control

INDIVIDUAL

Oral, subcutaneous or intravenous rehydration.

COMMUNITY

High standards of personal hygiene and sanitary practices should be employed, although these may not be entirely successful because the virus survives in contaminated water, on hands and is resistant to commonly used disinfectants. It is inactivated by chlorine. An effective vaccine was produced but has recently been withdrawn because of unexpected and serious adverse effects. Newer vaccines are being evaluated.

POLIOMYELITIS

Occurrence:	Indian subcontinent; Africa
Organisms:	Poliovirus I, II, III
Reservoir:	Humans
Transmission:	Person to person, faeco-oral, pharyngeal spread, food
Control:	Notification
	Isolation
	Safe disposal of faeces
	Hygiene
	Immunization
	Surveillance of acute flaccid paralysis (AFP)

Until recently, poliomyelitis was the most important enterovirus in the tropics but widespread immunization programmes have greatly reduced the incidence of the disease (Plates 19 and 20).

Indeed hopes are high that the disease will be eradicated within the next 5 years. At present, the only countries still experiencing the disease are those engulfed in civil strife, war, dispersed populations, difficult geography and/or impoverished states (Plate 21). The final stages of the polio eradication are expected to be the most difficult. Although the disease has been eradicated throughout the western hemisphere, wild virus is still circulating in many other regions of the world.

The incubation period varies from 3 to 21 days, with an average of about 10 days. Poliomyelitis is a notifiable disease. It is characterized by fever and a flaccid asymmetrical paralysis.

Epidemiology

The disease is now limited to a few countries in the tropics. All of the known types of poliomyelitis (1, 2 and 3) are prevalent although the virus strains responsible for paralytic illness in any area may vary, and at different periods in the same area one type or other may predominate. Large-scale epidemics may result if virulent wild-type virus (commonly type 1) is reintroduced into a community with breakdown in vaccine delivery and poor socio-economic and environmental conditions.

In the tropics, a seasonal peak occurs in the hot and rainy season. In 1999, 7086 cases were reported worldwide, of which 2814 were in India.

RESERVOIR

Humans are the reservoir of infection. The poliovirus is excreted in the stools of infected cases, convalescent patients and health carriers.

TRANSMISSION

Poliomyelitis is a highly infectious disease and the alimentary tract is of prime importance as a portal of entry and exit of the virus, as it is with other enteroviruses. The virus is transmitted from person to person by the faecal–oral route or pharyngeal secretions, rarely by foodstuffs contaminated by faeces.

HOST FACTORS

The incidence rates in males and females are similar. Trauma, excessive fatigue and pregnancy during the period of acute febrile illness, and intramuscular injections some time before the acute episode, all seem to be provoking factors leading to paralysis. Tonsillectomy increases the risk of bulbar poliomyelitis. The mechanism of these various stresses is not clear.

The factor of greatest importance in determining the incidence of paralytic poliomyelitis is the state of immunity of the affected population. In many tropical countries where sanitation is primitive and living conditions are crowded and poor, conditions for the spread of poliovirus are good. Consequently, infants have the opportunity of coming into contact with all three types of poliomyelitis virus early in life, and few of them reach preschool age without having been infected with at least one strain, although, clinically, the infection is in most cases unapparent. Immunity is acquired early: serum antibody surveys carried out among children in many parts of the tropics have shown that by the time they are 3 years old 90% have developed antibodies against at least one type of poliomyelitis. In countries where the sanitary arrangements are good, the risk of contact with the virus at an early age is diminished and older persons are affected. Thus, the most significant difference between the occurrence of poliomyelitis in the well-developed countries of the temperate zone and the less-developed areas of the tropics is in the distribution of cases in the various age groups.

Virology

There are three distinct types of poliovirus, that invade the central nervous system: type 1 (Brunhilde), type 2 (Lansing) and type 3 (Leon). The viruses grow well in tissue culture, they resist desiccation but are killed in half an hour by heat (60°C). Most outbreaks are due to type 1 poliovirus.

Laboratory diagnosis

The virus is isolated from specimens of faeces, throat swabs or from throat and nasopharyngeal washings. Clinically, the most important differential diagnosis is Guillain–Barée syndrome, in which the paralysis is usually symmetrical and progresses for longer periods – 10 days instead of 3–4 days as in poliomyelitis.

Control

High standards of hygiene and mass immunization are the two most important measures of control.

THE INDIVIDUAL

The disease is notifiable and isolation of individual cases is highly desirable. This measure itself is not enough to control an epidemic because of the large numbers of asymptomatic carriers. All pharyngeal and faecal discharges of patients should be treated with disinfectants and disposed of as safely as possible. Contacts should be protected with oral polio vaccine and kept under observation for a period of 3 weeks from the date of their last known contact. Tonsillectomy and dental extractions should be deferred when a poliomyelitis epidemic is present in the community and injections of any kind reduced to a minimum. Individuals should avoid over-exertion such as games, swimming, etc.

THE COMMUNITY

Crowds should be avoided during epidemics. Sanitary disposal of faeces should be encouraged. Health education aimed at raising the standards of personal hygiene should be rigorously carried out. Education on the advantages of childhood immunization should be enhanced.

Rehabilitation for paralysed persons is essential. A 'lameness register' for all children entering school from the time an immunization programme is initiated (see below) may serve as an indicator of the impact of the programme.

IMMUNIZATION

Immunization provides the most reliable method for the prevention of poliomyelitis and for controlling rapid spread during an epidemic. Two types of poliomyelitis vaccines are currently available: killed 'Salk' vaccine (IPV), which is given by injection, and the attenuated 'Sabin' vaccine, which is given by mouth (OPV). The advantages and disadvantages of each vaccine are compared in Table 4.1.

Most countries in the tropics use OPV alone, given at the same time as DTP and/or during national immunization days, regardless of immunization status. A limited number of countries use IPV alone and a few a combination of both OPV and IPV. Although other enteroviruses may

Table 4.1: Comparison of polio vaccines

Vaccine	Advantages	Disadvantages
Live, Sabin	Less expensive Oral administration Herd immunity Possible immediate protection by interfering with poliovirus	May cause paralytic polio Less stable, especially in tropical climates Interference by enteric viruses
Killed, Salk	Safe Stable Reliable humoral immunity not affected by other viruses	More expensive Administration by injection Wide coverage needed to protect populations

interfere with a satisfactory antibody response to OPV in a percentage of recipients, in practice the Sabin vaccine has afforded protection against the disease when used in mass immunization campaigns in tropical countries.

In countries undertaking polio eradication each case of Acute Flaccid Paralysis (AFP) in children under 15 years has got to be reported. Their surveillance performance has to meet the following criteria: (i) a non-polio AFP rate of at least 1/100 000 children under 15 years of age; (ii) two specimens of faeces collected 24–48 hours apart from at least 60% of detected AFP cases; and (iii) all specimens must arrive in 'good condition' (no leakage, no desiccation, presence of ice) and must be processed in a WHO-accredited laboratory.

National immunization days are used to supplement coverage of regular EPI programmes.

ERADICATION

In 1988 WHO declared the goal of eliminating poliomyelitis in the world due to wild-type virus by the year 2000. The strategy is four-pronged comprising: (i) high routine immunization coverage with OPV; (ii) supplementary immunization in the form of national immunization days (NIDs); (iii) effective surveillance; and (iv) in the final stages, door-to-door immunization campaigns in areas where the virus persists.

In 1996, 400 million children – two-thirds of the world's children under 5 years – were immunized during national immunization days; 118 million children were immunized in India on a single day.

Countries with continuing political unrest such as Afghanistan, Sudan, Somalia remain problem areas in achieving global eradication.

In 2002 WHO declared the European region poliomyelitis-free.

VIRAL HEPATITIS

There are six types of viral hepatitis – A and E, which are transmitted by the faeco-oral route, and B, C, D and G, which are blood-borne infections.

Viral hepatitis A (HAV)

Occurrence:	Worldwide
Organism:	Hepatitis A virus (HAV)
Reservoir:	Humans
Transmission:	Faeco-oral route, person to person, water, food
Control:	Personal hygiene
	Adequate disposal of faeces
	Safe drinking water
	Immunization

The disease is characterized by loss of appetite, jaundice, enlargement of the liver and raised levels of liver enzymes. The incubation period varies from 15 to 40 days with an average of around 20 days.

EPIDEMIOLOGY

The disease is widespread but is more common in the tropics and subtropics; in these areas, most infections are acquired in childhood and many are subclinical.

Four distinct epidemiological patterns are recognized related to the quality of public health sanitation, sewage disposal and population density. Thus in Africa, Asia and Central America infection occurs predominantly in children under 10 years of age; in the emerging countries of Eastern Europe, the republics of the former Soviet Union and China HAV infections tend to occur in adolescents and young adults, in the USA and Western Europe the infection affects older individuals resulting in substantial absence from work and economic loss, while in the Scandinavian countries where standards of hygiene are extremely high autochthonous transmission of HAV is rare. Changing economic conditions (e.g. in the tiger economies of South East Asia) will result in changing epidemiological patterns.

Reservoir

Humans are the reservoir of infection, excreting the organism in the faeces and possibly urine. Viraemia is present within a few days of exposure and virus shed in the faeces continues until the onset of clinical symptoms.

Transmission

Faeco-oral spread is the most important mode of transmission by direct or indirect contact. Sporadic cases are probably caused by person to person contact, but explosive epidemics from water and food occur. Food handlers can disseminate the infection. The ingestion of shellfish grown in polluted waters is attended by a risk of acquiring hepatitis A.

Host factors

Although in most parts of the tropics infective hepatitis is essentially a childhood disease, many adult patients are also seen. In many countries the incidence of infectious hepatitis is rising. Factors affecting the severity of the disease include:

- Age – children tolerate the infection and recover more rapidly than adults.
- Sex – men take longer than women to recover from an equivalent degree of liver damage.
- Pregnancy – exacerbates hepatitis.
- Strenuous exercise – in the early stages of the disease.
- Glucose-6-phospate deficiency – a high frequency of G6PD deficiency has been found among patients with hepatitis and those with this genetic enzyme defect have a longer and more severe course.

Hepatitis is a recognized hazard for 'overlanders' who return from tropical countries by bus or hitchhiking. Hepatitis A infection is more common among male homosexuals, especially those who practice oral–anal sex.

Hepatitis has many epidemiological similarities to poliomyelitis and is a sensitive indicator of poor community hygiene. A high incidence of acute coma and an increased death rate was associated in Accra (Ghana) with immigration, shantytown residency and lower socio-economic status.

VIROLOGY AND LABORATORY DIAGNOSIS

HAV is in the range of 25–28 nm and is identified by electron microscopy. Elevation of serum levels of liver enzymes is invariably found. The diagnosis is confirmed by the demonstration of IgM antibodies to the virus measured by solid phase, IgM capture immunoassays.

CONTROL

Control depends on high standards of personal and environmental hygiene, for example proper sewage disposal, safe drinking water.

Individual

If patients are in hospital they should, if possible, be barrier nursed as for any faeces-carried infection. Food handlers should not resume work until 3 weeks after recovery.

Immunization

Inactivated HAV vaccine is now available. A double-dose vaccine has been licensed which, if followed by a booster dose 6–12 months later, is expected to provide at least 10 years' protection. It induces antibodies in over 90% of individuals within 2 weeks and protects against infection. The vaccine should be given intramuscularly in the deltoid region.

Unfortunately, HAV vaccines are at present too expensive for use on a population-wide basis in most tropical countries. Passive immunity may be conferred using human immunoglobulin (IG). Even when it does not prevent infection it does modify the severity of the disease. It is useful in protecting family contacts during epidemics (0.2 ml/kg intramuscularly). For those going to the tropics a 0.2–0.5 ml/kg gives passive protection for

about 6 months. Recovery from a clinical attack creates a lasting active immunity.

Viral hepatitis E (HEV)

Like HAV, HEV causes malaise, anorexia, jaundice and liver enzyme serum elevation. The first outbreak occurred in India in 1955 involving over 30 000 people and was associated with a breach in the city's water supply system. The incubation period is around 40 days, a case fatality rate of 20% occurred in pregnant women in India, while 60% of sporadic cases of fulminant hepatitis seen in the country are all due to HEV.

EPIDEMIOLOGY

Subsequent to the Indian epidemic, hepatitis E has been reported from a number of countries in the tropics ranging from China to Mexico. The source of infection has been contaminated drinking water. The peak age specific sero-prevalence in endemic countries is in the over-16 years group – unlike hepatitis A, which usually occurs before the age of 5 years. Clinical manifestations occur in persons 25–40 years of age. Autochthonous cases of hepatitis E are rare in Western Europe and the USA.

CONTROL

As for HAV, provision of safe drinking water and sanitary disposal of faeces is required to prevent the infection. No vaccine is as yet available.

Hepatitis B (HBV)

Occurrence:	Worldwide
Organism:	Hepatitis B virus (HBV)
Reservoir:	Humans
Transmission:	Blood and blood products
Control:	Counselling
	Hygiene
	Blood screening
	Vaccination

Hepatitis B is not transmitted by the faeco-oral route but is a blood-borne agent, transmitted by inoculation. It is only included here for convenience.

Hepatitis B virus causes long-incubation hepatitis. It also gives rise to one of the 10 most common cancers, heptocellular carcinoma. There is evidence that HBV is the aetiological agent in up to 80% of cases.

EPIDEMIOLOGY

The carrier state (defined as the presence of HbsAg for more than 6 months – see below) rises from 0.1% in parts of Europe to 15% in several tropical countries. Globally, early childhood infections are the most common and most important. In China, Taiwan and Hong Kong, a large number of infections are acquired in the perinatal period, usually from a carrier mother.

Transmission may occur by:

- transfusion of blood or blood products;
- accidental inoculation, e.g. repeated use of hypodermic needles without adequate sterilization, in particular: drug addicts, mass immunization, tattooing and ritual sacrification;
- insect bites;
- perinatally – from a carrier mother;
- sexual intercourse – hetero- and homosexual;
- serous exudates of skin ulcers;
- injury-associated sports or jobs.

VIROLOGY

HBV possesses at least three separate antigens: surface antigen (HbsAg); core antigen (HbcAg) and enzyme antigen (HbeAg). The HbcAg is a valuable marker of potential infectivity of HbsAg positive serum. Subdeterminants of both surface antigen and c antigen occur.

CONTROL

Control is carried out by a combination of: (i) counselling; (ii) hygiene practices in high-risk areas; (iii) vaccination of at-risk individuals; and (iv) selective use of hepatitis B immunoglobin (HbIG). A recombinant HbsAg vaccine is now widely used. Three doses (at 0, 1 and 6 months) are required for complete protection. Vaccination is required for groups at high risk of infection (e.g. health-care staff in contact with blood or patients, homosexuals, drug users, etc.) depending on epidemiological patterns, socio-economic factors, cultural and sexual practices. In areas of the world where perinatal infection is common, immunization of susceptible women of childbearing age and of infants, particularly those born to carrier mothers, is desirable. Administration of HbIG confers extra protection to these infants and those individuals accidentally exposed (e.g. health workers following needle-stick injuries and sexual partners of acute cases).

WHO has recommended that all children should be vaccinated during the first year of life. In countries where perinatal transmission is frequent, vaccination should be done at or soon after birth.

Hepatitis C (HCV)

Hepatitis C virus was discovered in 1989, and contains six different genotypes (1–6) which vary in their geographical destination (e.g. type 4 predominates in the Middle East, North and Central Africa). The incubation period from exposure to liver function abnormalities is usually 8 weeks. Chronic infection is generally asymptomatic at first, later a large proportion of cases progress to cirrhosis of the liver and some to hepatocellular carcinoma.

EPIDEMIOLOGY

HCV has a worldwide distribution. The route of infection is parenteral (e.g. intravenous drug users, blood transfusion). Donor HCV sero-prevalence is high in Egypt. Transplanted organs may also transmit the infection. Unsterile needles in medical and dental procedures, tattooing and other perisubcutaneous procedures are also responsible.

CONTROL

- For the individual, interferon is now generally prescribed for the treatment of chronic hepatitis associated with HCV infection.
- Screening of blood donors has proved effective in reducing transmission of HCV.
- Education, greater availability of disposable needles, and for drug abusers, needle-exchange programmes could prevent the infection.
- No vaccine is currently available.

Hepatitis delta (HDV)

HDV is a small, incomplete virus incapable of independent replication, which can exist only in the presence of HBV. It gives rise to a more severe form of hepatitis. Two forms of infection have been recognized and are referred to as: *coinfection* together with acute HBV (i.e. HDV + HBV) and *superinfection* of an HBV carrier (i.e. DV + HbsAg). Like HBV, HDV is a blood-borne pathogen. Delta hepatitis is endemic in the Eastern Mediterranean, the Middle East, North Africa, the Amazon basin and some Pacific islands, but occurs worldwide.

CONTROL

- HBV vaccination also protects against HDV.
- Screening of blood has reduced the risk of infection.

Hepatitis G (HGV)

HGV has a similar role to HCV and should be sought in haemophilia, thalassaemia, dialysis patients, intravenous drug addicts and those handling blood. Co-infection with HCV is frequent.

BACTERIAL INFECTIONS

The most important bacterial infections that gain entry through the gastro-intestinal tract are:

- the enteric fevers;
- the bacillary dysenteries;
- cholera;
- brucellosis;
- food-poisoning bacteria.

ENTERIC FEVERS

Occurrence:	Worldwide
Organisms:	*Salmonella typhi*, *S. paratyphi* A, B
Reservoir:	Sick patient, convalescent, carrier (faecal, urinary)
Transmission:	Water, food, flies
Control:	Isolation, notification, search for source of infection
	Supervision of carriers
	Sanitary disposal of excreta, purification of water, control of flies, food hygiene
	Immunization

These infections are caused by members of the salmonella group: *Salmonella typhi* and *S. paratyphi* A, B or C. Paratyphoid fevers are food-borne rather than water-borne and both rates of infection and fatality are much lower than for typhoid fever. In other respects the diseases are very similar, and the same preventative measures are applicable to both. They are one of the most common causes of apyrexia of unknown origin. The incubation period is usually from 10 to 14 days.

Typhoid fever

BACTERIOLOGY

S. typhi is a Gram-negative, aerobic, non-sporing, rod-like organism. It can survive in water for 7 days, in sewage for 14 days and in ice-cream for 1 month. In warm dry conditions most of the bacilli die in a few days. Boiling of water or milk destroys the organism.

There are many phage types of *S. typhi* and these have proved of great value in tracing the source of an epidemic. Outbreaks of chloramphenicol-resistant *S. typhi* Vi-Phage Type E1 have occurred in Mexico, South East Asia, Pakistan and India. Molecular methods may be used to supplement phage typing. Multidrug resistance is causing increasing concern particularly in India and Pakistan (Plate 22).

EPIDEMIOLOGY

The enteric fevers have a worldwide distribution although they are endemic in communities where the standards of sanitation and personal hygiene are low. Typhoid fever presents one of the classical examples of a water-borne infection. All ages and both sexes are susceptible.

Reservoir

Humans are the only reservoir of infection. This may be an overt case of the disease, an ambulatory 'missed' case or a symptomless carrier. About 2–4% of typhoid patients become chronic carriers of the infection. The majority are faecal carriers. Urinary carriers also occur and seem more common in association with some abnormality of the urinary tract and in patients with *Schistosoma haematobium* infection. Although in most patients the focus of persistent typhoid infection in carriers is in the gall bladder, in some, the deep biliary passages of the liver have also been incriminated. This seems particularly so in Hong Kong, where an association between *Clonorchis sinensis* and *S. typhi* carriers has been demonstrated. An association between *Schistosoma mansoni* infections and *S. typhi* has been reported.

Transmission

Food handlers, especially if they are intermittent carriers, are particularly dangerous and have been responsible for many outbreaks of the disease. Close contact with a patient whether family or otherwise (e.g. nurse) may result in infection being transmitted by soiled hands or through fomites such as towels.

Contamination of water – the cause of major outbreaks – can occur through cross-connection of a main with a polluted water supply, faecal spread, by shellfish, particularly oysters which mature in tidal estuaries and are thus exposed to contaminated waters. Milk-borne outbreaks occur either by direct contamination from a carrier or indirectly from utensils. Ice-cream, other milk products, ice, fruit, vegetables and salads may be infected directly from a carrier or indirectly. Flies or infected dust may be sources of infection. Food (e.g. tinned meat, vegetables infected from human faeces used as manure) can also cause epidemics.

LABORATORY DIAGNOSIS

A leucopenia with a relative lymphocytosis is often seen. *S. typhi* is isolated from blood or 'clot' culture in the first week of disease, from faeces in the second and following weeks and from urine in the 3rd and 4th weeks. It can also be found in bile by duodenal aspirate culture and marrow cultures. A probe technique as well as the polymerase chain reaction (PCR) have been used. After about the 10th day the Widal test (0 and H agglutinations) becomes positive and rises progressively, a rising titre rather than absolute values is necessary for diagnosis. The diazo test is a red coloration given by the froth of the urine of typhoid patients when mixed with the diazo reagents. Despite its definite limitations it is a simple and useful diagnostic test in areas where laboratory facilities are minimal. It becomes positive during the 2nd and 3rd weeks.

The Vi reaction is of help in the detection of the carrier state, particular if one avoids denaturing the antigen in the procedure for an induced haemoglobination test.

CONTROL

The ultimate control of typhoid fever in a community depends on the sanitary disposal of excreta, which will stop the dissemination of faecal matter from one person to another, the introduction of a permanent method of purification of water, and raising the standards of personal hygiene. In any outbreak of typhoid fever every attempt should be made to trace it to its ultimate source by the use of phage-typing, and serological tests, particularly for the presence of Vi antibody, to detect the chronic carrier.

The individual

Cases

All typhoid patients should be barrier nursed in a general hospital or removed to an infectious diseases hospital. Cases should be immediately notified and, if possible, the room from where they came should be cleansed and disinfected. All fomites should be likewise disinfected. The treatment of choice is still chloramphenicol 2 g daily for 14 days, while trimethoprim–sulphamethoxazole is a valuable substitute. Other effective drugs are amoxycillin, the cephilasporisis and the fluoroquinolones. The patient should remain in hospital until, following treatment, stools and urine are bacteriologically negative on three occasions at intervals of not less than 48 hours. The above measures are not all feasible in many parts of the tropics and a compromise must often be found. Recent contact with a patient with the disease was found to be a risk factor in Vietnam. Strategies directed towards the persons in contact with a patient reduce the incidence of secondary cases of typhoid fever.

Carriers

The chronic carrier is a difficult problem, especially in the tropics. Each should be assessed in relation to his/her occupation and kept under as much surveillance as possible. In patients in whom the gall bladder is the definite site of infection, surgery (cholecystectomy) should be carried out. The prolonged administration of ampicillin (4 g daily for 1–3 months) or amoxycillin has given good results as have the fluoroquinolones. For urinary carriers treatment of the underlying condition or associated schistosomiasis has been successful.

The community

If the water supply is suspect (e.g. by the simultaneous occurrence of a large number of cases in a limited area) boiling or hyperchlorination is required. If food is implicated, it should be traced back to its source and enquiries made as to any recent illness among persons handling the food; samples of the food should be taken for medical examination. Milk should be pasteurized or boiled. The use of fresh human manure as fertilizer should be actively discouraged and vegetables boiled or cooked before consumption. Food should be protected from flies, the numbers of which should be reduced to a minimum.

Two vaccines are available – an injectable Vi vaccine, a single dose of which protects for 3 years, or an oral live attenuated vaccine, three doses of which must be taken at intervals of 2 days between doses and which effects protection for 1 year.

Escherichia coli

Five groups of *E. coli* are known to cause diarrhoea: (i) enteropathogenic (EPEC); (ii) enterotoxigenic (ETEC); (iii) verocytoxin-producing (VTEC); (iv) enteroaggregative (EAggEC); and (v) diffusely adherent *E. coli* (DAEC).

ENTEROPATHOGENIC E. COLI (EPEC)

EPEC strains are among the most frequent causes of diarrhoea in infants in the tropics. The clinical picture ranges from a syndrome of watery diarrhoea, vomiting and fever to a cholera-like disease. It is a significant cause of mortality in children under 5 years of age and a common cause of traveller's diarrhoea. The incubation period is short (12–24 hours). The reservoir of infection is humans. The peak age-specific prevalence is between 2 and 3 years. The mode of transmission is contaminated food, particularly contaminated weaning foods and contaminated water or hands.

ENTEROTOXIGENIC E. COLI (ETEC)

In developing countries this is a common cause of diarrhoea in children around 2 years of age.

A prospective study in Bangladesh estimated that ETEC was responsible for 2 out of 6–7 episodes of attacks of diarrhoea per child per year. Outbreaks have occurred on cruise ships and travellers are susceptible to infection when they visit endemic countries.

The reservoir of infection is humans. The incubation period is about 10–12 hours; contaminated food, particularly weaning foods, and contaminated water are the mode of transmission.

VEROCYTOXIN-PRODUCING E. COLI (VTEC)

VTEC produces diarrhoea and a haemorrhagic colitis that may progress to haemolytic–uraemic syndrome (HUS). It seems to be a problem in Chile, Argentina and Uruguay but has not been recognized as a significant cause of diarrhoea in many of the developing countries.

Cattle are the main reservoir of infection but human to human spread also occurs. The incubation period is 3–8 days. Transmission occurs by consumption of contaminated food (e.g. inadequately cooked beef especially minced beef 'hamburgers', unpasteurized milk), water-borne outbreaks have also occurred.

ENTEROAGGREGATIVE E. COLI (EAGGEC)

The incubation period is 20–48 hours. Studies in India, Mexico and Brazil have reported an association between EAggEC and persistent diarrhoea in children under 2 years.

DIFFUSELY-ADHERENT E. COLI (DAEC)

An association between DAEC and diarrhoea has been reported from Chile in children between 4 and 5 years of age.

CONTROL

- See control of diarrhoeal diseases (p. 51).
- For VTEC, good management of abattoirs; irradiation of minced meat; pasteurization of milk.

Campylobacter

Two species of *Campylobacter*, *C. jejuni* and *C. coli*, are the causative agents of *Campylobacter* enteritis. The average incubation period is 3 days.

Abdominal pain and diarrhoea are the common presenting symptoms.

EPIDEMIOLOGY

Poor-quality drinking water, poor sanitation and intimate contact with animals are responsible for the hyperendemicity of this infection in developing countries. Several episodes of diarrhoea occur in the first 3 years of life.

C. jejuni and *C. coli* are widely distributed in the intestines of a wide variety of birds and animals – it is a zoonotic infection.

Indirect transmission occurs through raw milk, raw meats (especially poultry) and contaminated water. Direct transmission occurs among occupational groups such as farmers, veterinarians and butchers, and in the home through contact with infected pets. Person to person infection is common.

DIAGNOSIS

Direct microscopy shows the characteristic rapid jerking movements in wet preparations or spiral morphology in stained smears. Culture, membrane filtration methods and serology can also be used.

CONTROL

- Good hygienic food practices, such as storing raw meat separately from other foods, and pasteurization of milk (see also p. 51).

BACILLARY DYSENTERY (SHIGELLOSIS)

Occurrence:	Worldwide
Organisms:	*Shigella* spp.
Source of infection:	Sick patient, convalescent, carrier (e.g. food handler)
Transmission:	Faecal contamination of food, water or fomites; flies
Control:	Adequate treatment of the patient
	Sanitary disposal of faeces
	Pure water supply
	Food hygiene
	Control of flies

Bacillary dysentery is characterized by diarrhoea (containing blood, mucus and pus), fever and a sudden onset of abdominal pain. The incubation period is 1–7 days. Shigellosis is a notifiable disease in some countries.

Bacteriology

Species and varieties of the genus *Shigella* (non-motile, Gram-negative bacilli) are numerous and they can be conveniently classified into four main subgroups:

- *Sh. dysenteriae* (10 serotypes);
- *Sh. flexneri* (8 serotypes);
- *Sh. boydii* (15 serotypes);
- *Sh. sonnei* (15 colicen types).

The proportion of infections due to individual serotypes varies from country to country, and within the same country at different times. Multiresistance (i.e. sulphonamides, tetracycline, ampicillin and chloramphenicol) is prevalent in many developing countries.

Epidemiology

Since 1968 several epidemics due to *Sh. dysenteriae* 1 have been recorded from various countries in the tropics. In Central America, the epidemic lasted about 4 years (1969–72) causing around half a million cases and 20 000 deaths. In Burundi between 1982 and 1985, there were 101 487 cases and more than 2000 deaths. Epidemic outbreaks continue to occur in developing countries (Plate 23).

SOURCE OF INFECTION

Infection is derived from cases of the disease, from healthy convalescents (who can excrete organisms for up to 2 months or more), and from symptomless carriers who keep up infection in the community.

TRANSMISSION

The organisms, which are excreted in the faeces, may gain access to food through the soiled fingers of patients or carriers. Owing to the low infectious dose of shigella, they may also pass from person to person by contact with inanimate articles or fomites (e.g. lavatory seats, door handles, crockery, bedding and clothes). Fly-borne infection is an important factor in the epidemiology of bacillary dysentery as well as of other faeces-transmitted disease.

HOST FACTORS

Young children are more liable than older persons to acquire shigella infections, and when infected to suffer from clinical disease. Diarrhoeal diseases surveys carried out in Mauritius, Sudan, United Arab Republic, Ceylon, Iran, Bangladesh and Venezuela showed that morbidity and mortality was highest among children under the age of 3 years. Diarrhoea was commonest during the weaning period and greater in bottle-fed than breast-fed infants. Shigellae were isolated both from children suffering from diarrhoea and from those having no diarrhoea.

Diagnosis

Diagnosis can be confirmed by the presence of faecal leucocytes, cultures, DNA–DNA hybridization and PCR.

Control

THE INDIVIDUAL

The patient should be treated at home or in hospital and barrier nursed if possible. Strict personal hygiene should be encouraged among the family contacts or nursing personnel looking after the case and the stools should be treated with a disinfectant before disposal, clothing and bed linen should be similarly treated. If the disease is notifiable, the Medical Officer of Health should be informed. Severe forms of shigellosis require appropriate antibiotic therapy with ampicillin, trimethoprim-sulphamethozale, nalidixic acid or ciprofloxacin, depending on the resistance position.

THE COMMUNITY

The most valuable community measures are provisions for the sanitary disposal of faeces, a pure water supply, food hygiene, and control of flies. Health education to increase the standards of personal hygiene and stop the transmission of the disease within a family and from food handlers is essential. Hands must be washed before food is handled and facilities for this must be made available. Specific strategies for the control

of *S. dysenteriae* 1 epidemics consist of their early detection, proper treatment of case, proper nutritional management, appropriate antimicrobial therapy, surveillance and education of contacts.

CHOLERA

Occurrence:	India/ Pakistan subcontinent, South East Asia, the Near East, Africa, Southern and Central Europe
Organisms:	*Vibrio cholerae* (classical, El Tor biotypes, 0139 Bengal)
Reservoir:	Humans
Transmission:	Water, food, flies
Control:	Diagnosis, isolation, notification and antibiotics
	Search for source of infection
	Concurrent and terminal disinfection
	Environmental sanitation
	Health education; personal hygiene
	International co-operation

This is a disease of rapid onset characterized by vomiting; profuse dehydrating diarrhoea with 'rice water stools' and marked toxaemia. Muscular cramps, suppression of urine and shock occur later. The incubation period is 1–7 days. Cholera is a notifiable disease.

Bacteriology

Vibrio cholerae 01 was discovered by Koch in 1883 and is a delicate Gram-negative organism. There are two biotypes, classical and El Tor. Each biotype contains three serotypes – Inaba, Ogawa and Hikojima. The El Tor biotype is named after the El Tor quarantine station in Egypt where it was first isolated in 1920 and has been responsible for most epidemics in recent years (Plate 24). In 1992, a new strain of *V. cholerae*, 0139 Bengal, appeared in India and caused an epidemic in a population that was largely immune to cholera caused by *V. cholerae* 01 strains.

Epidemiology

Cholera of the classical biotype is now virtually limited to the Indo-Pakistan subcontinent and notably in the deltas of the Ganges and Brahmaputra rivers.

The first outbreak of cholera El Tor was originally confined to a limited geographical area in the Celebes in Indonesia but has been spreading in a pandemic form since 1961 across Asia, through the whole of Africa into the Mediterranean, Europe and now even to the Gulf coast of the USA – a total of 93 countries have so far been affected. The disease is now established in Africa, with sporadic outbreaks occurring in the other zones affected (Fig. 4.2).

Cholera El Tor has been proved capable of speedy and extensive spread over much wider areas than classical cholera, and in several such areas cases due to cholera El Tor have displaced those of classical cholera. In Calcutta, for instance, by the end of 1964 there was only one case of classical cholera for every 10 or more cases of cholera El Tor. This epidemiological phenomenon is explained by the demonstration that the El Tor biotype eliminates the classical biotype in a few hours both *in vitro* and *in vivo*. In 1991, an El Tor epidemic started in Peru and spread rapidly to other countries in Latin America. Epidemic cholera continues to occur in refugee camps and elsewhere in Africa. As a result of the massive migration of Ruwandan Hutus to Zaire, a massive epidemic occurred in 1994 involving 30 000 people with crude mortality rates ranging between 19.5–31.2 per 10 000. *V. cholera* 0139 is at present limited to Asia. Cholera occurs rarely in the cooler months of the year. Cholera has a seasonal pattern but the season varies from locality to locality and can change dramatically.

RESERVOIR

The reservoir of infection is a sick person, a convalescent patient or a carrier (through the faeces or vomit). For every typical case of the disease there may be 10–100 other symptomless persons excreting the vibrio. The El Tor biotype produces a higher carrier:case ratio than that of the classical variety.

TRANSMISSION

Cholera may begin suddenly as a water-borne disease. In Calcutta, where cholera is endemic, the supply of filtered water falls short in summer and the people are found to use both unfiltered and tank water. Cholera also spreads by contaminated food (e.g. dates or shellfish), infected inanimate objects and by flies. Intrafamilial spread also occurs. Between outbreaks, several mechanisms of *V. cholerae* persistence are postulated:

- continuous transmission by asymptomatic carriers or persons with mild disease;
- an aquatic reservoir, e.g. seafood, plankton or water plants;

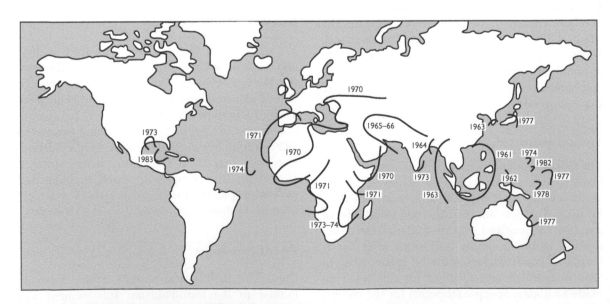

Figure 4.2: The spread of Cholera El Tor from 1961–82.

- seasonal movement of people or infected seafood.

Person to person spread is uncommon.

HOST FACTORS

Gastric acidity is a major factor in host resistance, the disease being more common in persons with hypochlorhydria. Because gastric acidity declines in old age, the elderly are more seriously ill than younger persons. In order to flourish, cholera requires a combination of dense population and poor sanitation (Plate 25). For many years there was a tendency to overlook the role of a symptomless carrier in the transmission of cholera, until it was shown that the carrier state in cholera El Tor may last for more than 12 years ('Cholera Dolores' in the Philippines) and that the vibrio can establish itself in the gall bladder. In areas where adults have developed some immunity, children are predominantly affected. In the Bengal epidemic with 0139 all age groups were affected.

Laboratory diagnosis

A definite diagnosis of cholera can be made only after isolation of *V. cholerae* from the faeces or rectal swabs of patients. The faeces should be transported to the laboratory as rapidly as possible in alkaline peptone water (pH 9.0). Four methods are available for the rapid recognition of cholera vibrios:

- selective enrichment/fluorescent-antibody technique;
- oblique-light technique;
- gelatin-agar method;
- microscopic examination of a fresh faecal specimen will reveal the 'shooting star' motility of the vibrios which halts abruptly if 01 antiserum is added to the slide;
- a rapid test based on colorimetric immunoassay detection of the 01 antigen is commercially available;
- serodiagnosis.

Control

During epidemics the clinical recognition of cases is relatively easy. Sporadic cases, however, can easily be missed and hence in endemic areas any case of severe gastro-enteritis must be considered as cholera until the contrary is proved.

THE INDIVIDUAL

Early diagnosis, isolation and notification of cases is very important. A search for the source of infection should be made and steps taken to deal with that source when found. Concurrent disinfection of stools, fomites, house, linen, clothing, etc. should be carried out.

Oral rehydration has revolutionized the treatment of cholera and other acute diarrhoeal diseases with a dramatic drop in mortality. A suitable fluid for oral and nasogastric use is a glucose–salt solution which contains in 1 litre of water:

sodium chloride (table salt)	2.6 g
sodium citrate (baking soda)	2.9 g
potassium chloride	1.5 g
glucose (dextrose)	13.5 g

Rice-based and maize starch solutions have been used successfully. A reduced osmolarity solution has proved better than the above*. Severe cases require intravenous Ringer's lactate or Dhaka solution.

The administration of antibiotics reduces the diarrhoeal period; the choice of antibiotics will depend on the status of resistance in the area. The potential for spread of resistant strains to neighbouring countries is a matter of concern. Before the patient is discharged from hospital, two negative stool cultures are required and terminal disinfection of bedding, etc. must be carried out.

Contacts

Attendants of patients must be instructed to observe scrupulous cleanliness and disinfection of their hands and should be forbidden to consume food or drink in the patient's room or to go into the kitchen. Selective chemoprophylaxis with a single dose of doxycycline to close family contacts is worth considering in situations where the secondary case rate is high. Detailed surveillance of every person who might have the disease is desirable but rarely feasible in most of the cholera-prone countries.

THE COMMUNITY

Sanitation

Immediate steps must be taken to raise the existing standards of environmental sanitation and in

---

*UNICEF reduced osmolarity and oral rehydration salts composition table available on pg 100.

particular to check all water supplies. Chlorination should be stepped up to 1.3 parts per million. Excreta and refuse disposal must be rigorously controlled and all other fly-breeding sources eliminated; if possible, houses should be sprayed with DDT.

Tracing the source

Bacteriological examination of pooled nightsoil has been used to detect infections in Hong Kong, and from this source the infection could be traced backwards to its origin. The same method applied to latrines in Calcutta was not as successful.

Hygiene

Food sanitation should be enforced and all public swimming pools closed. People should be instructed to boil water, to eat only cooked foods and to raise their standards of personal hygiene. Close attention to ice production should be ensured.

Minimizing contact

Camps and hospitals for isolation of cases should be improvised. Congregations of persons (e.g. in markets, places of prayer, etc.) should be discouraged during epidemics. Control of travellers and pilgrims, especially from endemic areas of cholera, should be rigidly and continuously enforced.

Treatment

The establishment of treatment centres for diarrhoeal diseases is advocated.

Co-operation

Countries must show a greater willingness to provide the WHO and their neighbours with a regular flow of information on their current status of cholera.

The vaccines available at present are not helpful in the control of cholera; indeed, a false sense of security is given to individuals and feelings of complacency to health authorities, who consequently often neglect the more effective precautions.

Realization of the limitations of vaccination has resulted in the abolition of the requirements of a certificate of vaccination against cholera in the international health regulations.

Two oral vaccines are available: Wc/rBs and CVD 103-HgR. They give 80–90% protection in persons under 2 years.

The complete sequencing of the *V. cholerae* genome will help to direct the development of a new vaccine and potential drugs in curing the disease.

Cholera control programme

Within a national Control of Diarrhoeal Diseases programme the following activities are considered important for cholera control:

- the formation of a national epidemic control committee;
- collection of stool specimens or rectal swabs from suspected cases;
- provision of local, regional, and reference laboratory services for the rapid identification of *V. cholerae* 01;
- training in clinical management of acute diarrhoea;
- continuing surveillance activities and maintenance of a diarrhoea case's record;
- early notification of changes in the pattern of diarrhoea;
- enforcement of basic principles of sanitation;
- continuing health education;
- establishment of mobile control teams in certain special circumstances;
- management logistics for supply and distribution requirements.

Cholera will ultimately be brought under control in the developing countries only when water supplies, sanitation and hygienic practices attain such a level that faeco-oral transmission of *V. cholerae* 01 becomes an improbable event.

BRUCELLOSIS

Occurrence:	Worldwide
Organisms:	Brucella abortus, Br. melitensis, Br. suis
Reservoir:	Animals (e.g. cattle, goats, sheep, camels, swine)
Transmission:	Ingestion, contact, inhalation, inoculation
Control:	Pasteurization of milk Vaccination of herds

Brucellosis is one of the most important zoonoses – infections of animals which can affect man. The human disease is characterized by fever, heavy night sweats, splenomegaly and weakness. The incubation period varies from 6 days to as long as 3 months.

Bacteriology

Human disease is attributed to *Brucella abortus*, *Br. suis* and *Br. melitensis* from cattle, swine and goat exposure respectively. Brucella are small, non-motile, non-sporing, Gram-negative coccobacilli. Apart from their different CO requirements, the members of this group resemble each other closely in their cultural characteristics.

Epidemiology

The infection is widely distributed but is particularly prevalent in the countries around the Mediterranean Sea and the Near East. Brucellosis is more prevalent in the tropics than is generally supposed and has been widely reported from Africa, South America, the Near East (Saudi Arabia, Kuwait) and India.

RESERVOIR

Many animals can serve as sources of infection for man, among which the most important are cattle, swine, goats and sheep.

TRANSMISSION

The modes of transmission from animals which are discharging brucella are ingestion, contact, inhalation and inoculation. Infection by ingestion may occur by the gastro-intestinal route and also by penetration of the mucous membrane of the oral cavity and throat. The transmission of brucella by ingestion of contaminated milk, milk products (soft cheeses), meat and meat products is well recorded. Viable brucella may be present in the viscera and muscles of infected carcasses for periods of over 1 month. Camel meat and milk and water are also vehicles of infection. Contact with infected material (e.g. placentae, urine, carcasses, etc.), is a common mode of infection and brucellosis is an occupational disease of veterinarians, farmers, etc. Air-borne infection through the mucous membranes of the eye and respiratory tract can occur, while accidental inoculation has been recorded among veterinarians and laboratory workers.

Brucellosis results in economic loss to animal husbandry; there is loss of protein food from animal abortion, premature births, infertility and reduced production of milk.

Laboratory diagnosis

The laboratory diagnosis of brucellosis includes bacteriological and serological methods as well as allergic tests. Brucella organisms can be cultured from the blood, bone marrow, synovial fluid, lymph nodes and other sources.

Numerous serological tests are available: standard tube-agglutination test (SAT); the rose bengal test; ELISA; 2-mercaptoethanol agglutination test; complement fixation test; Coombs antiglobulin test; radioimmunoassay; Western blotting and PCR. More than one of these tests should be used to confirm a diagnosis. Rising titres or titres that decline after appropriate antibiotic treatment indicate recent active infection. Titres of 640 or more are usually indicative of acute bucellosis. Lower titres are difficult to interpret in endemic areas. The intradermal test indicates previous exposure to infection and is of doubtful significance, especially in endemic countries.

Control

The main control of human brucellosis rests in the pasteurization of milk and environmental sanitation of farms.

THE INDIVIDUAL

Those having direct contact with herds should observe high standards of personal hygiene. Exposed areas of skin should be washed and soiled clothing renewed. Employees in the slaughter houses should wear protective clothing when handling carcasses and these should be removed and disinfected after use. The antibiotics of choice for the specific treatment of brucellosis are tetracycline plus streptomycin or rifampicin with doxycycline.

THE COMMUNITY

Pasteurization of milk is the most important method of prevention of human brucellosis; when this is not possible all milk should be boiled before use. Health education and propaganda should be carried out. Infected animals should be segregated and possibly slaughtered. High standards of animal husbandry must be encouraged and, when possible, animals should be vaccinated.

Immunization

HUMANS

Vaccination in man is dangerous. However, a living vaccine 19-BA (a derivative of *Br. abortus* strain 19) has been used in the USSR in persons at high risk of brucella infection.

ANIMALS

Vaccination of animals can result in control and even eradication of brucellosis among them. Living attenuated vaccines of *Br. melitensis* and *Br. abortus* have been widely and successfully used. Killed vaccines are also available.

BACTERIAL FOOD POISONING

Food poisoning in the tropics is commonly due to three species of bacteria: *Salmonella* spp. (the most important), *Staphylococcus aureus* and *Clostridium perfringens*.

Food-borne bacterial gastro-enteritis may be of three types: (i) infectious type (e.g. salmonella or *Vibrio parahaemolyticus*), when bacteria infected with food multiply in the individual; (ii) toxin type (e.g. *Staphylococcus aureus*) when food is ingested that already contains a toxin; and (iii) intermediate type (e.g. *Clostridium perfringens*, which releases a toxin in the bowel).

Salmonella food poisoning

Occurrence:	Worldwide
Organism:	*Salmonella* spp.
Reservoir:	Animals
Transmission:	Meat, meat products and eggs

Control:	Personal and food hygiene
	Inspection of abattoirs
	Health education of caterers and food handlers

Salmonella food poisoning typically presents with diarrhoea, vomiting and fever. The incubation period is usually 12–24 hours.

BACTERIOLOGY

Salmonellae have been subdivided into as many as 17 000 serotypes, the majority being named after the place where they were first isolated. The commonest type causing food poisoning is *S. typhimurium*, which is widely distributed in the mammal, bird and reptilian kingdoms.

EPIDEMIOLOGY

This is worldwide, but infection is commoner in tropical communities with low hygiene standards.

Reservoir

The source of infection is usually salmonella-infected animals, for example cattle, poultry, pigs, dogs, cats, rats and mice.

Transmission

Meat is the common mode of transmission, either as a result of illness in cattle or by contamination from intestinal contents in unhygienically maintained abattoirs. Other vehicles of infection are eggs and egg products (as a result of faecal contamination of the shell) and milk and milk products. Foodstuffs can be infected at any stage from the abattoir to the home by rats and mice, and by subclinically infected human carriers during the processing or preparation of food. Typically, infection occurs as explosive small epidemics among groups of people who have eaten the same food.

LABORATORY DIAGNOSIS

Serological agglutination methods are needed to identify the type of salmonella, but the genus is readily recognized by standard bacteriological techniques.

CONTROL

This is essentially a matter of food hygiene to be applied from the abattoir to the home.

The individual

Fluids and electrolytes should be replaced. No individual should handle foodstuffs except after thorough washing of hands. Any person suffering from diarrhoea should be debarred from handling or preparing food. High standards of personal hygiene must be maintained by any person connected with food, whether cooked or uncooked.

The community

Veterinary inspection of abattoirs must be thoroughly and scrupulously carried out and inspection of animals done both before and after slaughter. Carcasses of animals suffering from salmonellosis must be condemned for human consumption. The abattoirs should be hygienically maintained in order to avoid infection or contamination from intestinal contents. Meat and meat products should be thoroughly cooked and if possible refrigerated if they are to be served cold. If no refrigeration facilities are available, foods should be carefully stored away from rats, mice and flies, and kept as cool as is feasible in the circumstances. Health education is needed to raise the general standard of personal and food hygiene.

Staphylococcus food poisoning

Occurrence:	Worldwide
Organisms:	Enterotoxin-producing staphylococci
Reservoir:	Humans
Transmission:	Semi-preserved foods
Control:	Personal hygiene of food handlers
	Food hygiene and refrigeration

Staphylococcus food poisoning is characterized by an abrupt onset with nausea and vomiting sometimes accompanied by diarrhoea and shock. The incubation period is from 1 to 6 hours (i.e. very short) which is a differential point from salmonella food poisoning. Seven serologically distinct enterotoxins A, B, C, D, E, G and H are recognized. Enterotoxin A is most often responsible in outbreaks of food poisoning.

EPIDEMIOLOGY

The disease is worldwide.

Reservoir

The source of infection is humans (i.e. food handlers) carrying the organism in the nose, throat, hand and skin lesions such as boils, carbuncles and whitlows. Food is contaminated either by droplet infection or by direct contact with infected cutaneous lesions.

Transmission

The mode of transmission is through manufactured semi-preserved foods eaten cold such as hams, tinned meats, sauces, custards, cream fillings of cakes and unpasteurized milk due to staphylococcal infection of cattle. A sudden outbreak of vomiting and diarrhoea in a group of persons who have partaken of the same meal within a few hours suggests staphylococcus food poisoning. Any occasion for mass feeding as occurs at funerals, weddings, schools and other institutions, is liable to result in staphylococcus food poisoning. In these instances food is often precooked, stored and then served cold or after rewarming.

LABORATORY DIAGNOSIS

If an unconsumed portion of the suspected food is still available this should be sent to the laboratory for examination of enterotoxin-producing staphylococci. ELISA and reversed passive late agglutination (RPLA) are used for the detection of staphylococcal enterotoxins in food.

CONTROL

This consists of the proper education of food handlers and high standards of food hygiene.

The individual

Oral or intravenous therapy results in a quick recovery.

All food handlers should be educated in personal hygiene and excluded from contact with foodstuffs if they suffer from purulent nasal discharges or pyogenic skin lesions until they are cured.

The community

High standards of catering should be maintained and hygienic techniques for handling, preparation and storage of foods used. Whenever possible, cooked foods should be refrigerated and the adequate heat treatment of all milk and milk products is essential.

Clostridium perfringens food poisoning

Occurrence:	Worldwide, New Guinea ('pigbel')
Organism:	Clostridium perfringens
Reservoir:	Humans, animals
Transmission:	Ingestion of meat
Control:	Cooking and storage of meat Vaccination

Clostridium perfringens food poisoning presents with diarrhoea and abdominal pain; vomiting is not very common. The incubation period is 12–24 hours.

BACTERIOLOGY

There are many serotypes of Cl. perfringens. The rod-like organisms require anaerobic conditions in which to grow. They are Gram-positive and produce endospores. In New Guinea Cl. perfringens is thought to be associated aetiologically with 'pigbel' (see below).

EPIDEMIOLOGY

The condition is worldwide. A diffuse sloughing enteritis of the jejunum, ileum and colon known as 'enteritis necroticans' or 'pigbel' is very common in New Guinea.

Reservoir and transmission

The source of infection can be human, animal or fly faeces, and the spores of Cl. perfringens survive for long periods in soil, dust, clothes and in the environment generally. The carrier rate in human populations varies from 2–30%. The mode of transmission is by ingestion of meat which has been pre-cooked and eaten cold, or reheated the next day prior to consumption.

In New Guinea the disease in both epidemic and sporadic forms is related to pig feasting, which is an integral and complex part of the indigenous cultures of all highland tribes. Males are affected more often than females. The fatality rates vary from nil to 85%.

LABORATORY DIAGNOSIS

Cl. perfringens can be isolated from the stools of individuals suffering from the disease and from food remnants. The detection of enterotoxin is done by ELISA, vero-cell assay, reserve passive late agglutination and DNA hybridization.

CONTROL

A proper standard of food hygiene is the most effective method of controlling Cl. perfringens food poisoning.

All meat dishes should be either cooked and eaten immediately or refrigerated until required. Reheating of foodstuffs should be avoided and in New Guinea special precautions should be taken when pig-feasting occurs. A successful vaccine has been developed with a clostridial toxoid prepared from C cultures.

Vibrio parahaemolyticus food poisoning

Vibrio parahaemolyticus food poisoning is characterized by acute diarrhoea, abdominal pain and nausea. The incubation period is 4–96 hours (usually 12–24 hours).

Outbreaks are associated with contamination of fish or shellfish. Incidence is highest in the warmer months when V. parahaemolyticus is most prevalent in aquatic environments.

PROTOZOAL INFECTIONS

The most important protozoal infections transmitted by the faeco-oral route are:

- amoebiasis;
- the flagellate infestations;
- balantidiasis;
- toxoplasmosis;
- cryptosporidiosis.

AMOEBIASIS

Occurrence:	Worldwide
Organism:	Entamoeba histolytica/E. dispar
Reservoir:	Humans
Transmission:	Contaminated hands, food
Control:	Personal hygiene
	Sanitary disposal of faeces

Amoebiasis is caused by the protozoan *Entamoeba histolytica*. The parasite lives in the large intestine causing ulceration of the mucosa with consequent diarrhoea. *E. dispar* is morphologically similar but non-pathogenic.

Applied biology

The amoeba lives in the lumen of the large intestine where it multiplies by binary fission. Under suitable conditions it invades the mucous membrane and submucosa. If red blood cells are available, the amoeba will ingest them. When diarrhoea occurs, amoebae are expelled to the exterior, and then are found in the freshly passed fluid stools. Amoebae are very sensitive to environmental changes, and so are short lived outside the body.

When there is no diarrhoea and other conditions are favourable for encystation, the amoebae cease feeding, become spherical, secrete a cyst wall and the nucleus divides twice to form the characteristic mature four-nucleate cyst. There are two other characteristic structures: a glycogen vacuole which acts as a carbohydrate reserve and chromatoid bodies which are a ribosome store. Cysts kept cool and moist remain viable for several weeks.

The cyst is the infective form, and when ingested hatches in the lower part of the small intestine or upper part of the large intestine. The four-nucleate amoeba undergoes a series of nuclear and cytoplasmic divisions, each multinucleate amoeba giving rise to eight uninucleate amoebae, which establish themselves and multiply in the large intestine. Cysts are 10–16 µm in diameter. *E. hartemanni* produces smaller cysts (<10 µm) and is non-pathogenic.

Epidemiology

Amoebiasis has a worldwide distribution, but clinical disease occurs most frequently in tropical and subtropical countries. In temperate climates the infection is often non-pathogenic and symptomless.

In certain areas of Africa, Asia and Latin America, the prevalence of asymptomatic infections ranges from 5% to more than 80%. Recent estimates suggest that 500 million people per year are infected with *E. histolytica* and approximately 8% will develop overt disease. Also, 40 000–100 000 deaths per year are attributable to invasive amoebiasis. Globally, amoebiasis is the third most common parasitic cause of death – after malaria and schistosomiasis.

RESERVOIR

The reservoir of disease is humans. Although several animals harbour *E. histolytica* (monkeys, dogs, pigs, rats, cats) they are thought to be of no epidemiological importance in human infections. The disease is spread by cyst passers, who may be divided into two main groups:

- convalescents who have recovered from an acute attack;
- asymptomic individuals who can recall no clinical evidence of infection.

The latter possibly are the more common source of infection, even in countries with high standards of hygiene. Bad sanitation is more important than climate in the predominance of overt infection in the tropics. Carrier rates of *E. dispar* among symptomless subjects have varied from 5% in temperate areas with good hygiene to 80% in some tropical communities.

TRANSMISSION

The parasite can be transmitted by direct contact through the contaminated hands of cyst carriers (e.g. in institutions); it is also transmitted indirectly by means of contaminated food, such as raw vegetables fertilized with fresh human faeces, and through the food infected by food handlers and flies. Amoebic dysentery is frequently a house or family infection. Infected water has occasionally been held responsible for the transmission of large outbreaks of the disease.

HOST FACTORS

Among the host factors influencing the epidemiology of the disease we have to consider the following:

Sex

Any differences that have been reported in the incidence of the disease between males and females are probably related to exposure rather than a true sex susceptibility to the infection. The disease seems to appear in fulminating form in pregnant and puerperal women. This may be a corticosteroid effect.

Age

Amoebiasis in childhood is not uncommon. It usually occurs in the age group nil to 6 years, as those between the ages of 7 and 14 years seem to enjoy a greater immunity to ill effects from *E. histolytica* infection than others.

Race

All races are susceptible to the disease. Although the infection is often milder in Europeans, this is probably related to sanitary standards, diet and freedom from debilitating disorders, rather than to a genuine racial factor. Reports from Madras indicate that amoebiasis was 20 times more frequent in Hindus than in Muslims, while in Durban the incidence and severity of amoebic dysentery is greater in Africans than in Indians or Europeans.

Immunity

There is no evidence that amoebiasis confers any protective immunity and the infection can persist for many years after its establishment. The general condition of patients plays an important role; thus, severe cases of amoebiasis are often seen among soldiers on active service.

Diet

Milk and iron supplementation can influence the invasiveness of *E. histolytica*.

Laboratory diagnosis

The clinical diagnosis of amoebiasis has to be confirmed by identification of *E. histolytica*.

MICROSCOPY

During an attack of amoebic dysentery the motions are loose, offensive, and contain mucus and blood; faecal elements are always present. On microscopical examination motile amoebae, some with engorged red cells, will be found in the freshly passed stool or in specimens removed at sigmoidoscopy or proctoscopy.

In asymptomatic infections, and during remission, the stool is semiformed and contains *E. histolytica* cysts. They can be seen to contain one or more bar-shaped chromatoid bodies and staining with iodine reveals one to four nuclei and a glycogen mass. Repeated stool examinations (six specimens collected at weekly intervals) should be made before absence of infection can confidently be assumed. Concentration techniques for cysts are available, and cultural methods may assist diagnosis in scanty infections.

IMMUNOLOGICAL AND BIOCHEMICAL IDENTIFICATION

ELISA can detect the presence of amoebic antigen in serum and faecal samples. Serological tests are particularly useful in extra-intestinal amoebiasis. Colorimetric PCR techniques have a high specificity and sensitivity.

Biochemical, immunological and genetic data differentiate between *E. histolytica* and *E. dispar*.

Control

The main method of control is the provision and use of facilities for the sanitary disposal of faeces coupled with personal cleanliness.

THE INDIVIDUAL

Raising the standards of personal hygiene through health education is the only method that can be applied to the individual, for example advice on washing of hands, especially after defecation. Food handlers, for example cooks, are an especially important group to train. Adequate treatment of individual infections with tissue and luminal amoebicides should be ensured.

THE COMMUNITY

The provision of a safe water supply and facilities for sanitary disposal of faeces are the main control measures applicable to the community. The use of human faeces as a fertilizer should be discouraged. In areas where a pure water supply is not available, water should be boiled and raw vegetables and fruit thoroughly washed and dipped in boiling water. Food should be protected from flies.

OTHER AMOEBAE

Infection of the human gut may occur with other amoebae, namely *Entamoeba coli*, *Dientamoeba fragilis*, *Endolimax nana* and *Iodamoeba butschlii*. There is controversy, however, concerning the actual pathogenicity of these organisms. *Naegleria fowleri* has been reported as causing a fatal necrotizing meningoencephalitis.

FLAGELLATE INFESTATIONS

A number of flagellate protozoa commonly parasitize the human intestine and genito-urinary tract:

- *Trichomonas hominis;*
- *Chilomastix mesnili;*
- *Trichomonas vaginalis;*
- *Giardia lamblia.*

The ones with real claims to pathogenicity are *G. lamblia* and *T. vaginalis*, which are found both in the tropics and in temperate countries. *T. vaginalis* urethritis is common in males: for an account of trichomoniasis see page 114. Giardiasis is described below.

Giardiasis

Occurrence:	Worldwide
Organism:	Giardia lamblia
Reservoir:	Humans and animals
Control:	Personal hygiene
	Sanitary disposal of faeces

Heavy infection with *Giardia lamblia* is often accompanied by diarrhoea or steatorrhoea.

The trophozoite lives in the upper part of the small intestine particularly the duodenum and jejunum. In appearance it resembles a half-pear split longitudinally measuring 12–18 μm in length.

It reproduces itself by a complicated process of binary fission. The cysts (which are the infective forms) occur in the faeces, often in enormous numbers. They are oval in shape, and contain at first two nuclei which divide, giving rise to four in the mature cyst.

EPIDEMIOLOGY

Reservoir

Humans are the source of infection. *G. lamblia* is harboured by many animals, and there is now compelling evidence that giardiasis is a zoonosis.

Transmission

The infection is transmitted by the direct ingestion of cysts between individuals, a result of insanitary habits, or contaminated food or water.

Host factors

It is common in children and in adults, sometimes causing symptoms of malabsorption in both, due to mechanical irritation rather than invasion of the mucous membrane. Giardia infections may persist for years and the parasite may invade the biliary tract. 'Overlanders' are particularly prone to acquire the infection.

Recent outbreaks have occurred in communities with the following features in common:

- surface water (streams, rivers, lakes) and well water;
- chlorination is the principal method for disinfecting water;
- water treatment does not include filtration.

These outbreaks exemplify the increasing frequency with which giardia is being implicated as the cause of water-borne outbreaks of diarrhoea. It is also evident that chlorine levels used in routine disinfection of municipal drinking water (0.4 mg/1 free chlorine) are not effective against giardia cysts, although hyperchlorination (5–9 mg/1 free chlorine residual) may be successful.

High-risk groups are infants and children, travellers and the immuno-compromised. Age-specific prevalence rises throughout childhood and begins to fall during adolescence. Prevalence rates in children have ranged from 20 to 45%. Malnutrition may be an additional risk factor.

LABORATORY DIAGNOSIS

Diagnosis of infection is made by finding cysts of the parasite in formed stools, cysts and vegetative forms in fluid stools or duodenal aspirates. Fluorescent labelled monoclonal antibodies techniques have a sensitivity of around 70–85%.

CONTROL

Individuals can be treated with nitromidazole derivatives.

The main control measures are the provision and use of a safe method of excreta disposal and the raising of personal standards of hygiene. Boiling is the most reliable method for killing giardia cysts in water. It is vital to ensure that water supplies are giardia-free.

BALANTIDIASIS

Occurrence:	Worldwide
Organism:	Balantidium coli
Reservoir:	Humans and animals, especially pigs
Transmission:	Contaminated hands, food
Control:	Personal hygiene
	Sanitary disposal of faeces

Balantidiasis in man has been recorded from most parts of the world, and is caused by infection with the ciliate protozoon, *Balantidium coli* which is a common parasite of the pig. Infection can cause severe diarrhoea.

The large ovoid cysts are passed in the faeces and contain the parasite, which may be seen moving actively. The enclosed balantidium then loses its cilia, and sometimes two individuals are found in the same cyst. *B. coli* reproduces asexually by transverse fission. Transmission of infection takes place by ingestion of cysts, but the subsequent life cycle is not known.

Epidemiology

The reported incidence in humans is very variable and depends on whether or not freshly collected specimens of faeces are examined. Epidemics have been reported from mental institutions, and in Papua New Guinea infection rates among swineherders and abattoir workers have been reported as high as 28%. In Muslim countries balantidiasis is uncommon.

RESERVOIR

B. coli has been found in the intestinal contents of humans and a large number of animals (wild boars, sheep, horses, rats, frogs, monkeys, etc.) but domestic pigs are much the most important reservoir hosts. Infection in man is comparatively rare despite man's close contact with pigs in many countries, and in more than 50% of human cases there may be no history of contact with pigs.

TRANSMISSION

It is possible that humans are most often infected by fingers, food, drinking water, or soil contaminated by pigs' faeces containing balantidia, usually in the encysted form. Handling of the intestines of infected animals or transmission by flies are other possible modes of spread. Furthermore, the possibility of infection from green vegetables grown in soil fertilized by pig excrement must be borne in mind, especially as cysts may remain viable for weeks in moist faeces.

Laboratory diagnosis

The stools are bloody and mucoid. Examination of faeces reveals the typical large ovoid cysts 45–75 μm in length, containing the parasite. The trophozoites may also be seen in freshly collected stools: the protozoon is oval in shape and of variable size (30–300 μm in length by 30–100 μm in breadth). The body is clothed with a thick covering of cilia arranged in longitudinal rows. Both the direct and indirect fluorescent antibody techniques have recently been applied in the diagnosis of *B. coli*.

Control

Individuals infected can be treated with tetracycline. High standards of personal hygiene must be maintained, especially among persons in close contact with pigs – gloves should be worn when handling the intestines of potentially infected animals. Green vegetables should be washed and dipped in boiling water. Environmental sanitation of piggeries should be encouraged. Sanitary disposal of faeces and purification of water are the main control measures for the community.

TOXOPLASMOSIS

Occurrence:	Worldwide
Organism:	*Toxoplasma gondii*
Reservoirs:	Humans, other mammals
Transmission:	Raw beef and pork
Control:	Personal hygiene
	Thorough cooking of meat

Toxoplasmosis is caused by the intracellular sporozoon *Toxoplasma gondii*. The infection may be congenital or acquired. Clinically, there are four types of acquired toxoplasmosis:

- asymptomatic;
- acute glandular;
- ocular;
- cerebral.

The life cycle of *T. gondii* is similar to that of coccidian parasites and its taxonomic status is now considered to be a coccidian parasite related to the genus *Isospora*. When extracellular, the organism is crescent shaped and about 6 μm long. The cytoplasm stains blue and the eccentric nucleus stains red with Giemsa. In the intracellular stages *T. gondii* appears singly or in clusters within the reticuloendothelial cells. Aggregations of the organisms may form pseudocysts. The cystic form of the parasite has reached 100 μm in diameter. Reproduction of the organism is by binary fission. Toxoplasma trophozoites and cysts characterize acute and chronic infections respectively, but cysts may form early in the acute stage and trophozoites may remain active for years in some chronic infections.

Epidemiology

Toxoplasmosis has a worldwide distribution. In the tropics it is probably commoner than is generally realized.

RESERVOIR AND TRANSMISSION

Humans

Humans are the main reservoir of human infection. The method of transmission of *T. gondii* from person to person is unknown except in congenital infections. Surveys of various populations have shown that a high incidence of asymptomatic infection occurs in the warm or hot humid areas, and a low incidence in the cold areas and hot dry areas. In general, there does not appear to be any difference in infection rate between urban and rural populations, between sexes or between races in the same environment. Toxoplasmosis is a serious infection in the immunocompromised host.

Animals

T. gondii is widely distributed in the animal kingdom, being particularly common in cats, dogs and rabbits. However, in spite of the circumstantial evidence indicating a possible transmission between animals and man, it is probable that both may become infected from a common source or sources. Ingestion of raw beef and pork meat are a recognized mode of infection and it has been demonstrated that infection was particularly high in a tuberculosis hospital in France, where the children were fed raw or underdone meat. Antibodies, however, are found just as frequently in vegetarians as in meat eaters in India. High infection rates have also been found in sewage workers, rabbit trappers, laboratory workers and nurses. The role of droplet infection and mechanical subcutaneous inoculation by biting, or bloodsucking arthropods, in the transmission of toxoplasmosis, has yet to be proved. Toxoplasma can be transmitted inside the egg of the cat roundworm *Toxocara cati,* but this is not likely to be the main mode of infection in man.

Laboratory diagnosis

HAEMATOLOGY

In the blood there may be a leucocytosis or leucopenia. An eosinophilia has been described. There may be a mild degree of anaemia and a leukaemoid reaction and atypical lymphocytes may be seen.

ISOLATION

Toxoplasma may be isolated from blood, cerebrospinal fluid, saliva, sputum, lymph nodes, skin, liver and muscle; by intraperitoneal injection of the biopsy or other material into mice, guinea-pigs or hamsters. Mice are the most suitable medium for culturing the organism as they do not suffer from toxoplasmosis.

SEROLOGY

A number of serological tests have been described for the detection of antibodies to *T. gondii*. The cytoplasm-modifying test of Sabin-Feldman (dyetest) is the one most widely used. It is a sensitive test which shows the presence of antibody in many members of the normal adult population. The most convincing method of diagnosing active toxoplasmosis is by the demonstration of at least a four-fold rise in titre, coupled with the isolation of toxoplasma in the tissues or body fluids by inoculation of mice.

Other serological tests in common use are the complement-fixation test, direct agglutination test, haemagglutination test and fluorescent antibody test. PCR has been successfully used.

Control

The most effective treatment for both humans and animals is a combination of pyrimethamine and sulphonamides. Intimate contact with sick animals should be avoided, and ingestion of raw meat discouraged. Serological surveillance during pregnancy is practical in some countries. A vaccine exists to control infection in cats and non-feline beasts.

CRYPTOSPORIDIOSIS

Occurrence:	Worldwide
Organism:	Cryptosporidium spp. particularly C. parvum
Reservoir:	Animals, especially calves
Transmission:	Faeco-oral
Control:	Avoid contact with animals Personal hygiene

Cryptosporidium causes intractable, profuse, watery diarrhoea in immunosuppressed and immunocompromised individuals. It is thought to be a major contributory cause of death in AIDS patients. It is probably a more important cause of diarrhoea in children in the tropics than has hitherto been realized.

Cryptosporidium is a coccidian parasite with an extracellular life cycle in mucoid material on the surface of the epithelial cells of the gut.

Epidemiology

Cryptosporidiosis has a worldwide distribution. It is a common cause of diarrhoea in children in the tropics, with heavy infections reported from Costa Rica, Guinea-Bissau and Bangladesh. Serosurveys reveal rates ranging from 70 to 100% in the tropics. The incidence of infection is highest in the warm humid months. In Gaza, it peaks in the hot dry months.

RESERVOIR AND TRANSMISSION

Cryptosporidiosis is a zoonotic infection. The main mode of transmission is by the faeco-oral route from calves and other animals through contamination of food. Person to person transmission, particularly between children and within households, also occurs. Water-borne infections are increasingly being reported. Heavy rainfall moves oocysts from manure systems in the watershed or sewage overflow due to failed systems, shellfish and vegetables are a source of infection. Molecular markers are able to predict the source of an outbreak – humans or cattle.

Most common causes of outbreaks are either deficiencies of treatment of water supplies or sewage overflow due to failed systems.

HOST FACTORS

In adults infected with AIDS, cryptosporidiosis is an opportunistic infection causing death from severe diarrhoea and malabsorption. Malnutrition increases the severity of infection.

Laboratory diagnosis

Diagnosis involves simple staining of faecal smears and examination by bright-field or fluorescent microscopy.

Control

Contact with animals, especially calves, should be avoided and improvement in personal hygiene at homes, schools and nurseries emphasized.

HELMINTHIC INFECTIONS (PLATE 26)

In the past, only heavy worm burdens have been associated with significant morbidity. In recent years, however, it has become apparent that lower worm burdens are associated with demonstrable clinical effects such as growth retardation, anaemia and possibly a detrimental effect on cognition and educational achievement. The fact that school children are a captive population provides an excellent opportunity to deliver mass treatments through an existing infrastructure. It has been demonstrated that in many countries of the developing world the education sector can deliver a simple health package including health education antihelminthics to millions of school children aged 5–14 years. These programmes will not only benefit the treated individual, but should also reduce overall levels of transmission, since this is the age group that is the major contributor to infection. The *Partnership in Child Development* aims at improving the health and education of school-age children in developing countries through the control of soil-transmitted helminths. However, the Cochrane review of the results of various such public health interventions, based on the expectation that there will be an improvement in growth and learning, has concluded that the results are not based on consistent or reliable evidence.

The WHO recommended drugs for the treatment of intestinal nematodes are albendazole, levamisole, mebendazole and pyartel.

Many important helminths are transmitted through the gastro-intestinal tract and the infections they give rise to can be classified as in Table 4.2.

NEMATODE (ROUNDWORM) INFECTIONS

Ascariasis

Occurrence:	Hot humid climates of the world
Organism:	*Ascaris lumbricoides*
Reservoir:	Humans
Transmission:	Contaminated hands, food, drink
Control:	Personal hygiene
	Sanitary disposal of faeces
	Chemotherapy

Table 4.2: Classification of important helminthic diseases transmitted through the gastro-intestinal tract

Roundworms (Nematodes)	Tapeworms (Cestodes)	Flukes (Trematodes)
Ascariasis	Taeniasis	Paragonimiasis
Trichuriasis	Diphyllobothriasis	(lung)
Enterobiasis	Hydatid disease	Chlonorchiasis
Toxocariasis	Hymenolepsiasis	(liver)
Trichinosis		Opistorchiasis
Dracontiasis		(liver)
(filarial worm)		Fascioliasis
		(liver)
		Fasciolopsiasis
		(intestine)

This disease, due to the large intestinal roundworm, *Ascaris lumbricoides*, is often symptomless and infection is discovered incidentally; occasionally it causes intestinal obstruction in children.

The adult worms of *A. lumbricoides* live in the small intestine. Their colour is yellowish-white and they may reach a length of 40 cm. The female is prolific, laying up to 200 000 eggs a day. The typical egg has a yellowish-brown mamillated appearance. Ascaris eggs are resistant to cold and to disinfectants in the strengths in normal use. They are killed by direct sunlight and by temperatures of about 45°C. Under optimum conditions, eggs may remain viable for as long as 1 year (Fig. 4.3).

EPIDEMIOLOGY

A. lumbricoides has a worldwide distribution, the incidence of which is largely determined by local habits in the disposal of faeces. Its highest prevalence is in the hot humid climates of Asia, Africa and tropical America.

Reservoir and transmission

Humans are the reservoir of infection which is spread by faecal pollution of the soil. The eggs are swallowed as a result of ingestion of soil or contact between the mouth and various inanimate objects carrying the adherent eggs. Contamination of food or drink by dust or handling is also a source of infection. Eggs of ascaris pass unaltered through the intestine of coprophagous animals and can thus be transported to locations other than human

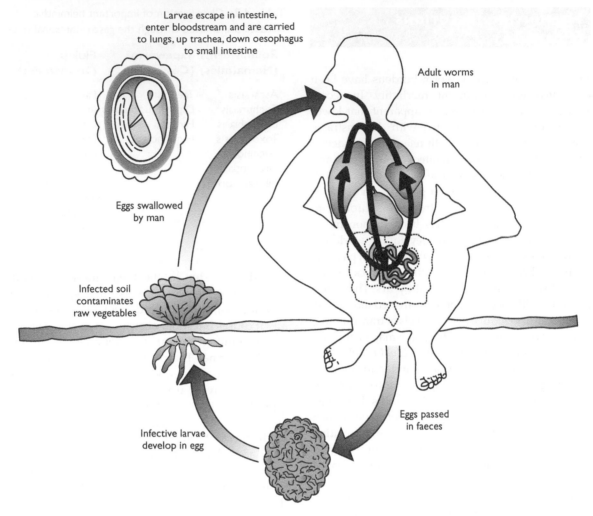

Larvae escape in intestine, enter bloodstream and are carried to lungs, up trachea, down oesophagus to small intestine

Adult worms in man

Eggs swallowed by man

Infected soil contaminates raw vegetables

Infective larvae develop in egg

Eggs passed in faeces

Figure 4.3: Life cycle of *Ascaris lumbricoides*.

defecation sites. The well-protected eggs withstand drying and can survive for lengthy periods.

A. suis, which infects pigs, is morphologically identical and can mature in humans, but cross-infection has not been proved.

Host factors

Although all age groups show infection in endemic areas, the incidence and intensity are highest in the younger age groups. Infants may be parasitized soon after birth by ova on the mother's fingers. The observed variation in incidence and intensity with age is probably due to differences in behaviour and occupational activities between children and adults, as well as to the development of acquired resistance. It has been claimed that ascaris infection retards

growth in children. Clinical signs of protein-energy malnutrition increase in ascaris-infected children and significantly decrease after deworming.

The prevalence of ascaris infection in children can be usefully used as an index of faeco-oral transmission in a community.

LABORATORY DIAGNOSIS

The microscopical diagnosis of ascariasis can be confirmed by examination of faeces samples. Because of their characteristic morphology and colour the ova can be found relatively easily in 'direct smears'. Concentration and quantitative techniques are available. The Kato–Katz cellophane quantitative technique is the WHO recommended method.

CONTROL

The main method of control is the sanitary disposal of human excreta, complemented by chemotherapy.

The individual

Health education should raise standards of personal hygiene and mothers should encourage young children not to defecate indiscriminately. Chemotherapy will reduce morbidity.

The community

Sanitation

A method of sanitary disposal of faeces (i.e. some type of latrine acceptable to the people and best suited to the terrain – see Chapter 1) should be introduced and its use encouraged. The provision and use of such facilities is particularly important for groups that spend long hours working out of doors (e.g. farmers). Human faeces should not be used as a fertilizer (Plate 27) unless previously composted so that the resulting high temperature can kill the eggs. Mass treatment of preschool and school children has been undertaken using a single dose of one of the broad-spectrum antihelminthics (see pp. 140–141).

Mass chemotherapy has been utilized as the medium-term approach to control, fortified by improvements in personal hygiene and sanitation as the long-term solution for ascaris and the other faeco-orally transmitted helminth infections. Whether this popular intervention (chemotherapy) is cost-effective has recently been challenged.

Trichuriasis

Occurrence:	Worldwide
Organism:	*Trichuris trichiura*
Reservoir:	Humans
Transmission:	Contaminated hands, food and drink
Control:	Personal hygiene
	Sanitary disposal of faeces
	Chemotherapy

This infection is due to the whipworm *Trichuris trichiura* and it is often symptomless. However, heavy infections of over 1000 worms may cause bloody diarrhoea with anaemia and prolapse of the rectum.

LIFE CYCLE

See Figure 4.4.

EPIDEMIOLOGY

Trichuriasis occurs throughout the world but is more prevalent in the warm humid tropics.

Reservoir and transmission

Humans are the reservoir of infection. Soil pollution is the determining factor in the prevalence and intensity of infection in a community, and clay soils are more favourable than sandy soils.

Transmission occurs through the insanitary habit of promiscuous defecation, and infection usually results from the ingestion of infective ova from contaminated hands, food or drink. Although trichuris infection of domestic and other animals occurs, it is unlikely that animal reservoirs play a part in the epidemiology of human infection. Coprophagous animals can transport trichuris eggs to locations other than human defecation sites, since the eggs are passed unaltered through their intestine.

Host factors

The high prevalence in children is probably due to greater exposure to infection.

LABORATORY DIAGNOSIS

Microscopy

Direct smear examination of faeces will reveal the characteristic lemon-shaped ova. An egg count on an ordinary wet faecal smear (containing about 2 mg of faeces) of more than 100 ova is indicative of a heavy infection. Concentration and quantitative techniques can be applied. The mucoid sticky stools may contain a preponderance of eosinophil cells and Charcot–Leyden crystals.

Haematology

Eosinophilia (10–20%) is usually present, especially in massive infections. An associated microcytic hypochromic anaemia may be seen.

CONTROL

- Mass treatment.
- Sanitary disposal of faeces.
- Personal hygiene.

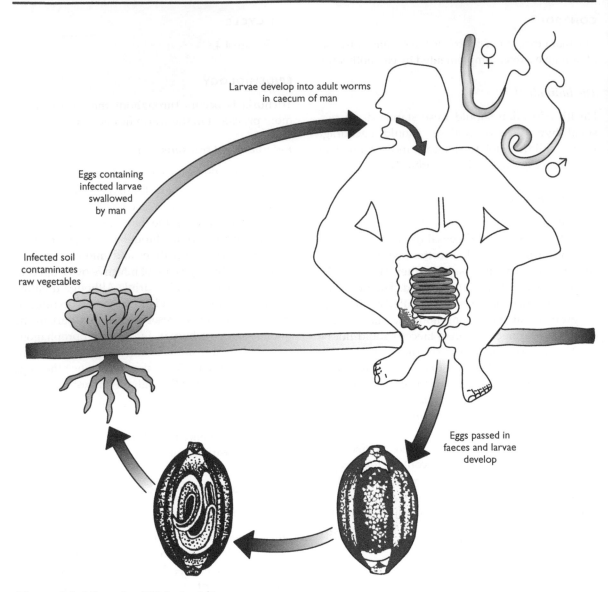

Figure 4.4: Life cycle of *Trichuris trichiura*.

Enterobiasis

Occurrence:	Worldwide
Organism:	*Enterobius vermicularis*
Reservoir:	Humans
Transmission:	Contaminated hands, dust
Control:	Personal hygiene
	Chemotherapy

This infection due to the pinworm *Enterobius vermicularis* may be symptomless or there may be mild gastro-intestinal discomfort and pruritus ani. It is prevalent throughout the world and is probably less common in the tropics than in countries of the temperate zone.

The female worm is about 8–13 mm long while the male worm (which is rarely seen) is only 2–5 mm. They both live in the caecum, where copulation takes place. The gravid females then migrate to the colon and rectum and at night pass through the anus to deposit their eggs on the perianal skin and genitocrural folds. Within a few hours larvae develop within the eggs, which are now infective. Upon ingestion by man, the larvae hatch in the duodenum and mature in the caecum. The life cycle from egg to adult lasts 3–7 weeks.

The survival of the ova depends upon temperature and humidity, viability being greatest in cool, moist surroundings.

EPIDEMIOLOGY

Enterobiasis is prevalent throughout the world and is probably less common in the tropics than in countries of the temperate zone.

Reservoir and transmission

Humans are the reservoir of infection. The ova from the perianal region are transferred to night clothes, towels and bedding, and infection may follow when these are handled. Infective ova may be present in the dust and infection can therefore take place by inhalation. The intense pruritus around the perianal regions results in scratching and the hands, especially beneath the finger nails, become contaminated. Ova are transferred directly to the mouth or indirectly through food and other objects which have been handled. Occasionally the larvae, after hatching in the perianal regions, re-enter the anus and migrate to the caecum, where they mature (retroinfection). The highest incidence of enterobiasis is in school children from 5 to 15 years. It is very prevalent in crowded districts with faulty hygiene, in institutional groups, and among members of the same family.

Host factors

There may be a racial susceptibility to infection, thus Puerto Rican children living in crowded conditions in New York had a lower incidence of infection than white, non-Puerto Rican children.

LABORATORY DIAGNOSIS

Adult female worms may be found in the faeces or penianal skin. The method of choice for making a diagnosis is the Scotch adhesive tape swab applied to the perianal region in the morning before bathing or defecation. Ova are identified by their asymmetrical shape and well-developed embryo when the tape is mounted on a slide for examination. The Scotch tape can be also applied to that part of the person's clothing which has been in contact with the perianal region. At least three examinations should be carried out before a negative diagnosis is made. Enterobiasis is very infectious and if one person is infected in a household all other members of the family should be suspect.

CONTROL

Because enterobiasis is an infection of families or institutions, all members should be examined and those positive treated simultaneously. Scrupulous cleanliness, frequent washing of the anal region, the hands and the nails, especially after defecating, controls the infection. Cotton drawers and gloves should be worn at night and boiled daily. Pyrantel compounds and the benzimidazoles are effective in a single dose.

Toxocariasis

Occurrence:	Worldwide
Organisms:	Toxocara canis and T. catis
Reservoir:	Dogs and cats
Transmission:	Handling infected household pets or their faeces
Control:	Personal hygiene Treatment of household pets

Evidence has now accumulated that human disease due to larval migration of Toxocara canis and T. cati constitutes an important public health problem, and although the majority of reports to date have emanated from the more developed countries, we believe that it is merely a question of time before these infections are widely reported from the tropics as a major cause of some of the otherwise unexplained clinical syndromes seen in these areas. The liver and eye are the most common organs involved, with an associated hypereosinophilia.

T. canis and T. cati are parasites of dogs and cats and their presence in the human host is an abnormal migration of their larval phase.

Under favourable conditions, the eggs passed in the dog's faeces become infective in 2–3 weeks. From the swallowed eggs emerge the second-stage larvae which penetrate the intestinal walls and reach the liver. The majority of larvae remain in the liver but others may pass on to the lungs or other organs of the body, including the central nervous system and the eye. Occasionally the larvae complete their cycle of development in the human host, resulting in infection with adult T. canis or T. cati.

It is possible that nematode larvae other than toxocara may be involved in visceral larva migrans. Viral encephalitis due to larval migration has been reported and the transmission of poliomyelitis virus by larvae of toxocara has been postulated.

EPIDEMIOLOGY

The majority of human cases have been reported from the eastern half of the United States, but the disease has been recognized in the Philippines, Mexico, Hawaii, Turkey, Puerto Rico and other countries. Toxocaral infection of dogs has been reported from Malta, Nigeria, Uganda, Kenya, Tanzania, Mexico and India.

Reservoir and transmission

The reservoir of infection is the dog, or less frequently the cat. Infection is acquired by ingesting soil which has been contaminated, usually by dogs' faeces.

Host factors

Young children are particularly susceptible to toxocariasis because of their habit of eating dirt, and of handling soiled fur of puppies and then putting their fingers in their mouths. The severity of the disease depends upon the numbers of worms that have invaded the body and the duration of infection. It has been shown that puppies are more infected than adult dogs and that the incidence among bitches is lower at all ages.

LABORATORY DIAGNOSIS

A high, stable persistent eosinophilia reaching levels of 60% is a prominent feature. Toxocara larvae can be identified in biopsy material and provide the most certain means of making a definite diagnosis. Unfortunately biopsies are often negative. ELISA and high levels of IgM are useful adjuncts to diagnosis.

CONTROL

Elimination of infection in puppies and dogs is the most effective way of controlling the disease. Puppies used as household pets should be regularly examined and treated with one of the piperazine compounds. Dog owners should avoid public parks

as defecation sites for their pets. Children should be instructed in habits of personal hygiene.

Dracunculiasis (guinea worm)

Occurrence:	Tropical Africa
Organism:	Dracunculus medinensis
Reservoir:	Humans
Transmission:	Water contaminated with cyclops
Control:	Filtration of water
	Boiling of water
	Provision of safe drinking water

The guinea worm *Dracunculus medinensis* has been known since ancient times. It results in the formation of skin ulcers, often in the ankles or legs, with extrusion of embryos on contact with water. The ulcers frequently become infected and are a cause of disability and school absenteeism.

The sexually mature female is up to 1 m long and 2 mm in diameter; the uterus, which occupies most of the body, contains millions of embryos. The male is small and its fate after copulation is not known.

LIFE CYCLE

See Figure 4.5.

EPIDEMIOLOGY

Contamination of fresh water with larvae from infected persons takes place when such persons share drinking water from shallow ponds (Plate 28) or wells. The water in these ponds, being stagnant with a high organic content, favours the presence of the vecta species of cyclops. In the dry seasons these ponds are much frequented since they often provide the only readily accessible source of water, thus creating a high cyclops:man contact ratio.

In other places, transmission may occur during the rainy season when surface pools exist which disappear in the dry season. Infection can also be contracted when drinking water while bathing in contaminated pools or during ritual washing of the mouth in the performance of religious ablutions.

CONTROL

Individual

Filtering the water through a gauze linen mesh will prevent infection by holding back the cyclops.

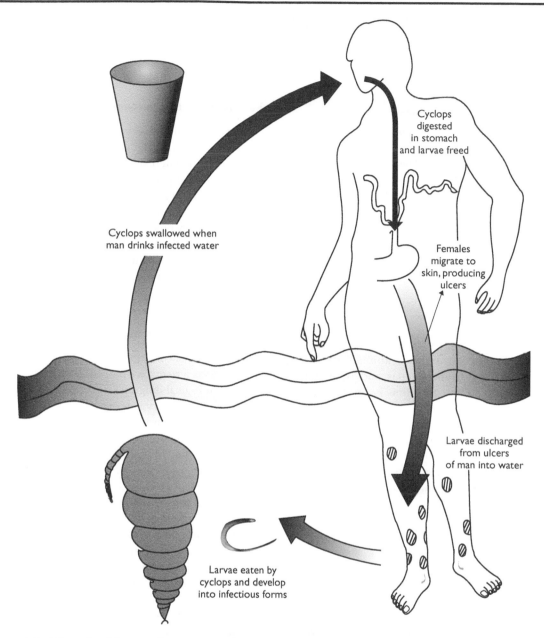

Cyclops swallowed when man drinks infected water

Cyclops digested in stomach and larvae freed

Females migrate to skin, producing ulcers

Larvae discharged from ulcers of man into water

Larvae eaten by cyclops and develop into infectious forms

Figure 4.5: Life cycle of *Dracunculus medinensis* (guinea worm).

Community

The eradication of guinea worm infection was adopted as a subgoal of the Clean Drinking Water Supply and Sanitation Decade (1981–90). The concept was further enhanced by other aid agencies by making the provision of safe drinking water a priority in rural areas of Africa and Asia.

Other interventions include filtering or boiling of water, especially the former by the use of monofilament nylon nets, which are long lasting and have a regular pore size and are able to sieve out cyclops. Treating water sources with temephos added to ponds is a useful adjunct in certain circumstances.

An international commission for the certification of dracunculiasis eradication monitors progress at regular intervals. The eradication of guinea worm infection is nearing completion (Plate 29). The only countries where a substantial number of cases still occur are the Sudan and Nigeria.

Trichinosis

Occurrence:	Worldwide
Organism:	Trichinella spiralis
Reservoir:	Pigs
Transmission:	Eating inadequately cooked pork or pork products
Control:	Adequate cooking of pork meat

Trichinosis is caused by encysted larvae of *Trichinella spiralis*. The disease is characterized by diarrhoea with abdominal pain, followed by a febrile illness with severe muscular pain.

APPLIED BIOLOGY

The adult worms are found in the small intestine of a number of carnivorous animals including the pig, bush-pig, rats, hyenas and other hosts. Their lifespan in the intestine is approximately 8 weeks.

After fertilization, the female worms bury themselves in the intestinal mucosa and each produces about 1500 larvae. The larvae migrate via the intestinal lymphatics to the thoracic duct and into the bloodstream, whence they are distributed to the muscles. Here they develop and become encysted between the muscle fibres in 4–7 weeks. Calcification occurs in about 18 months but the encysted larvae remain alive for many years. When food containing encysted larvae is ingested by a suitable host the larvae are released by the action of the digestive juices on the capsule and the cycle is repeated in the new host. In susceptible animals the larvae grow into sexually differentiated adults which on mating produce larvae which then invade striated muscle. In man, infection terminates at the cystic stage.

EPIDEMIOLOGY

This parasite is more prevalent in temperate than in tropical countries and is mainly confined to those countries where pork is eaten. Serological tests have shown that in many communities the incidence of infection is apparently higher than the number of clinically diagnosed cases, and

it is obvious that many light infections pass unnoticed. In recent years small and large epidemics have occurred. Congenital trichinosis has been reported.

Reservoir and transmission

Pigs are the main 'reservoir' of infection although many other animals harbour the infection. Trichinosis in man results from eating raw or inadequately cooked pork or pork products, for example sausage meat. In Kenya, the bush-pig is a common source of infection. Pigs become infected chiefly from eating uncooked slaughterhouse refuse containing infected meat scraps; occasionally rats, which have a high natural infection rate of trichinosis, can be a source of infection when they are eaten by pigs.

LABORATORY DIAGNOSIS

One of the most constant, single, diagnostic aids in trichinosis is a rising eosinophilia of 10–40%.

Parasitological diagnosis is based on the finding of the encysted larval worms in a thin piece of muscle biopsy compressed between two glass slides and examined under a low magnification of the microscope. In light infections, when direct examination is negative, the biopsy specimen should be incubated overnight in an acid–pepsin mixture and the centrifuged deposit examined for larvae. Immunological tests such as ELISA and countercommunoelectrophoresis are positive as early as 2 weeks after infection.

The CFT can provide a diagnosis in the first week of the disease – the specificity of the test is high. The bentonite, latex, and cholesterol agglutination tests are excellent tests for diagnosing recent infections but are unreliable in chronic infections.

CONTROL

Adequate cooking of pork and other meats (e.g. hare, polar bear, dog, etc.) will essentially protect the individual. Legislation compelling all pig feed containing meat to be cooked virtually stops transmission of trichinosis to the pig.

Mebendazole or albendazole kills or sterilizes trichinella adult worms and may prevent trichinellosis.

Angiostrongyliasis

Occurrence:	South East Asia and Oceania
Organism:	Angiostrongylus cantonensis
Reservoir:	Rodents
Transmission:	Snails
Control:	Adequate cooking and cleaning of vegetables

Angiostrongyliasis is an eosinophilic meningitis due to the nematode worm *Angiostrongylus cantonensis*.

APPLIED BIOLOGY

A. cantonensis is essentially a parasite of rats and only occasionally infects man. The eggs hatch in the faeces of the rat in which they are expelled, and the infective larvae invade certain snails or slugs. These are later eaten by rats, which thereby become infected. The life cycle in man is unknown, but young adult worms have been found in the cerebrospinal fluid and the brain where they measured 8–12 mm in length.

EPIDEMIOLOGY

Sporadic, small epidemics occur in certain Pacific Islands, including Tahiti and Hawaii, and in South East Asia including Vietnam and Thailand. It has been suggested that *A. cantonensis* originated in the islands of the Indian Ocean (Madagascar, Mauritius, Ceylon) and then spread eastwards to South East Asia and so to the Pacific area, and that the giant African snail *Achatina fulica* might have been instrumental in the spread of the parasite.

Reservoir and transmission

Rats are the reservoir. Human infection results from the accidental ingestion of infected snails, slugs and land planarians (worm-like creatures) found on unwashed vegetables, such as lettuce. The peak incidence of eosinophilic meningitis occurs in the cooler, rainy months between July and November, the period of highest consumption of lettuces and strawberries which when unwashed lead to infection. It is also the season when fresh-water prawn may become infected from snails and slugs washed into rivers and estuaries. This was thought to be the main source of local, human infection in Tahiti.

Eating raw or pickled snails of the genus *Pila* is considered the mode of infection in Thailand; the percentage of positive snails for *A. cantonensis* infections varying from 1.8 to 72%. In Malaysia, the shelled slug *M. malayanus* has been shown to shed infective third-stage larvae, but no human cases have yet been reported.

Host factors

In Thailand, males are affected twice as frequently as females, the highest attack rate occurring in the second and third decade.

LABORATORY DIAGNOSIS

Examination of the cerebrospinal fluid reveals increase in protein and a strikingly high eosinophilia (60–80%). Larval worms are sometimes found in the CSF and can be identified as *A. cantonensis* on microscopy.

CONTROL

The infection is prevented by not eating unwashed vegetables and strawberries and uncooked snails, slugs and prawns infected with larvae. Efficient rat control will reduce the reservoir of infection.

Gnathostomiasis

Occurrence:	Thailand
Organism:	Gnathostoma spinigerum
Reservoir:	Domestic and wild cats
Transmission:	Eating or preparing raw fish or chicken
Control:	Adequate cooking

Gnathostoma infection may present as 'creeping eruption', transitory swellings or eosinophilic meningitis.

APPLIED BIOLOGY

The life cycle in the definitive animal hosts (felines, dogs and foxes) is well known, and involves two intermediate hosts – a cyclops and a fish or an amphibian. Man is an unnatural host and the immature worms may locate either in the internal organs or near the surface of the body. As the larvae rarely develop into adults the life cycle in man is not known. Adults have, however, been reported in the intestine and ova have been found in human faeces.

EPIDEMIOLOGY

Reservoir

The normal hosts for *Gnathostoma spinigerum* are domestic and wild felines, dogs and foxes. Human infections have, however, been reported from Israel, the Sudan, India and the Far East. The majority of human cases to date have occurred in Thailand, where a substantial animal reservoir has been reported. The parasite has been isolated from cats, dogs, domestic pigs, freshwater fish, eels, snakes, frogs, leopards, chickens and fish-eating birds. One per cent of dogs in Bangkok is infected with gnathostomiasis. In Thailand, human infection usually results from eating fermented fish, which is a Thai delicacy much liked by women. The dish known as Somfak is made up of raw freshwater fish, cooked rice, curry, salt and pepper and then wrapped in banana leaves. Recently it has been shown experimentally that penetration of the skin by the third-stage infective larva can occur.

There is a possibility therefore that in addition to ingestion, human infection is possible during the preparation of raw fish dishes or raw chicken dishes by the third-stage larva penetrating the bare skin of the hands of individuals preparing these meals. Other ways for man to acquire the infection is by eating other forms of raw fish, frogs, and possibly snakes infected with encysted larvae.

Human infection has occasionally been attributed to *G. hispidum,* the definitive host in this instance is the pig.

LABORATORY DIAGNOSIS

Diagnosis in human infections depends on finding the immature worms and identifying them. Cutaneous tests with antigens from larval or adult worms as well as precipitin tests have been used for diagnosis. Eosinophilia is present.

CONTROL

The infection is prevented by not eating uncooked fish and meats of other animals infected with encysted larvae. Ancylol (disophenol) kills both the larval and adult forms of gnathostoma in dogs and cats. Unfortunately the compound is too toxic for man.

Cestode (tapeworm) infections

Taeniasis

Occurrence:	Worldwide
Organisms:	*Taenia solium, T. saginata, Cysticercus cellulosae*
Reservoir:	Humans
Transmission:	Uncooked meat
	Auto-human infection (cysticercosis)
Control:	Personal hygiene
	Individual specific treatment
	Sanitary disposal of faeces
	Thorough cooking of meat

Taeniasis occurs in all countries where beef or pork are eaten. The larval stage of *T. solium* produces cysticercosis. Clinical features of taeniasis are often absent, the patients only becoming aware of the worm infection when segments are passed in the stool.

The life cycles of *T. saginata* and *T. solium* are shown in Figures 4.6 and 4.7.

Direct infection of man by larval worms of *T. solium* produces a condition known as cysticercosis. For this to occur, man must be exposed to a source of ova from water and food contaminated by faeces; unclean hands transferring eggs from the adult worm carrier; auto-infection by carrying eggs from the anus to the mouth on the fingers; and, rarely, by auto-infection by massive regurgitation of ova from the small intestine into the stomach.

The liberated larvae penetrate the intestinal mucosa and are then carried by the bloodstream to various parts of the body where they encyst, the commonest sites being the subcutaneous tissues, skeletal muscles and the brain. The cysticercus takes about 4 months to develop and becomes enveloped in a fibrous capsule, which eventually calcifies and may be seen radiologically.

The life cycle of the cysticercus ranges from a few months up to 35 years.

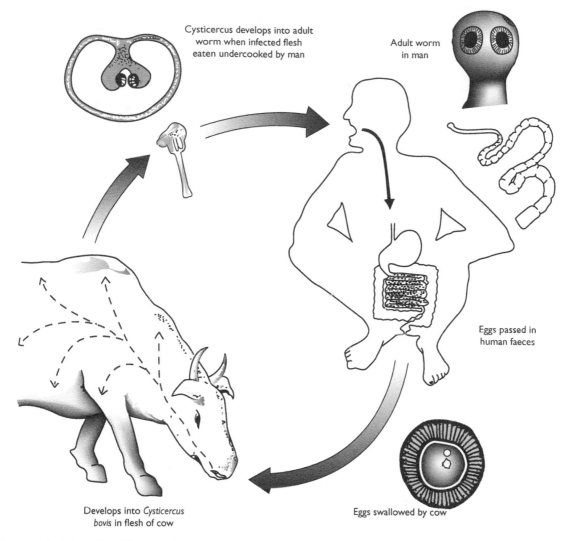

Cysticercus develops into adult worm when infected flesh eaten undercooked by man

Adult worm in man

Eggs passed in human faeces

Eggs swallowed by cow

Develops into *Cysticercus bovis* in flesh of cow

Figure 4.6: Life cycle of *Taenia saginata*.

EPIDEMIOLOGY

The beef tapeworm *Taenia saginata* has a cosmopolitan distribution and is particularly common in the Middle East, Kenya and Ethiopia. The world incidence of *T. saginata is* much higher than that of *T. solium* and it is estimated that in some parts of Kenya infection rates of taeniasis in man may approach 100% and that 30% of cattle may harbour cysticerci.

The pork tapeworm *T. solium* is also widely distributed in Central and South America, Africa and South East Asia and its larval stage, *Cysticercus cellulosae*, produces cysticercosis in man. In several countries (e.g. Ecuador) the prevalence of human neurocysticercosis is high and constitutes a serious public health problem.

Reservoir and transmission

Humans are the only reservoir of infection. Humans acquire *T. saginata* infection by eating raw or partially cooked beef, while cattle are infected by grazing on pastures fertilized by human faeces or which are flooded with sewage-laden water. The role of birds in the transmission of the disease is not clear.

T. solium is spread by the insanitary disposal of faeces, thus providing the pigs with a ready opportunity for infection when they ingest human

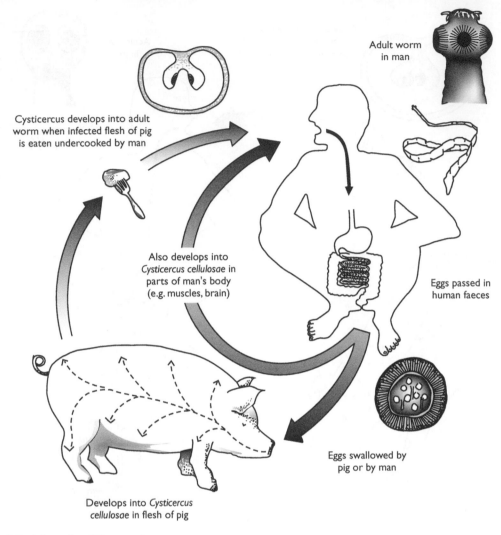

Adult worm in man

Cysticercus develops into adult worm when infected flesh of pig is eaten undercooked by man

Also develops into *Cysticercus cellulosae* in parts of man's body (e.g. muscles, brain)

Eggs passed in human faeces

Eggs swallowed by pig or by man

Develops into *Cysticercus cellulosae* in flesh of pig

Figure 4.7: Life cycle of *Taenia solium*.

excreta. Man is infected when eating uncooked or insufficiently cooked pork (Plate 30).

Host factors

Taeniasis is uncommon in young children and the incidence increases with age. The sexes are equally susceptible.

LABORATORY DIAGNOSIS

'Direct smear' examination of the faeces occasionally reveals the typical taenia ova. The intact segments that are usually passed can be compressed between two glass slides and the branches of the uterus at their origin from the main uterine stem can be counted and a differentiation easily made between *T. saginata* (20–35 branches) and *T. solium* (7–12 branches). A coproantigen ELISA has recently been developed as well as a PCR technique for identification of *T. saginata* proglotids and eggs.

CYSTICERCOSIS DIAGNOSIS

Calcified cysts can be seen radiologically, while computerized axial tomography (CAT) and magnetic resonance have replaced older methods. Complementary procedures are ELISA and Western blotting (WT).

Biopsy of palpable subcutaneous nodules may be diagnostic.

CONTROL

Transmission of taeniasis and cysticercosis can be controlled by the sanitary disposal of human faeces, the thorough cooking of meat and raising the standards of personal hygiene.

The individual

All persons suffering from taeniasis should be dewormed with niclosamide (given in a single dose of 2 g) or praziquantel (a single dose of 5–10 mg/kg after a light meal). The thorough cooking of all beef and pork meat affords personal protection and health education should be carried out to raise the standards of personal hygiene, especially among persons harbouring *T. solium*.

The treatment of cerebral cysticercosis includes praziquantel, albendozole, steroids and surgery.

The community

Sanitary disposal of human excreta is essential. Untreated human faeces should not be used as fertilizer and if possible human faeces should be avoided altogether as a means of manuring crops.

Strict abattoir supervision resulting in adequate inspection of carcasses and condemnation of infected meat should be carried out. If meat containing cysticerci has to be consumed it should be thoroughly cooked under the close supervision of a health officer.

Recently, community-oriented chemotherapy of *T. solium* taeniasis with praziquantel has been introduced in order to prevent local endemic neurocysticercosis.

Diphyllobothriasis

Occurrence:	Commoner in temperate zones
Organism:	*Diphyllobothrium latum*
Reservoir:	Humans, fish-eating mammals
Transmission:	Eating raw fish
Control:	Thorough cooking
	Sanitary disposal of faeces
	Control of fishing and export of raw fish

Infection by the fish tapeworm *Diphyllobothrium latum* is characterized by a megaloblastic anaemia due to vitamin B12 deficiency.

APPLIED BIOLOGY

The adult, which may be 10 m long, lives in the ileum of humans or other mammals, and may have as many as 4000 segments. The gravid segments disintegrate and the ova are passed in the faeces. On reaching water the ciliated embryo escapes and is swallowed by the first intermediate host – a freshwater crustacean (*Cyclops* or *Diaptomus* species) – in which it develops as a procercoid. When the infected crustaceans are swallowed by various freshwater fishes (salmon, pike, etc.) further development takes place in the musculature of these second intermediate hosts to form plerocercoids. When man and other animals eat raw fish the plerocercoid is liberated and attaches itself to the small intestine, where it grows into an adult in about 6 weeks.

EPIDEMIOLOGY

Diphyllobothriasis is more common in the temperate zones than in the tropics where it has been reported from the Philippines, Madagascar, Botswana, Uganda and southern Chile.

Reservoir and transmission

Man and a number of fish-eating mammals (e.g. dog, cat, fox, pig, bear, seal, etc.) are the reservoir of infection. Man is infected by eating raw or insufficiently cooked fish; the latter having acquired their infections in waters contaminated by faeces containing ova of *D. latum*. As with the other tapeworms, the adult fish tapeworm is long-lived. The export of raw fish may cause infection outside the endemic areas.

LABORATORY DIAGNOSIS

If segments are passed in the faeces or vomitus, diagnosis can be made by seeing the typical rosette-shaped uterus when the segment is crushed between two glass slides. More commonly, however, 'direct smear' examination of the faeces will reveal the characteristic operculate ova.

CONTROL

Thorough cooking of fish affords personal protection, all infected persons should be treated with niclosamide (Yomesan) or praziquantel in the same dosage as for taeniasis. Control of export of raw or smoked fish should be exercised. Sanitary disposal of the human faeces will reduce infection of fish, and fishing should be forbidden in infected waters.

Hymenolepiasis

Occurrence:	SE United States, S. America, India
Organism:	Hymenolepsis and Drepanido taemia spp.
Reservoir:	Humans, rodents
Transmission:	Contaminated water, food
Control:	Personal hygiene
	Sanitary disposal of faeces

Three dwarf tapeworm infections can occur in man due to *Hymenolepis nana*, *H. diminuta* and *Drepanido taemia lanceolata* respectively. They all occur in the tropics and subtropics.

EPIDEMIOLOGY

H. nana is a common tapeworm of man in the southeastern United States, parts of South America, and India. Humans become infected by ingesting the ova in food or water that has been contaminated by human or rat faeces. The infection can also be transmitted directly from hand to mouth. Although rats and mice are commonly infected, man is the chief source of human infections, infection being spread directly from patient to patient without utilizing an intermediate host. Owing to their unhygienic habits, *H. nana* is more prevalent in children, with the highest incidence occurring between 4 and 9 years.

H. diminuta is an infection of rats and mice, humans being an incidental host. The principal source of infection is food contaminated by rat and mice droppings on which the intermediate insect hosts also thrive. When persons eat food containing these insect vectors they get accidentally infected. Human infection is chiefly in children who ingest rat fleas.

LABORATORY DIAGNOSIS

A moderate eosinophilia (4–16%) occurs in both *H. nana* and *H. diminuta* infections. Diagnosis is made by finding the characteristic ova in the faeces.

CONTROL

Personal hygiene, sanitary disposal of faeces and food hygiene will control these infections with dwarf tapeworms. The treatment of the individual is as for taeniasis, but it is advisable to repeat the dose after an interval of 3 weeks to kill any further tapeworms which may have emerged from their larval state in the intestinal villi.

Hydatid disease

Occurrence:	Worldwide
Organism:	Echinococcus spp.
Reservoir:	Dogs
Transmission:	Ingestion of infective ova
Control:	Personal hygiene
	Albendazole
	Deworming of dogs (praziquantel)
	Abattoir hygiene

This disease can be caused by any one of three species of the genus *Echinococcus*: *E. granulosus*, *E. multilocularis* and *E. oligaettas*. Since the epidemiological and pathological features of these three tapeworms are very similar, only a detailed description of *E. granulosus* is given here.

LIFE CYCLE

See Figure 4.8.

EPIDEMIOLOGY

Hydatid disease, caused by the larval form of *E. granulosus*, has a cosmopolitan distribution, being particularly prevalent in the sheep- and cattle-raising areas of the world.

Reservoir and transmission

Dogs are the main reservoir of human infection. Humans acquire hydatid disease when they swallow infected ova as a result of their close association with dogs, and the insanitary habit of not washing hands before ingesting food. The ova may live for weeks in shady environments but they are quickly destroyed by sunlight and high temperatures. The dog faeces contaminating fleeces of sheep can also be an indirect source of human infection.

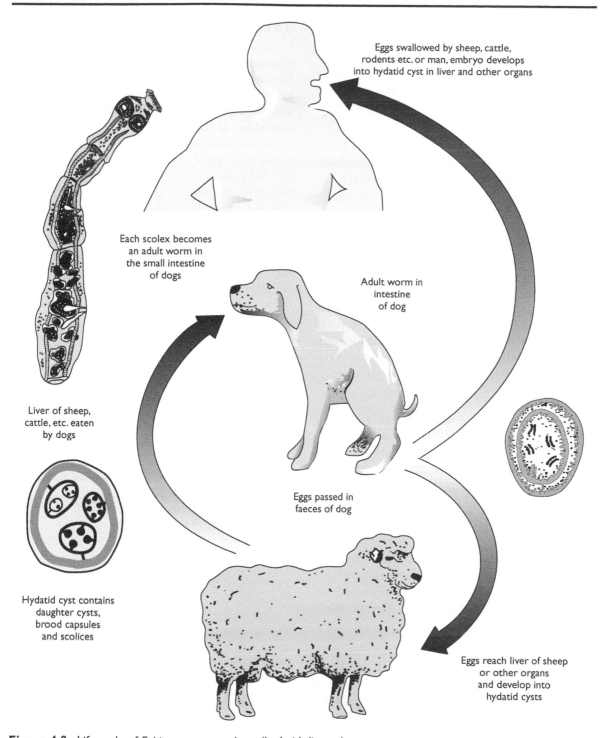

Figure 4.8: Life cycle of *Echinococcus granulosus* (hydatid disease).

The main cycle of transmission in Kenya is between dogs and domestic livestock (Plate 31). It has been shown that in Kenya hydatid cysts are present in more than 30% of cattle, sheep and goats, though the disease in humans occurs infrequently, except in the areas of Turkana. Canines are heavily infected while light infections have been recorded in wild carnivores, for example jackals and hyenas. Turkana tribesmen are the most heavily infected people in Kenya because of the intimate contact between children and the large number of infected canines in the area – here dogs are used to clean the face and anal regions of babies.

Host factors

Although infection is usually acquired in childhood, clinical symptoms do not appear until adult life.

LABORATORY DIAGNOSIS

If the hydatid cyst ruptures, its contents (hooklets, scolices, etc.) may be found in the faeces, sputum or urine. Eosinophilia is present but is usually moderate in degree (300–2000/mm^2) and there may be hypergammaglobulinaemia. Ultrasound technology, MR and CT scanning are often used in diagnosis. ELISA and indirect haemaglutination are procedures of choice in initial screening of sera.

CONTROL

This depends on raising the standards of personal hygiene, deworming of infected dogs with praziquantel (Droncit) and adequate supervision of abattoirs. Infected offal and meat should be destroyed, dogs excluded from slaughterhouses, and infected carcasses deeply buried or incinerated.

The individual

People must be warned of the danger of handling dogs or sheep and the importance of washing their hands immediately afterwards. The results of treatment with albendazole have shown great promise.

The community

Deworming of all infected dogs, if possible, is the best means of getting rid of the main reservoir of infection. The most suitable drug for this purpose is praziquantel (Droncit). In addition, all meat or offal containing hydatid cysts should be disposed of and thus be made inaccessible to dogs. Abattoir supervision and hygiene will exclude dogs from the premises and infected carcasses should be incinerated. In sheep-rearing areas burial or incineration of dead sheep should be carried out. Stray dogs should be eliminated.

TREMATODE (FLUKE) INFECTIONS

Throughout the world over 40 million people have food-borne trematode infections and 750 million are at risk. They are particularly prevalent in South East and East Asia. The factors determining the epidemiology of these infections are: (i) food related (e.g. consumption of raw fish or food plants); (ii) social or cultural determinants; (iii) aquaculture; and (iv) water resources development. All of these factors are indirectly influenced by poverty, pollution and population growth.

National strategies for control must include the following components: (i) a national co-ordinating body to set up a 'horizontal' programme; (ii) training; (iii) health education; (iv) food control; (v) improvement in sanitation; and (vi) intersectional collaboration with agriculture and fisheries departments.

Immunodiagnostic tests (e.g. ELISA, complement fixation and precipitin tests) are useful in the diagnosis of extraintestinal and tissue-dwelling trematode infections. DNA detection and the polymerase reaction are available but not in general use.

Paragonimiasis

Occurrence:	East and South East Asia and West Africa
Organism:	*Paragonimus westermani*
Reservoir:	Humans
Transmission:	Eating uncooked crab and crayfish
Control:	Adequate cooking of crab and crayfish
	Sanitary disposal of faeces

The infection is characterized by cough, expectoration of bloody sputum and later signs of bronchiectasus or lung abscess.

LIFE CYCLE

See Figure 4.9.

EPIDEMIOLOGY

Paragonimiasis is due to the lung fluke *Paragonimus westermani*, which has a worldwide geographical distribution. It occurs focally throughout the Far East, South East Asia, the Pacific Islands, West Africa

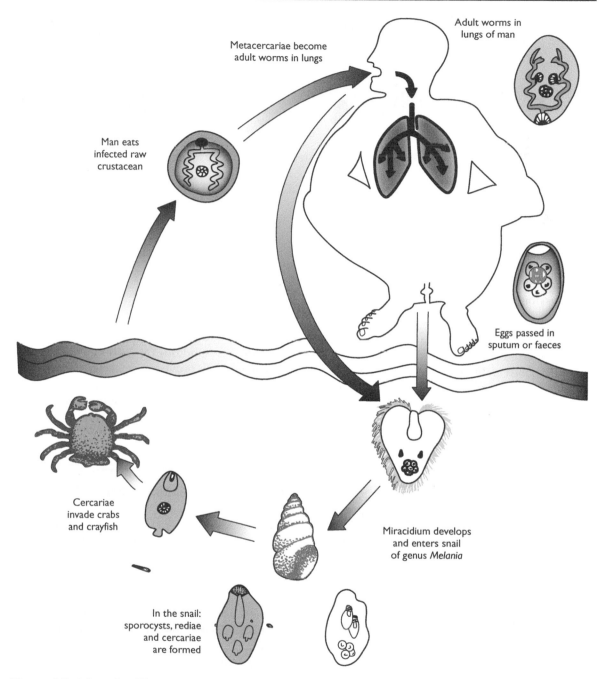

Figure 4.9: Life cycle of *Paragonimus westermani*.

and parts of South America (Fig. 4.10). A new species, *P. africanus,* which is considered to be a local causative agent of paragonimiasis, has been described from the Cameroons. Other species responsible for human infections are *P. heterotremus* and *P. szechuanensis.*

Reservoir

Humans are the reservoir of infection. Although a considerable domestic and wild animal reservoir of paragonimus infection exists, the part it plays in the epidemiology of human disease has yet to be fully determined.

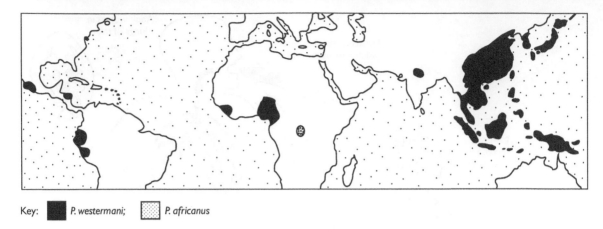

Key: ■ *P. westermani*; ▨ *P. africanus*

Figure 4.10: Distribution of paragonimiasis.

Transmission

Transmission is maintained by faecal and sputum pollution of water in which the appropriate snails and vector crustaceans live, and by the custom of eating uncooked crabs and crayfish soaked in alcohol, vinegar, brine or wine. Infection can also occur during the preparation of such food, when encysted cercariae can be left on the knife or other utensils.

Host factors

Although in most areas infection is higher in males than in females, in the Cameroons women are infected three times as often as men. The peak age of incidence is between 11 and 35 years of age. It has been reported that during a measles epidemic in Korea, 80% of paragonimus infections were produced by the administration of the fluid extract of crushed crabs given medicinally to the patients.

The infection may persist for many years after leaving endemic areas.

LABORATORY DIAGNOSIS

The infected sputum is characteristically sticky and bloody, usually of a dark, brownish red colour. The characteristically shaped eggs are usually found in the sputum or in the faeces on 'direct smear' examination or by concentration techniques. In the first year of infection eggs are seldom found but there is usually an eosinophilia of about 20–30%. ELISA is a sensitive and practical immunological test. Radiography may show patchy foci of fibrotic change, with a characteristic 'ring shadow'.

CONTROL

Crabs and crayfish should be cooked before eating. Faecal pollution of water should be prevented. Elevation of standards of personal and public hygiene and the provision of latrines will reduce transmission. Praziquantel has been used both for individual treatment and community control.

Clonorchiasis

Occurrence:	East Asia
Organism:	*Clonorchis sinensis*
Reservoir:	Humans
Transmission:	Eating raw or undercooked fish
Control:	Adequate cooking of fish
	Chemotherapy
	Sanitary disposal of faeces

This infection is caused by the oriental liver fluke *Clonorchis sinensis* and may be symptomless or result in severe liver damage with the possibility of malignant change.

LIFE CYCLE

See Figure 4.11.

EPIDEMIOLOGY

Clonorchiasis is mainly found in the Far East. Endemic foci occur in Japan, South Korea, South East China, Taiwan and Vietnam (Fig. 4.12).

Adult worms in bile ducts of man and animals

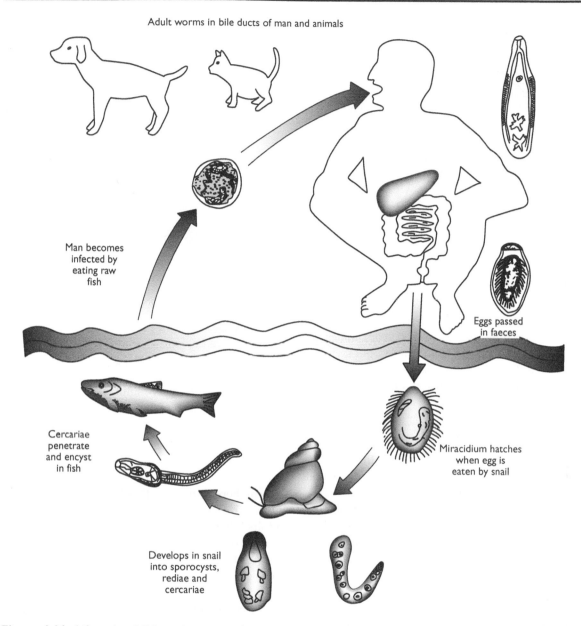

Man becomes
infected by
eating raw
fish

Eggs passed
in faeces

Cercariae
penetrate
and encyst
in fish

Miracidium hatches
when egg is
eaten by snail

Develops in snail
into sporocysts,
rediae and
cercariae

Figure 4.11: Life cycle of *Chlonorchis sinensis*.

Reservoir

Humans are the reservoir of infection. As with paragonimiasis many animals harbour *C. sinensis*, but their importance in the epidemiology of the human disease has yet to be fully assessed.

Transmission

Humans and other mammals are infected by eating raw or undercooked fish containing metacercariae.

Fish ponds fertilized with fresh human faeces are a common source of infection (Plate 32). Infected fish exported to other countries can result in the spread of the disease to areas where the parasite is not normally found.

Host factors

Clonorchiasis is rare in infants under 1 year of age. It begins, however, at about 2 years, rising to 65% in

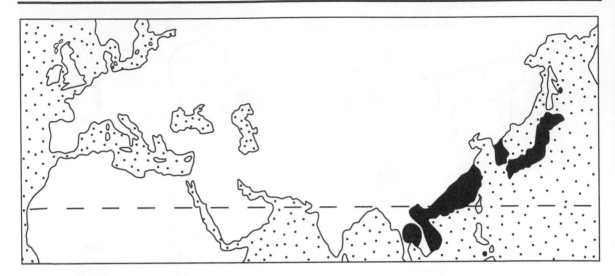

Figure 4.12: Distribution of *Chlonorchis sinensis*.

those aged 21–30 years and to a peak of 80% in those dying between the ages 51 and 60 years. Males are more frequently infected than females, but there are no social differences in the prevalence of the disease because of the universal custom of eating raw fish. The lifespan of the worm is 25–30 years.

LABORATORY DIAGNOSIS

A definitive diagnosis is made by finding the typical operculated ova by 'direct smear' examination of the faeces or duodenal aspirate.

There is usually a leucocytosis (23 000–48 200) with eosinophilia. In severe cases with secondary infection of the bile ducts there may be severe hypoglycaemia and a raised alkaline phosphatase.

CONTROL

Fish should not be eaten raw and the use of human faeces in fish ponds should be avoided. Sanitary disposal of faeces and raising the standards of personal and community hygiene will reduce transmission. Praziquantel has been successfully used both for individual treatment, and community control.

Opisthorchiasis

Occurrence:	South East Asia
Organism:	*Opisthorchis viverrini, O. felineus*
Reservoir:	Humans and animals

Transmission:	Eating raw fish
Control:	Adequate cooking of fish
	Chemotherapy

This infection is very similar to clonorchiasis, resulting in enlargement of the liver and eventually malignant change.

APPLIED BIOLOGY

The life cycle and pathogenesis of the two human hepatic trematodes *Opisthorchis felineus* and *O. viverrini* are similar to that of *C. sinensis*. The adults inhabit the distal bile ducts and the ova are passed out in the faeces. After ingestion by the appropriate snails (e.g. *Bithynia*) the miracidia develop into cercariae, which in turn penetrate the flesh of suitable species of freshwater fishes (e.g. cyprinoid family) in which they encyst and develop into metacercariae. When the metacercariae are ingested by a suitable host (man, domestic, wild and fur-bearing animals) they encyst in the duodenum and migrate to the distal bile ducts particularly those of the left lobe of the liver. The entire life cycle takes about 4 months.

EPIDEMIOLOGY

In the tropics *Opisthorchis felineus* is prevalent in the Philippines, India, Japan and Vietnam, while *O. viverrini* is endemic in North and North East Thailand and Laos. The largest number of human infections occur during the latter portion of the rainy season and the first part of the dry season (i.e. from September to February).

Reservoir

Humans, domestic, wild and fur-bearing animals are the reservoir of infection. The chief reservoir of *O. felineus is* the cat.

Transmission

Humans and the reservoir hosts are infected by the consumption of raw or insufficiently cooked fish (Plate 33). Snails and fish are infected by faeces deposited on the sandy shores and washed into the streams.

In North East Thailand 90% of people over the age of 10 years are infected with *O. viverrini* and it is estimated that over 7 million persons in Thailand harbour the parasite. The source of infection is a popular dish called 'Koi-pla', consisting of raw fish, roasted rice, and vegetables seasoned with garlic, lemon juice, fish sauce and pepper (Plate 34). Chinese residents of Thailand who do not eat raw fish are free from infection.

LABORATORY DIAGNOSIS

This is made by finding the ova on 'direct smear' examination of faeces or duodenal aspirate.

CONTROL

Fish should be eaten only if cooked. The sanitary disposal of faeces and a raised standard of personal and public hygiene will reduce transmission. Praziquantel given as a single dose is effective for individual treatment and a large community chemotherapy control scheme involving 1.5 million people has been carried out in North East Thailand, combining chemotherapy, health education and environmental hygiene measures.

Fascioliasis

Occurrence:	Worldwide
Organism:	*Fasciola hepatica*
Reservoir:	Ruminants, especially sheep
Transmission:	Eating contaminated lettuce or water cress
Control:	Avoid eating wild lettuce or water cress

This infection by the trematode *Fasciola hepatica* (sheep-liver fluke) may be silent or may present with symptoms of chronic liver disease and portal hypertension.

APPLIED BIOLOGY

The adult worm, which is large (30 mm long and 13 mm broad), flat and leaf-shaped, lives in the bile ducts or liver parenchyma of sheep, cattle, goats and other mammals, and man. The eggs are passed in the faeces and hatch in a moist environment. The released miracidia then enter the appropriate species of snails (*Limnaea*), and develop successfully into sporocytes, rediae and cercariae. The cercariae then leave their snail host and encyst on various grasses and water plants. When this water vegetation is ingested by the appropriate hosts, the larvae excyst in the intestine, penetrate the mucosa, enter the liver through the portal circulation, and eventually reach the bile ducts, where they mature in about 3 months. *F. hepatica* obtains its nourishment from the biliary secretions and can absorb simple carbohydrates.

EPIDEMIOLOGY

Fascioliasis has a worldwide distribution in ruminants, being especially prevalent in the sheep-rearing areas of the world. It is a widespread problem in Bolivia, Ecuador, Egypt, Iran and Peru. In some areas, for example Hawaii, the causative agent of fascioliasis is *F. gigantica*.

Reservoir and transmission

The reservoir of infection is ruminants, especially sheep. Humans usually contract infection by eating lettuce or water cress contaminated by sheep or other animals' faeces. The highest incidence of infection occurs in low, damp pastures where the grasses and the water are infected with encysted cercariae.

LABORATORY DIAGNOSIS

The finding of the typical operculated eggs in faeces (150 × 90 g) is diagnostic, but unfortunately these do not appear until about 3 months after infection. Duodenal intubation may reveal the ova in biliary secretions at an earlier stage of the disease. There may be a leucocytosis (12 000–40 000/ml) and an eosinophilia of 40–85%.

CONTROL

Lettuce or water cress should be sterilized by momentary immersion in boiling water; this will destroy the encysted cercariae. The unique biology and life cycle of *F. hepatica* make it amenable to effective use of geographical information systems (GIS). Individuals can be treated with triclabendazole.

Fasciolopsiasis

Occurrence:	East and South East Asia
Organism:	*Fasciolopsis buski*
Reservoir:	Humans and pigs
Transmission:	Eating raw water plants
Control:	Adequate cooking of water plants

Fasciolopsiasis is caused by the large, fleshy fluke, *Fasciolopsis buski*. Infection is often symptomless, but with heavy infections abdominal pain with alternating diarrhoea and constipation may occur.

LIFE CYCLE

See Figure 4.13.

EPIDEMIOLOGY

Fasciolopsiasis is found mainly in China, but also in India, Indo-China, Thailand, Malaysia, Indonesia, Taiwan and Europe.

Reservoir and transmission

Humans, who are a source of infection, are infected when they eat raw water plants contaminated with encysted cercariae. Pigs are also an important animal reservoir, infecting the stagnant ponds in which edible water plants grow. The commonest source of infected edible water plants are the water caltrops (Plate 35) and water chestnuts which are often cultivated in ponds fertilized by human faeces. In China, these tubers are eaten raw and fresh from July to September and, as they are peeled with the teeth, an easy entry of the cercariae to the mouth is provided.

LABORATORY DIAGNOSIS

The diagnosis can be made by finding the characteristic operculated ova in the faeces. There may be a leucocytosis and eosinophilia. Occasionally, adult flukes are vomited or found in the faeces.

CONTROL

This consists of adequate cooking of the potentially infected foods and prevention of faecal pollution of water in which they grow. Provision of latrines and the raising of standards of personal and public hygiene by health education helps to reduce transmission. Praziquantel is the drug of choice for individual treatment.

HETEROPHIASIS AND METAGONIMIASIS

These conditions are due to infection by two very minute flukes, *Heterophyes heterophyes* and *Melagonimus yokogawai*. The pathogenicity of these parasitic infections is very low, unless aberrant ova enter the circulation when the spinal cord may be affected. Both flukes have similar life cycles and epidemiology.

LIFE CYCLE

The adults live in the upper part of the small intestine embedded in mucus or in the mucosal folds. The eggs containing miracidia are passed in the faeces and, on ingestion by suitable snails, develop into sporocysts, rediae and cercariae. The cercariae then leave the snails and enter the appropriate fish, in which they encyst into infective metacercariae. When the fish are eaten raw or partially cooked the metacercariae are liberated and the larvae develop into adult worms in the small intestine.

The first snail intermediate hosts for *H. heterophyes* are brackish water snails (e.g. *Pirinella conica*), while the second intermediate hosts are mullets; for *M. yokogawai* the hosts are snails of the *Semisukospira* species and salmonoid and cyprinoid fishes.

EPIDEMIOLOGY

In the tropics the *H. heterophyes* is found in Egypt, Tunisia, South China, India and the Philippines, while *M. yokogawi* occurs in the Far East and Indonesia. In addition to humans, other mammals are also infected and, like clonorchis infection, heterophiasis and metagonimiasis are acquired by eating raw or partially cooked infected fish.

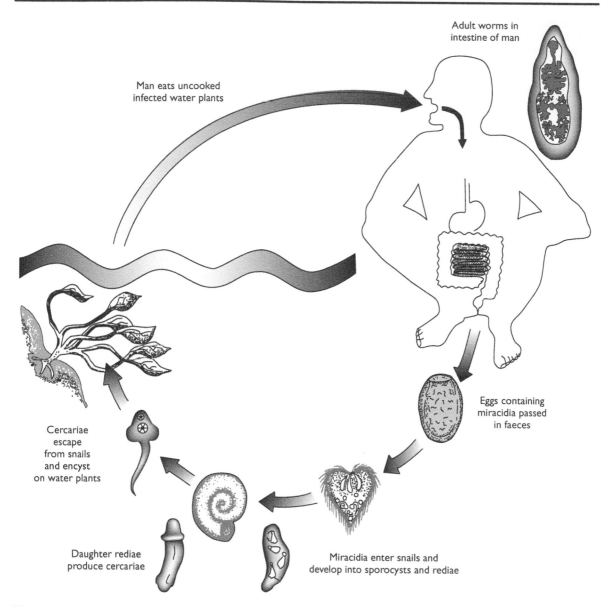

Figure 4.13: Life cycle of *Fasciolopsis buski*.

Diagnosis is made by finding the characteristic ova in the faeces. There may be eosinophilia. Praziquantel is the drug of choice.

REFERENCES AND FURTHER READING

Griffin G. & Krishnas (1998) CME. Infectious diseases. *Journal of the Royal College of Physicians, London* 32 (3 & 4).

OkeKe In. & Nataro J.P. (2001) Enteroaggregative *E. coli*. *Lancet*: Infectious Diseases 1: 304–307.

WHO (1995) *The Treatment of Diarrhoea*. WHO/CDR/ 95.3. WHO, Geneva.

WHO (1995) *Control of Foodborne Trematode Infections*. WHO Technical Report Series No. 849. WHO, Geneva.

WHO (1996) *Report of the WHO Informal Consultation on the Use of Chemotherapy for the Control of Morbidity due to Soil-transmitted Nematodes and Helminths*. WHO/ CTD/SIP. 96.2. WHO, Geneva.

WHO (1998) *Guidelines for the Evaluation of Soil-transmitted Helminthiasis and Schistosomiasis at Community Level.* WHO/CTD/SIP/98.1. WHO, Geneva.

WHO (1999) *Report of the WHO Informal Consultation on Monitoring of Drug Efficiency in the Control of Schistosomiasis and Intestinal Nematodes.* WHO/CDS/ SIP. 99.1. WHO, Geneva.

WHO (1999) *WHO Recommended Surveillance Standards.* WHO/CDS/CSR/ISR/99.2. WHO, Geneva.

WHO (2000) *Overcoming Antimicrobial Resistance.* WHO/ CDS/ 2000.2. WHO, Geneva.

contd from page 65

Formulation of UNICEF reduced osmolarity Oral Rehydration Salts (ORS)
Each sachet contains the equivalent of:

	grams/litre		mmol/litre
Sodium chloride	2.6	Sodium	75
Glucose, anhydrous	13.5	Chloride	65
Potassium chloride	1.5	Glucose, anhydrous	75
Trisodium citrate, dihydrate	2.9	Potassium	20
		Citrate	10
		Total Osmolarity	245

± flavouring dissolved in one litre of drinking water.

CHAPTER FIVE

INFECTIONS THROUGH SKIN AND MUCOUS MEMBRANES

- The infective agents
- The eradication of smallpox
- Infections transmitted through human contact

- Infections acquired from non-human sources
- References and further reading

Infections transmitted through skin and mucous membranes may be divided into two groups:

- Transmission requires human contact either direct (person to person) or indirect (through fomites). These are often called 'contagious' diseases.
- Infection is acquired from various non-human sources: (i) infected soil (hookworm); (ii) water (schistosomiasis, leptospirosis); (iii) animal bites (rabies); or (iv) through wounds (tetanus).

THE INFECTIVE AGENTS

The agents include viruses, bacteria, fungi and arthropods, as listed in Table 5.1.

PHYSICAL AND BIOLOGICAL CHARACTERISTICS

Some of the agents that require direct person to person contact are notably delicate organisms which do not survive long outside the human host and cannot become established in any part of the environment outside the human body, either in an alternate host or in an inanimate object such as soil or water. The sexually transmitted diseases such as gonorrhoea and syphilis are the best examples of this group; the usual mode of infection is therefore through intimate contact, mucous membrane to mucous membrane, or skin to skin.

The infective agents that can survive in the environment for relatively longer periods may be spread indirectly through the contamination of soil and other inanimate objects.

In most of these infections humans are the sole reservoir of infection, although some of the superficial fungal infections may be acquired from lower animals.

TRANSMISSION

Infection by *direct contact* may result from touching an infected person; or more intimate contact through kissing and sexual intercourse may be required, especially in the case of sexually transmitted diseases.

Indirect contact through the handling of contaminated objects such as toys, handkerchiefs, soiled clothing, bedding or dressings may be sufficient for the transmission of some infections. High population density as in urban areas, overcrowding within households and poor environmental and personal hygiene facilitate the transmission of these infections.

Patterns of spread

A contact infection would tend to spread from an infected source to susceptible persons in the same household and to others who make contact at work and in other places. There is, therefore, a tendency

Table 5.1: The infective agents

HUMAN CONTACT

Viral infections
Chickenpox (varicella-zoster virus)
Viral haemorrhagic fevers (Lassa fever virus,
   Marburg virus, Ebola virus)
Acquired immune deficiency syndrome
   (Human immunodeficiency viruses)*

Protozoal infections
Trichomoniasis (*Trichomonas vaginalis*)*

Bacterial infections
Lymphogranuloma venereum
   (*Chlamydia trachomatis*, serotypes L1-3)*
Soft chancre (*Haemophilus ducrei*)*
Granuloma inguinale*
   (*Calymmatobacterium granulomatis*)
Gonorrhoea (*Neisseria gonorrhoeae*)*
Sexually transmitted syphilis*
   (*Treponema pallidum*)
Yaws (*Treponema pertenue*)
Pinta (*Treponema carateum*)
Endemic syphilis (*Treponema pallidum*)
Trachoma (*Chlamydia trachomatis*,
   serotypes A–C)
Inclusion conjunctivitis (*Chlamydia trachomatis*,
   serotypes D–K)
Leprosy (*Mycobacterium leprae*)

Fungal infections
Superficial fungal infections (*Epidermophyton* spp.,
   Trichophyton spp., *Microsporon* spp.,
   Mallassezia furfur)
Candidiasis (*Candida albicans*)

Arthropod infections
Scabies (*Sarcoptes scabei*)

OTHER SOURCES

Viral infection

Rabies (rabies virus)

Bacterial infections
Tetanus (*Clostridium tetani*)
Buruli ulcer (*Mycobacterium ulcerans*)
Leptospirosis (*Leptospira* spp.)
Anthrax (*Bacillus anthracis*)

Helminthic infections
Hookworm (*Ankylostoma duodenale*,
   Necator americanus)
Strongyloidiasis (*Strongyloides stercoralis*)
Schistosomiasis (*Schistosoma* spp.)

---

*Sexually transmitted infections.

for cases of contact infections to occur in clusters among household contacts, and within groups in children's nurseries, schools and factories. In the case of sexually transmitted diseases, the clustering occurs in relation to those who are in sexual contact.

Host factors

The behaviour of the human host is an important factor in the occurrence of certain contact infections. For example, a high level of personal cleanliness discourages the spread of some superficial infections. Age is another important factor, as for example in such infections as scabies and tinea capitis to which children are generally more susceptible than adults. The occurrence of sexually transmitted diseases is largely determined by the sexual behaviour of the host.

In some of the infections, for example measles, one attack confers lasting immunity but this is not a general rule for all the contact infections. Thus, repeated attacks of gonorrhoea may occur. The herd immunity that is derived from the high frequency of an endemic treponemal infection such as yaws may protect the community, though not the individual, from sexually transmitted syphilis.

Control of contact infections

1   The infective agent
    - elimination of the reservoir by case finding, selective or mass treatment.
2   The route of transmission
    - improvement of personal hygiene;
    - elimination of overcrowding;
    - avoidance of sexual promiscuity.
3   The host
    - specific immunization, e.g. tetanus;
    - chemotherapy and chemoprophylaxis, e.g. yaws.

THE ERADICATION OF SMALLPOX

In May 1980, the World Health Assembly formally declared the eradication of smallpox from the world. This unique achievement was the result of a global campaign, initiated and co-ordinated by the World Health Organization (WHO) in collaboration with national health authorities and governments. The final certification of eradication was based on a stage by stage, country by country, region by region examination of evidence which led to the final conclusion that the transmission of smallpox is no longer occurring in the world. This declaration was based on the following facts:

- no new cases reported for over 2 years;
- the dormant virus becomes uninfectious within 1 year;
- no animal reservoir;
- mutation of the virus is very unlikely.

VACCINATION POLICY

It is generally agreed that it is no longer desirable to vaccinate populations routinely against smallpox nor is it necessary for governments to require a certificate of smallpox vaccination from international travellers.

Laboratory stocks of variola virus

By international agreement, a few centres which provide adequate security against accidental infection have been designated for holding stocks of variola virus. The genomic structure of the virus has been determined. Using modern molecular biological methods, scientists are generating more detailed knowledge about the organism. The World Health Assembly passed a resolution (WHA 52.10) in 1999 extending the date of destruction of all remaining variola virus stocks until the end of 2002 to allow these studies to be completed.

Vaccine stocks

Even though most people are firmly convinced that smallpox has been eradicated, stocks of vaccine are still being held. This is a wise precaution in support of the policy of suspending routine vaccination. Furthermore, there is some concern that because populations are now not immunized, the variola virus may be a tempting candidate for biological warfare.

LESSONS LEARNED FROM THE ERADICATION OF SMALLPOX

Co-operation

First and foremost, this successful campaign illustrates the value of international collaboration. Governments throughout the world contributed to the success through generous donations in cash and in kind, through various forms of technical co-operation including the free exchange of information, and through the co-ordinating function of the WHO.

Technical improvement

Technical improvements in the vaccine (freeze drying) and in vaccination (the bifurcated needle), aided the eradication of smallpox.

Surveillance

More important than the technical advances was the development of a revised strategy for the application of these tools. At first, smallpox campaigns were largely based on repeated rounds of immunization of the population. In the course of the eradication programme, the importance of epidemiological surveillance was recognized. The systematic tracing of foci of infection through surveillance techniques proved to be a powerful measure in the campaign. The value of epidemiological surveillance is a most important lesson that has since been applied in the control of other communicable diseases.

INFECTIONS TRANSMITTED THROUGH HUMAN CONTACT

VIRAL INFECTIONS

Chickenpox

Occurrence:	Worldwide
Organism:	Varicella-zoster virus (VZV)
Reservoir:	Humans
Transmission:	Contact, droplets, fomites
Control:	Immunization of high-risk groups
	Notification

Chickenpox is an acute febrile illness with a characteristic skin rash. The incubation period is usually from 10 to 21 days. The aetiological agent is the varicella-zoster virus (VZV).

EPIDEMIOLOGY

Chickenpox is a common infection all over the world.

Reservoir and transmission

The reservoir of infection is exclusively human. Transmission is from person to person, either directly through contact with infectious secretions from the upper respiratory tract and through droplet infection or indirectly through contact with freshly soiled articles. The patient remains infectious 1–2 days before the rash appears and until all blisters have formed scabs.

Host factors

Host factors play an important part in determining the clinical manifestations of this infection. In most cases, it is a mild, self-limiting disease. It tends to be more severe in adults than in children. The overall case fatality rate is low, but it is high in cases complicated with primary viral pneumonia. Severe infections may occur in immunocompromised patients. One attack of chickenpox usually confers lifelong immunity; the patient may subsequently exhibit a recrudescence of infection in the form of herpes zoster from latent infection.

LABORATORY DIAGNOSIS

The organism may be cultured or identified immunologically from the early skin lesions or from throat washings. A rising titre of antibodies in acute and convalescent sera is also diagnostic.

CONTROL

The disease is usually notifiable, the main interest being in investigating cases and outbreaks to exclude smallpox. Infected persons may be isolated from other susceptibles. New antiviral agents, viradabine and acyclovir, are effective in the treatment of zoster and immunocompromised patients.

IMMUNIZATION

In some developed countries, a live attenuated varicella virus (Oka strain) vaccine is now available and is routinely offered to non-immune children 12 months to 12 years. High-risk groups including immunocompromised persons may be protected passively with varicella-zoster immunoglobulin made from plasma of healthy volunteer blood donors with high levels of antibody to VZV.

Viral haemorrhagic fevers

Several viral haemorrhagic fevers that affect humans are listed in Table 5.2. This section deals

Table 5.2: A classification of haemorrhagic fevers

Arenaviruses	Bunyaviruses	Filoviruses	Flaviviruses
Argentine haemorrhagic fever	Crimean–Congo haemorrhagic fever (CCHF)	Ebola haemorrhagic fever	Yellow fever
Bolivian haemorrhagic fever	Rift Valley fever	Marburg haemorrhagic fever	Kyasanur forest disease
Sabia-associated haemorrhagic fever	Hantavirus pulmonary syndrome (HPS)	Akhurma virus	Omsk haemorrhagic fever
Lassa fever	Haemorrhagic fever with renal syndrome (HFRS)		Tick-borne encephalitis
Lymphocytic choriomeningitis (LCM)			
Venezuelan haemorrhagic fever			

For the arbovirus infections see Chapter 7.

with Lassa fever, Marburg virus disease and Ebola virus disease. A common feature of these infections is that transmission requires intimate exposure to the patient or contact with blood or other bodily secretions.

PREVENTION OF TRANSMISSION IN HOSPITAL

Risk factors for nosocomial or person to person spread are:

- care of an infected individual;
- contact with infected needles;
- contact with blood or secretions;
- preparation of a body for burial;
- sexual contact.

Nosocomial infections have followed obstetric care, laparotomy, and resuscitation procedures. Patient management by barrier nursing techniques should be adopted rigorously to prevent nosocomial transmission. Ideally, patients should be managed at the hospital where they are first admitted, as they do not tolerate the stress of transfer well, and evacuation increases the potential for secondary transmission.

LASSA FEVER

Lassa fever is an acute febrile disease caused by a virus belonging to the arenavirus group. It was first described in the 1950s and the virus was isolated in 1969. Outbreaks of varying size and severity have occurred in Nigeria, Guinea, Liberia and Sierra Leone. Lassa virus has been isolated from blood, pharyngeal secretions and urine.

Reservoir and transmission

The multimammate rat, *Mastomys natalensis*, is the reservoir host of Lassa fever. The rodent virus is primarily transmitted to man by contamination of soil, food and other objects with their excreta. Person to person transmission occurs especially in the hospital environment, by direct contact with blood (e.g. contaminated needles), pharyngeal (throat) secretions or urine of a patient, or by sexual contact.

Host factors

No seasonal, yearly, sex or age pattern has been seen. In West Africa, there are an estimated 300 000–500 000 cases of Lassa fever each year, with a case fatality of 1–2%. Subclinical infections are, however, quite frequent and in some villages in West Africa as many as 50% of the population have antibody to Lassa fever virus (i.e. evidence of past infection). The disease is particularly severe in pregnant women.

Control

Patients suspected of Lassa fever should be isolated. High-risk contacts should be identified and kept under active surveillance. Postexposure prophylaxis with ribavirin is now recommended for persons known to have been exposed to Lassa virus (e.g. by needlestick injury). Strict barrier nursing procedures must be observed with hospitalized patients including the wearing of protective gear when taking specimens from the patient. Restriction of entry of rodents into homes, contamination of foods and other rodent-control measures may also be useful.

MARBURG VIRUS DISEASE

The first documented outbreak of Marburg virus disease occurred in 1967 in Marburg, West Germany and Belgrade, Yugoslavia. Contact with the blood, organs and cell cultures of imported African green monkeys was responsible for the epidemic. A total of 31 people were affected and seven died; all secondary cases survived. The disease appeared again in a young Australian man who was admitted to a Johannesburg hospital in February 1975 after having toured Rhodesia and Zambia. His female travelling companion and one female attendant nurse were also infected. The index case died, the other two survived. Two cases were reported from Kenya in 1980.

Although in the 1967 epidemic the immediate source of infection was the African green monkey no reservoir–host–vector chain has yet been consistently identified in nature. The incubation period is estimated to be between 3 and 9 days.

Control

- Barrier nursing of infected patient as for Lassa fever.

EBOLA VIRUS DISEASE

First recognized in 1976, sporadic outbreaks of Ebola haemorrhagic fever have been reported in humans from the Democratic Republic of the Congo, Gabon, Sudan, the Ivory Coast and Uganda and in non-human primates – monkeys and chimpanzees (USA). The causative agent is an RNA virus of the family Filoviridae, the same family as the Marburg virus. Three species of the virus have been associated with human disease: Ebola–Zaire, Ebola–Sudan, and Ebola–Ivory Coast. The fourth, Ebola–Reston, was responsible for an outbreak in non-human primates, but so far, not in humans.

Transmission

Humans can transmit the virus by direct contact with the blood or secretions of an infected person. It spreads through the families and friends who take care of infected persons. The fatality rate is high (between 30 and 50%) but subclinical infections do occur; thus 11% of case contacts in hospital and in the local community had antibodies to Ebola virus. No animal reservoir has yet been identified and the cycle of transmission is not known.

Control

Since the reservoir of infection is not known, there is no primary preventive intervention available. Precautions outlined for Lassa fever equally apply to Ebola but the latter does not respond to treatment with ribavirin.

SEXUALLY TRANSMITTED DISEASES

These are infections which are specifically transmitted during sexual intercourse. Although various other infections may be transmitted during sexual intercourse, the commonly recognized sexually transmitted diseases include:

1   Viral and rickettsial infections
    - HIV/AIDS;
    - herpes genitalis.
2   Bacterial infections
    - lymphogranuloma venereum;
    - soft chancre;
    - granuloma inguinale;
    - gonorrhoea;
    - sexually transmitted syphilis.
3   Protozoal infections
    - trichomoniasis.

Infective agents

The infective agents include viruses, bacteria and protozoa, but most of them share the characteristic of being delicate, being easily killed by drying or cooling below body temperature, and with the reservoir exclusively in man. Hence, transmission is mainly through direct close contact but rarely indirectly through fomites.

Transmission

Lesions are generally present on the genitalia, and the infective agents are also present in the secretions and discharges from the urethra and the vagina. Extragenital lesions may occur through haematogenic dissemination as in syphilis or through inoculation of the infective agent at extragenital sites. Transmission occurs through:

- genital contact;
- extragenital sexual contact, e.g. kissing;
- non-sexual transmission, e.g. mother to child transmission (MTCT) of HIV infection and syphilis, gonococcal ophthalmia neonatorum, or accidental contact as when doctors, dentists or midwives handle tissues infected with syphilis;
- fomites, e.g. soiled moist clothing such as wet towels, may transmit vulvovaginitis to prepubescent girls;
- blood and blood products, e.g. HIV infection.

It is not uncommon for patients to claim that they contracted the sexually transmitted infection through some indirect contact such as the lavatory seat; such a mechanism is extremely unlikely and the patient will usually admit to sexual exposure once confidence has been established.

Host factors

The most important host factor is sexual behaviour, the significant feature being sexual promiscuity. The transmission of a sexually transmitted disease almost always implies sexual activity involving at least three persons. For if A infects B, it implies that A has also had sexual contact with at least one other person X, who infected A. The highest frequency of sexually transmitted diseases occurs in those who are most active sexually, particularly those who indulge in promiscuous sexual behaviour – unprotected sex with multiple partners. Promiscuity before marriage and infidelity after marriage represent the major behavioural factors underlying the occurrence of sexually transmitted diseases. On the other hand, sexual abstinence and marital fidelity are protective. Young adult males away from home (sailors, soldiers, long-distance lorry drivers, migrant labourers, etc.) are often at high risk.

Cultural factors

Cultural attitudes to sex also play an important role. In some communities sexual matters are treated on a system of double standards in that whilst young unmarried girls are expected to remain chaste, young men are permitted or even encouraged to indulge in promiscuous sexual activities often with a small group of notorious women including commercial sex workers. Even after marriage, similar standards may apply: married women may be veiled, confined to special quarters in the household, or chaperoned on outings, but with little or no restrictions on the extramarital sexual activities of the male. In recent decades, a more permissive attitude to sexual relations has developed in some communities. There is increasing endorsement of recreational sex as a legitimate leisure activity and there is a tendency to regard all forms of sexual relations as being equally acceptable, regardless of the sex or the marital status of the partners.

Changing patterns of sexual behaviour

The pattern of sexual behaviour is undergoing major changes in developing countries as they evolve from rural traditional societies to modern urban industrial communities. There is also greater mobility from community to community, and easier communication through books, the cinema, television and the internet. The overall effect of these changes is to challenge and destabilize traditional values and customs, especially with regard to sexual behaviour. On the one hand, those who fear and respect sexual mores dictated by religious beliefs, strict parents, public opinion and the law, are less likely to indulge in promiscuous sexual behaviour than those who are no longer

bound by these considerations. The risk of unwanted pregnancy and of contracting sexually transmitted diseases also discourages sexual promiscuity. Self release through masturbation avoids these two risks. On the positive side, interest in work and absorbing leisure pursuits also tend to diminish promiscuity. The use of sex for gain encourages sexual promiscuity and increases the risk of spread of these infections.

Control

The general guidelines for the control of sexually transmitted diseases include action at the level of agent, transmission and host.

INFECTIVE AGENT

Eliminate the reservoir of infection

The reservoir is exclusively human; it includes untreated sick patients but for some infections, inapparent infection, especially in women, represents the most important part of the reservoir. The identification and treatment of the promiscuous female pool is of great importance: regular medical examination and treatment of known commercial sex workers, inhabitants of brothels, and other places where promiscuous sexual behaviour is known to occur. Such medical supervision of commercial sex workers cannot entirely eliminate the risk of infection.

For the control of HIV/AIDS, voluntary counselling and testing is used as a means of identifying infected persons who may be guided on how to prevent them from infecting others and they may be offered available antiretroviral chemotherapy.

TRANSMISSION

Discourage sexual promiscuity

Through sex education, make the community aware of the dangers of sexual promiscuity. One objective would be to influence young persons before their sexual habits become established. Promote abstinence as a desirable lifestyle for single persons or during temporary separations from spouses and regular partners. Encourage stable family life by providing married quarters in work camps, etc.

There are conflicting views about the best way to deal with the problem of prostitution in relation to sexually transmitted disease. At the one extreme it is suggested that prostitution is a social evil that should be totally abolished, if necessary, by imposing severe penalties. An alternative view holds that whilst it may be desirable to abolish prostitution, it is not feasible to do so, and that harsh laws merely drive the practice underground and discourage the commercial sex workers and their partners from seeking appropriate medical treatment. In place of clandestine prostitution, licensed brothels are allowed to operate under the close supervision of the health authorities. Neither method provides a satisfactory solution.

Local protection

The use of the male condom diminishes, but does not eliminate, the risk of infection. Female condoms have also been recently introduced and may similarly diminish the risk of acquiring sexually transmitted diseases.

It has also been suggested that careful toilet of the genitals with soap and antiseptic creams immediately after sexual exposure may give partial protection.

HOST

Specific prophylaxis

Specific immunization is not available against any of the sexually transmitted diseases. Although a measure of protection can be obtained by using antibiotic chemoprophylaxis, this approach can be dangerous for the individual and the community. Chemoprophylaxis may suppress the acute clinical manifestations but the disease may remain latent and progress silently to late complications. The widespread use of a particular antibiotic in subcurative doses may encourage the emergence and dissemination of drug-resistant strains.

Early diagnosis and treatment

Patients

This is one of the most important measures for the control of sexually transmitted diseases. Facilities for the diagnosis and treatment of those diseases must be freely accessible to all infected persons. Experience has shown that in order to reach the whole community everyone must have access to a free and confidential service.

Contacts

In addition to treating the patient, sexual contacts must be investigated and treated. In highly promiscuous groups where sexual activities occur in association with the use of alcohol or drugs, the details of the chain of transmission may be difficult to unravel. In such cases, one may use the technique of 'cluster tracing'. Apart from seeking a list of sexual exposures with dates, the patient is asked to name friends of both sexes whom he feels may profit from investigation for sexually transmitted diseases.

HIV infections and acquired immune deficiency syndrome (AIDS)

Occurrence:	Worldwide (high concentrations in Africa and other developing countries) (Plate 36)
Organism:	Human immunodeficiency viruses – different strains of HIV-1, HIV-2
Reservoir:	Humans
Transmission:	Sexual contact, blood transfusion, contaminated needles, perinatal infection
Control:	Education, safe blood supplies, counselling of patients, specific chemotherapy

During the past two decades, the world has been affected by the massive infection with the human immunodeficiency virus (HIV) which causes the clinical syndrome of acquired immune deficiency syndrome (AIDS). The aetiological agents of the disease are strains of two related retroviruses, human immunodeficiency viruses HIV-1 and HIV-2.

CLINICAL FEATURES (TABLE 5.3)

A few weeks after infection, some patients have a brief, self-limiting mononucleosis-type of illness in the course of which specific antibodies to the virus appear in the blood. Next follows a long period, usually lasting several years, during which

Table 5.3: The clinical spectrum of HIV infections

Stage	Disease	Clinical features
Initial	Acute infection	Mononucleosis-type illness Seroconversion
Intermediate	Asymptomatic infection AIDS-related complex (ARC)	None Fever, weight loss, persistent lymphadenopathy
Late	Full-blown AIDS	Opportunistic infections: ■ *Pneumocystis carinii pneumonia* ■ disseminated cytomegalovirus (CMV) infection ■ CNS toxoplasmosis ■ atypical mycobacterial infection ■ oesophageal candidiasis ■ cryptosporidium infection ■ herpes virus infection Secondary cancers: ■ Kaposi's sarcoma Neurological disease: ■ AIDS dementia complex

Table 5.4: Antiretroviral drugs

Reverse transcriptase inhibitors		Protease inhibitors
Nucleoside reverse transcriptase inhibitors (NRTIs)	**Non-nucleoside reverse transcriptase inhibitors (NNRTIs)**	
Zidovudine (AZT, ZDV) Didanosine (ddI) Zalcitabine (ddC) Stavudine (d4T) Lamivudine (3TC) Abacavir (ABC)	Nevirapine (NVP) Efavirenz (EFV) Delavirdine (DLV)	Saquinavir (SQV) Ritonavir (RTV) Indinavir (IDV) Nelfinavir (NFV) Amprenavir (APV) Lopinavir/ritonavir

the patient is asymptomatic but can transmit the infection to others. At this stage, a positive serological test is a marker of exposure to infection.

The full-blown clinical picture of AIDS is characterized by the occurrence of otherwise unexplained opportunistic infections (i.e. infections with organisms, normally benign in healthy individuals, but which cause severe pathology in persons whose immune systems are depressed), certain cancers (notably Kaposi's sarcoma), and neurological manifestations including dementia. An intermediate phase, the AIDS-related complex (ARC), includes fever, loss of weight and persistent lymphadenopathy. The immune deficiency in this disease results mainly from reduction in the number of T4 lymphocytes, the helper T cells. The T4 cell count has been used as an additional criterion for classifying the course of the infection.

There is much variation in the pace of progress of the disease and it is influenced by the coexistence of modifying factors.

ANTIRETROVIRAL CHEMOTHERAPY (TABLE 5.4)

Treatment with Zidovudine, the first specific drug for the treatment of HIV/AIDS, gave clear but limited benefits to patients with advanced disease and those who were immunocompromised. Newer drugs, reverse transcriptase and protease inhibitors, used in combination significantly reduce mortality and confer other clinical benefits, more substantial and more durable than monotherapy with AZT (see Table 5.4). It also significantly reduces the risk of vertical transmission from an infected pregnant woman to her child. In summary:

- ART using triple therapy is beneficial but the regimes are complex;
- ART has major side-effects; safe use of the drugs demands careful supervision and monitoring of patients;
- ART poses major problems in maintaining the compliance of patients;
- resistance to ART drugs is an important problem;
- currently available antiretroviral drugs cannot eradicate the virus from the host, but it significantly reduces the viral load in treated patients.

ART is indicated for patients with the acute HIV syndrome, those within 6 months of HIV seroconversion, for infected pregnant women and for patients who have symptoms ascribable to HIV infection. The indication for the treatment of asymptomatic patients is less clear-cut; it raises questions about compliance and the risk of selecting resistant strains of the virus.

The incubation period is long and variable and is currently estimated to be 2–10 years but may be longer.

VIROLOGY

Two retroviruses have been identified as the aetiological agents of AIDS. (A retrovirus is characterized by coding its genetic material in RNA instead of in DNA. Other retroviruses have been associated with immunodeficiency and cancers in animals.) Human immunodeficiency virus, HIV-1, formerly called the lymphadenopathy-associated virus (LAV) or the human T-lymphocyte virus type III was discovered in 1983. More recently, a new strain, HIV-2 was discovered in West Africa. HIV binds specifically to CD4 lymphocytes and eventually destroys them. The virus also invades other cells and lies dormant in them for long periods.

EPIDEMIOLOGY

HIV/AIDS has developed into a massive global pandemic (Plate 36). Sub-Saharan Africa is the most severely affected region with prevalence rates among adults in some communities of the

---

Box 5.1: Global statistics of HIV/AIDS

UNAIDS (the Joint United Nations Programme on HIV/AIDS) noted the following trends of HIV/AIDS as of the end of 2000:

- 36.1 million people are estimated to be living with HIV/AIDS. Of these, 34.7 million are adults; 16.4 million are women; and 1.4 million are children under 15 years.
- An estimated 21.8 million people have died from AIDS since the epidemic began; 17.5 million were adults, including 9 million women; 4.3 million were children under 15 years.
- During 2000, AIDS caused the deaths of an estimated 3 million people, including 1.3 million women and 500 000 children under 15 years.
- Women are becoming increasingly affected by HIV. Approximately 47%, or 16.4 million, of the 34.7 million adults living with HIV or AIDS worldwide are women.
- The overwhelming majority of people with HIV – approximately 95% of the global total – now live in the developing world.

---

order of 20–30%. As the epidemic evolves, foci of high prevalence are developing in Asia and other regions (Box 5.1).

Reservoir

The reservoir of infection is in human beings. Although there are related viruses in animals, there is no evidence of naturally occurring zoonotic infection. The infective agent is present in blood and is excreted in various body fluids (saliva, semen, breast milk) of infected persons even during the latent phase when the patient is asymptomatic.

Transmission

The best epidemiological evidence confirms that infection is not transmitted through casual contact in the household, office or school nor during other normal social activities. Biting insects do not seem to play a role in the transmission of the infection. Transmission occurs through the transfer of body fluids by four main routes:

Sexual

The disease was initially associated with male homosexual practices. Homosexual or bisexual men remain the predominant high-risk group in western Europe and North America where cases show a male/female ratio of 10 to 1. In Africa and in many other developing countries, however, heterosexual transmission is common and the infection occurs with equal frequency in men and women.

Perinatal infection

Children born to infected women acquire infection and progress to clinical disease. This mother to child transmission (MTCT) accounts for most of the cases in children less than 15 years. The United Nations agencies recommend a three-pronged strategy to prevent transmission of HIV to infants:

- primary prevention of HIV among parents-to-be;
- prevention of unwanted pregnancies among HIV-infected women;
- prevention of HIV transmission from HIV-infected women to their infants through the provision of antiretroviral drugs to HIV-infected pregnant women and their infants, safe delivery practices, and counselling and support for safer infant feeding practices.

Blood transfusion and tissue transplantation

Some patients, especially haemophiliacs, have acquired infection through receiving contaminated blood or blood products. The infection can also be transmitted by tissue transplantation.

Intravenous drug abusers

Drug addicts become infected by sharing unclean needles and other paraphernalia with infected persons.

Patterns of spread

There are two main epidemiological patterns of spread:

Pattern I

In western Europe, North America, Australia, New Zealand and most areas of South America, occurrence is mainly in homosexual/bisexual men and in intravenous drug abusers. Limited heterosexual transmission occurs mainly in the contacts of iv drug abusers. Transmission through blood transfusion has been virtually eliminated in developed countries by excluding high-risk donors and screening blood.

Pattern II

This is found in parts of Africa, the Caribbean, in Asia and some areas of South America. Transmission is mainly heterosexual. Both sexes are equally affected and perinatal transmission to the infant is a significant problem. Homosexual transmission is not a major factor but transfusion of contaminated blood remains a public health problem.

Host factors

Some host factors which facilitate infection have been identified, notably the presence of genital ulcers and co-infection with other sexually transmitted diseases. Cases of direct inoculation, as in blood transfusion, suggest that most persons are susceptible to infection and that once it is established, there will be progression to clinical disease and fatal outcome. However, there are interesting exceptions. For example, prospective study of commercial sex workers in Kenya led to the identification of individuals who, despite repeated exposure to unprotected sex, remained apparently uninfected. Immunological study of this refractory group indicated that they developed cytotoxic T lymphocytes (CTL) against epitopes not recognized by most infected people.

There is, as yet, no effective vaccine but there are promising leads and some candidate products are currently being evaluated.

HIV AND MALARIA

See page 204.

LABORATORY DIAGNOSIS

Antibody antigen detection

Serological tests are widely used to detect antibodies; they are simple to perform, sensitive and specific at most stages of the infection, and relatively inexpensive. The presence of the specific antibody to HIV-1 or HIV-2 is confirmation of exposure to the infection. ELISA tests are commonly used for screening sera and more specific tests (e.g. Western blot technique) for confirmation. Some rapid screening tests including home collection kits have been developed but these require confirmation by formal laboratory tests. The antibody tests are negative in the early stages of the infection but infection can be diagnosed by detecting HIV RNA in blood samples. The HIV RNA test is used to measure the viral load, usually stated as the number of HIV RNA copies in 1 ml of plasma. Together with monitoring of the CD4 lymphocyte count, it helps predict the clinical status of the patient and progression of the disease. The viral load is also used to measure the response of the patient to antiretroviral therapy.

Blood cell count

As infection progresses, there is a fall in the blood count of the CD4 lymphocytes from the normal level of about $800/mm^3$. When the CD4 count falls below $200/mm^3$, the patient becomes vulnerable to tuberculosis and a variety of opportunistic infections such as *Pneumocystis carinii*, *Cryptococcus neoformans*, *Histoplasma neoformans*, *Coccidioides immitis* and *Aspergillus* spp.

Delayed hypersensitivity reaction

Defects in the delayed hypersensitivity reaction occur in the later stages of the disease.

Associated disorders

Laboratory tests are used to identify opportunistic infections which affect these patients, to diagnose Kaposi's sarcoma and to evaluate the neurological damage.

CONTROL

The most logical approach to the control of the infection is to reduce transmission whilst providing humane care for patients. The role of chemotherapy in the control of the disease is expanding but it is limited in developing countries because of the high cost of the drugs and the complexity of the schedules as well as the demanding close monitoring of the patients. The most important tool is modification of human behaviour through education directed at each of the four modes of transmission:

Sexual behaviour

Avoidance of exposure

Ideally, sexual activities should be confined to persons who are in permanent monogamous relationships – one man, one wife, for life.

Reducing the risk of infection

Whenever sexual activity does not conform to the ideal, measures should be taken to reduce the risk of infection, for example by the use of male or female condoms. Such measures do not assure absolute protection.

Perinatal infection

Infected women of childbearing age should be counselled on avoidance of pregnancy through the use of contraceptives. There is a clear indication for using antiretroviral therapy, either the protocols based on triple therapy or the more affordable treatment based on nevirapine. One difficult issue is the feeding of the baby. Breast-feeding significantly increases the risk of mother to child transmission. Current recommendations are summarized in Box 5.2.

Box 5.2: Recommendations about breast-feeding by HIV-positive mothers

- Exclusive breast-feeding should be protected, promoted and supported for 6 months. This applies to women who are known not to be infected with HIV and for women whose infection status is unknown.
- When replacement feeding is acceptable, feasible, affordable, sustainable and safe, avoidance of all breast-feeding by HIV-infected mothers is recommended; otherwise, exclusive breast-feeding is recommended during the first months of life.
- To minimize HIV transmission risk, breast-feeding should be discontinued as soon as feasible, taking into account local circumstances, the individual woman's situation and the risks of replacement feeding (including infections other than HIV and malnutrition).
- HIV-infected women should have access to information, follow-up clinical care and support, including family planning services and nutritional support.

Blood transfusion

Donors who belong to high-risk groups and their sexual partners should be excluded. Donated blood should be screened to avoid transfusing infected specimens.

Contaminated needles and other equipment

Great care should be exercised in handling blood and other human specimens which are potentially infected. Instruments should be carefully disinfected and whenever feasible disposable needles and syringes should be used. Intensive education should be given to drug abusers to avoid the sharing of contaminated needles. If economically possible, free needles should be provided.

PRACTICAL PROGRAMMES

These theoretical considerations have to be translated into practical programmes. Many countries have set up national programmes for the control of the disease.

Surveillance

The HIV/AIDS control programme should be based on a good surveillance system for collecting and analysing relevant data about:

- the prevalence and the distribution of the infection;
- the high-risk groups;
- patterns of behaviour, especially sexual activities;
- the state of knowledge of the population about AIDS and other sexually transmitted infections;
- community attitudes to AIDS and the patients.

Serological surveys should be used to gather information about the distribution of latent infection.

Education

A strategy should be developed to educate the public about 'safe sex', promoting abstinence in young persons and stable monogamous relationships among adults but advising the use of the condom where people deviate from the ideal. Major efforts should be made to reduce the use of blood transfusion to the absolute minimum and to ensure that all transfused products are safe. In developed countries some patients store some of their own blood for use during planned surgery or childbirth, but most developing countries do not have the appropriate infrastructure to use this approach. Programmes for the control of drug abuse should be intensified.

Public education should seek to replace irrational fears with sound knowledge about the infection. Patients should be sympathetically counselled and protected from unfair discrimination.

A multisectoral approach to control

Although the health sector must play a leading role in tackling the HIV/AIDS epidemic, national programmes should involve other sectors. Table 5.5 summarizes major elements in the control of HIV/AIDS.

PROTOZOAL INFECTION

Trichomoniasis

Occurrence:	Worldwide
Organism:	Trichomonas vaginalis
Reservoir:	Humans
Transmission:	Sexual contact, indirect contact through fomites
Control:	As for other sexually transmitted diseases
	Improvement in general hygiene

This is a chronic infection of the genital tract of both sexes. In the female it presents with vaginitis accompanied by copious discharge; in the male, with urethritis.

The incubation period is from 1 to 3 weeks.

PARASITOLOGY

The causative agent is *Trichomonas vaginalis*, a protozoan flagellate.

LABORATORY DIAGNOSIS

Microscopy of wet film preparation of vaginal or urethral discharge may show the motile organism. The organism can also be identified in stained smears.

EPIDEMIOLOGY

Trichomoniasis has a worldwide distribution.

The reservoir of infection is exclusively in humans, the infected genital discharges being the

Table 5.5: Major elements in national programmes for the control of HIV/AIDS

Item	Comment
Health education	■ Promote community wide awareness of the problem of HIV/AIDS ■ Inform people how they can protect themselves against infection with emphasis on sexual abstinence and monogamous relationships ■ Promote safe sex including the use of male and female condoms ■ Promote safer habits among illegal drug users
Control sexually transmitted diseases	■ Promote safe sexual habits (see above) ■ Ensure access to inexpensive condoms ■ Prompt diagnosis and treatment of other sexually transmitted diseases
Establish and manage surveillance programme	■ Promote voluntary counselling and testing ■ Collate and analyse data from sentinel sites and groups to determine trends ■ Identify high-risk groups including commercial sex workers
Prevent mother to child transmission	■ General prevention of HIV infections ■ Voluntary screening of pregnant women ■ Prevent unwanted pregnancies in infected persons ■ Use antiretroviral therapy to protect the child and care for the mother
Provide and manage antiretroviral therapy	■ Give high priority to treatment of pregnant woman and her child ■ Define feasible chemotherapeutic programme in view of the complexity of the schedules, the need for close monitoring of patients including laboratory support, and the high cost of drugs

source of infection. Transmission is by sexual intercourse or by indirect contact through contaminated clothing and other articles. Clinical manifestations occur more frequently in males than in females. The flagellate is commonly found in women during the reproductive period, and vaginal infection may be associated with lowered vaginal acidity.

CONTROL

Although the general principles for the control of sexually transmitted diseases apply, the main approach is the treatment of infected persons and their sexual partners. Improvement in personal hygiene is also important.

BACTERIAL INFECTIONS

Lymphogranuloma venereum

Occurrence:	Tropics and subtropics mainly
Organism:	*Chlamydia trachomatis* (serotypes L1–3)
Reservoir:	Humans
Transmission:	Genital sexual contact, indirect contact

Control:	As for other sexually transmitted diseases Sulphonamides and broad-spectrum antibiotics

This is a chronic infection of the genitals which spreads to involve regional lymph nodes and the rectum. Typically it produces ulcerative lesions on the genitalia with induration of the regional lymph nodes ('climatic bubo'). Anal and genital strictures may occur at a late stage; so also may elephantiasis of the vulva. Extragenital lesions and general dissemination occasionally occur.

VIROLOGY

Lymphogranuloma venereum (LGV) is one of a range of diseases caused by *Chlamydia trachomatis* (see p. 122). Unlike trachoma and inclusion conjunctivitis (see p. 122) the serotypes of Ll, L2 and L3 cause systemic disease rather than being restricted to the mucous membrane surfaces.

LABORATORY DIAGNOSIS

Stained smears of pus and other pathological material may show virus particles. The organism can be identified on culture in the yolk sacs of embryo-nated eggs. Serological tests become positive some 2–4 weeks after the onset of the illness. A skin test, the Frei test, is available, but cross-reactions with other viral infections of the psittacosis group may occur depending on the purity of the antigen. It tends to remain positive for long periods.

EPIDEMIOLOGY

The infection is endemic in many parts of the trop-ics and subtropics.

Reservoir and transmission

The reservoir of infection is in humans, the source being the open lesions in patients with active dis-ease. Transmission is mainly by sexual contact but also by indirect contact through contaminated clothing and other fomites.

Host factors

As with other sexually transmitted diseases, the sexual behaviour of the host is a major factor deter-mining the distribution and spread of this infec-tion. Recovery from a clinical attack does not confer immunity.

CONTROL

The main principles are as for other sexually transmitted diseases. The early stages of infection respond to antibiotics including doxycycline, eryth-romycin and tetracycline.

Soft chancre (chancroid)

Occurrence:	Tropics, especially seaports
Organism:	Haemophilus ducreyi
Reservoir:	Humans
Transmission:	Sexual contact, accidental infection through non-sexual contact
Control:	As for other sexually transmitted diseases Chemotherapy with antibiotics

This is an acute sexually transmitted infection which typically presents as a ragged painful ulcer on the genitalia (known as soft chancre in contrast to the hard chancre of syphilis). The inguinal lymph nodes become enlarged and may suppurate (buboes). Extragenital lesions may be found on the abdomen, fingers or other sites.

The incubation period is usually from 3 to 5 days but it may be very short (24 hours) where the lesion affects mucous membranes.

BACTERIOLOGY

The causative agent is *Haemophilus ducreyi*, a Gram-negative non-sporing bacillus.

EPIDEMIOLOGY

The infection occurs in many parts of the world, especially in tropical seaports.

Reservoir

The reservoir of infection is in human beings. The open lesions are the most important source of infection.

Transmission

Sexual contact is the usual mode of transmission but extragenital lesions may occur from non-sexual infection of children or accidental infection of doctors, nurses or other medical personnel who come into contact with infected lesions.

LABORATORY DIAGNOSIS

Microscopy of the stained smear of the exudate from ulcers or pus from the regional lymph nodes may show a mixed flora including Gram-negative bacilli. The organism can be isolated on culture of pus from the ulcer or bubo. An intradermal skin test is available but it does not differentiate active infections from previous attacks. Biopsy of the regional lymph nodes may also provide useful information.

CONTROL

The general measures for the control of sexually transmitted diseases apply to the problem of chan-croid. Active infections usually respond to treat-ment with antibiotics.

Granuloma inguinale

Distribution:	Tropics and subtropics
Organism:	Calymmatobacterium granulomatis
Reservoir:	Humans
Transmission:	Contact, including sexual contact
Control:	General hygienic measures as for other sexually transmitted diseases

This is a chronic infection which presents with granulomatous lesions of the genitalia; regional lymph nodes may be affected and metastatic lesions occur. The incubation period is 1 week to 3 months.

ORGANISM

The aetiological agent is *Calymmatobacterium granulomatis* (formerly *Donovania granulomatis*).

EPIDEMIOLOGY

The infection occurs in various parts of the tropics and subtropics, particularly in poorer communities. The reservoir of infection is in human beings. Transmission may be by sexual contact, but transmission through non-sexual contact also occurs.

LABORATORY DIAGNOSIS

Stained smears from active lesions show the typical Donovan bodies. A skin test is available and the complement fixation test can also be used in diagnosis.

CONTROL

General hygienic measures are important. Known cases should be treated with antibiotics (streptomycin, tetracycline, chloramphenicol or erythromycin). Contacts should be examined and treated if indicated.

Gonorrhoea

Occurrence:	Worldwide
Organism:	Neisseria gonorrhoeae
Reservoir:	Humans
Transmission:	Sexual contact, rarely through fomites
	Eye infection during delivery
Control:	As for other sexually transmitted diseases
	Toilet to the eyes of newborn babies

In the male, this disease usually presents as an acute purulent urethritis with spread in some cases to involve the epididymis and testis. Late complications include urethral stricture, urethral sinuses and subfertility.

A high proportion (80–90%) of infected females are unaware of the infection; the others present with symptoms of urethritis and urethral or vaginal discharge. Complications in the female include bartholinitis, salpingitis, pyosalpinx and pelvic inflammatory disease. Late complications include subfertility resulting from tubal obstruction.

The incubation period is usually between 2 and 5 days, occasionally shorter (1 day), but may be as long as 2 weeks. It is usually notifiable nationally.

BACTERIOLOGY

Neisseria gonorrhoea is a Gram-negative diplococcus, with a characteristic bean shape. It dies rapidly outside the human body, being susceptible to drying and heat.

EPIDEMIOLOGY

The distribution is worldwide with particular concentrations at seaports, and in areas having a high concentration of migrant labour or military personnel.

Reservoir

The reservoir of infection is in human beings; the most important component is the female pool with asymptomatic infection.

Transmission

Transmission of the infection is mostly by:

Sexual genital contact

- *Indirect contamination* This may produce infection in prepubertal females. Vulvovaginitis may occur in a young girl who is infected by sharing towels or other clothing with an infected older relative. Postpubertal girls do not become infected in this way; some cases of vulvovaginitis in young girls are the result of sexual contact with infected males.

- *Ophthalmia neonatorum* This infection occurs in the course of delivering the baby of an infected mother.

Host factors

All persons are susceptible. There is no lasting immunity after recovery: repeated infections are common. As with other sexually transmitted diseases, the most important host factor is sexual behaviour.

LABORATORY DIAGNOSIS

Clinical diagnosis can be confirmed by bacteriological examination of stained smears of urethral discharge, cervical discharge or other infected material: the characteristic diplococci, some within pus cells, can be seen. The organisms can also be cultured on chocolate agar as a form of enrichment medium or on selective media such as the Thayer–Martin medium which contains antibiotics which suppress the growth of other organisms. Fluorescent antibody techniques are also available for diagnosis.

CONTROL

The control of gonorrhoea is posing a difficult problem in most parts of the world. Various factors have contributed to this difficulty:

- revolutionary change in sexual mores;
- replacement of the condom by effective contraceptive techniques which do not provide a mechanical barrier to infection;
- emergence of drug resistant strains (Plate 37).

The control of gonorrhoea is based on the principles set out in the section on sexually transmitted diseases. Gonococcal ophthalmitis can be prevented by treating all infected pregnant women and by toilet to the eyes of all newborn babies. The latter consists of instilling one drop of 1% silver nitrate into the eyes of every newborn baby. Alternatively, tetracycline ointment may be used with the added advantage of protection against chlamydial infection.

Table 5.6: The trepanomatoses

Venereal	
Sexually transmitted syphilis	*Treponema pallidum*
Non-venereal	
Yaws	*Treponema pertenue*
Pinta	*Treponema carateum*
Non-sexually transmitted syphilis	*Treponema pallidum*

Treponematoses

The treponematoses are diseases caused by spirochaetes which belong to the genus *Treponemata*. The most important diseases in this group, both sexually transmitted and non-venereal, are shown in Table 5.6.

There has been much speculation about the origin and differentiation of these organisms. One view regards the organisms as being virtually identical but apparent differences in clinical manifestations result from epidemiological factors; the other view regards the organisms as separate but related entities. In practical terms, the pattern of treponemal diseases is still evolving with the elimination of the non-sexually transmitted treponematoses from endemic areas and with the rise in the frequency of sexually transmitted syphilis in some areas where the disease was previously not recognized as an important public health problem.

SEXUALLY TRANSMITTED SYPHILIS

Occurrence:	Worldwide
Organism:	*Treponema pallidum*
Reservoir:	Humans
Transmission:	Sexual contact, non-sexual contact, transplacental
Control:	Education
	Control of sexual promiscuity
	Early detection and treatment of infected persons, including serological screening

This is a chronic infection which is characterized clinically by a localized primary lesion, a generalized secondary eruption involving the skin and mucous membranes, and a later tertiary stage with involvement of skin, bone, abdominal viscera, cardiovascular and central nervous systems.

The incubation period is usually 2–4 weeks but may be from 9 to 90 days. The primary lesion is usually a painless sore associated with firm enlarged regional lymph nodes. The initial lesion tends to heal spontaneously after a few weeks. Six weeks to 6 months or even a year later, secondary lesions appear usually as a generalized non-itchy, painless and non-tender rash, shallow ulcers on the oral mucosa, widespread lymphadenopathy and mild systemic disturbance, including fever. These manifestations regress spontaneously and the infection enters a latent phase which may last for 10 years or more before the tertiary lesions appear, although spontaneous healing may occur during the latent stage.

Bacteriology

The spirochaete *Treponema pallidum* is a thin organism, 1–15 μm long with tapering ends; there are about 5–20 spirals. Fresh preparations under darkground illumination show its characteristic motility. The organism is delicate, being rapidly killed by drying, high temperatures (50°C), disinfectants such as phenolic compounds, and by soap and water. It may survive in refrigerated blood for 3 days and may remain viable for several years if frozen below $-78°C$.

Epidemiology

Although sexually transmitted syphilis was previously unknown or was not recognized in some parts of the world, its distribution is now virtually worldwide.

Reservoir

The reservoir of infection is human, the sources of infection being moist lesions on the skin and mucosae, and also tissue fluids and secretions such as saliva, semen, vaginal discharge and blood.

Transmission

Transmission is mainly sexual, through genital or extragenital contact, but it may be non-venereal.

Sexual transmission Genital contact may lead to infection, the organisms penetrating normal skin and mucous membranes. In the male, the infection may be quite obvious in the form of a primary chancre on the penis but the infective female may be unaware of a similar lesion on her cervix. Inapparent infection in the female, especially the promiscuous female, is an important source of infection.

Infection may also be transmitted during sexual play from extragenital sites such as the mouth during kissing; the infected partner may develop primary lesions on the lips, tongue or breast.

Non-sexual transmission This may be accidental, through touching infected tissues as in the case of dentists or midwives.

Congenital infection may occur in a child who is born to an infected mother, even though the mother is at a latent phase. Intrauterine syphilitic infection may be associated with repeated abortions, stillbirths, or congenital infection in a live child. Lesions may be present at birth, but more commonly clinical signs appear later.

Host factors

The most important host factor in the epidemiology of syphilis is sexual behaviour, a high frequency of infection being associated with sexual promiscuity. A current infection with syphilis may provide some immunity, but if super-infection occurs, the clinical manifestations may be modified. There is some degree of cross-immunity to syphilis in persons infected with the other non-sexually transmitted treponematoses but such immunity is not absolute.

Laboratory diagnosis

Dark-field microscopy

Examination of exudates from primary and secondary lesions under a dark-ground microscope usually reveals the characteristic shape and movements of the spirochaete.

Serological tests

Blood and cerebrospinal fluid may be tested for syphilis using a variety of serological tests. They fall into two main groups:

Non-treponemal antigen These tests are based on the presence of the antibody complex (reagin) in syphilitic infections. This complex may be detected by using a flocculation test, for example VDRL, slide test, Kahn test, Mazzine cardiolipin, or Kline cardiolipin. Alternatively, a complement-fixation

Table 5.7: Diseases associated with false-positive reactions in serological tests for syphilis

Spirochaetal	Leptospirosis
	Relapsing fever
Protozoal	Malaria
	Trypanosomiasis
Bacterial	Leprosy
	Tuberculosis
Viral	Atypical pneumonia
	Glandular fever
	Lymphogranuloma venereum
Other	Collagen vascular disease
	Vaccination for smallpox,
	yellow fever

test may be used, for example Kolmer test. These non-specific tests are prone to false-positive reactions associated with certain diseases (Table 5.7).

Treponemal antigen tests These include the *Treponema pallidum* immobilization test (TPI), fluorescent treponemal antibody (FTA) and the reiter protein complement-fixation test (RPCFT). These tests specifically detect antitreponemal antibody and are therefore less likely to give false-positive reactions.

Neither type of test can differentiate syphilis from other treponemal infections. A positive serological test therefore indicates the probable presence of a specific treponemal infection, the nature of which can be determined on clinical and circumstantial evidence.

Serological tests usually become positive 1–2 weeks after the appearance of the primary lesions, and are almost invariably positive during the secondary stage of the illness but may later become negative spontaneously or after successful chemotherapy at any stage.

Control

The general principles for the control of sexually transmitted diseases apply to the control of syphilis.

General health promotion Through health and sex education make the population aware of the danger of promiscuous sexual activity. Young persons especially should be encouraged to take up diversional activities in the form of games, hobbies and other absorbing interests. Although the provision of good recreational facilities is highly desirable, it cannot by itself produce a significant change in sexual habits.

Control of commercial sex and promiscuous sexual behaviour The role of commercial sex workers in the transmission of syphilis varies from community to community. In some societies, professional commercial sex workers make a major contribution but, in others, much of the transmission results from promiscuous behaviour not involving immediate financial gain.

As for other sexually transmitted diseases, modification of sexual behaviour is an important goal of public health action.

Early diagnosis and treatment Serology plays an important role in the detection of cases of syphilis, especially in the latent phase. Whenever feasible, there should be routine serological screening of pregnant women, blood donors, those who are about to get married, immigrants, hospital patients, prisoners and other groups. Where there is a high probability that a person has been infected, such as the contact of a patient with open lesions, epidemiological treatment (i.e. treatment on the basis of presumptive diagnosis) should be given. Penicillin is the drug of choice: given early and in appropriate doses, syphilitic infection can be eradicated. Other antibiotics (e.g. erythromycin, tetracyclines) may be used if the patient is allergic to penicillin. There is, as yet, no effective artificial immunization against syphilis.

YAWS

Occurrence:	Tropics and subtropics. Now well controlled or eradicated from most areas
Organism:	*Treponema pertenue*
Reservoir:	Humans
Transmission:	Direct contact
Control:	Mass survey and chemotherapy Improvement of personal hygiene

This non-sexually transmitted treponemal infection mainly affects skin and bones, rarely if ever affecting the cardiovascular or the nervous system. The skin lesions may be granulomatous, ulcerative or hypertrophic, destructive lesions of bone and hypertrophic changes are late lesions of bone.

The incubation period is usually about 1 month, varying from 2 weeks to 3 months.

Bacteriology

The infective agent, *Treponema pertenue*, cannot be distinguished from *T. pallidum* on microscopy (light, phase-contrast or electron).

Epidemiology

The disease was highly endemic in many parts of the tropics and subtropical zones of Africa, South East Asia, the Pacific, the Caribbean and Central and South America. There has been a marked fall in the incidence of the disease, but constant surveillance is required to detect resurgence and institute prompt and energetic treatment.

Reservoir and transmission

The reservoir of infection is in human beings, the source of infection being the often moist skin lesions in the early phase of the disease. Transmission is mainly by direct contact, but flies, especially *Hippelates pallipes*, may carry the infection from a skin lesion to a susceptible host. Transplacental transmission does not occur.

Host factors

Most early cases are seen in children under 15 years. The disease occurs predominantly in rural communities where there is the combination of poverty, low level of personal hygiene, warm humid climate, and where children, especially, usually wear little clothing.

Laboratory diagnosis

Dark-field microscopy

Exudates from moist lesions will reveal the spirochaete which is morphologically indistinguishable from *T. pallidum*.

Serological tests

Blood serology becomes positive at an early stage of the infection, but tends to become negative when the disease has been latent for several years. None of the serological tests can differentiate syphilis from other treponemal infections.

Control

Yaws has been successfully controlled and virtually eliminated from some parts of the world where it had been highly endemic. The successful programme, backed by the World Health Organization, consisted of:

- an epidemiological survey by clinical examination of the entire population;
- mass chemotherapy – patients including those with latent infection and contacts were treated with a single intramuscular injection of long acting penicillin in oil with 2% aluminium monostearate (PAM);
- surveillance – periodic clinical and serological surveys.

Apart from such specific campaigns, general improvement in personal hygiene and in the level of living standards has contributed greatly to the disappearance of the disease.

PINTA

Occurrence:	Tropics and subtropics (America, Africa, Middle East, India, Philippines)
Organism:	*Treponema carateum*
Reservoir:	Humans
Transmission:	Direct and indirect contact
Control:	As for yaws

This is a spirochaetal infection which initially presents as a superficial non-ulcerating papule. Later flat, hyperpigmented skin lesions develop, and these may become depigmented and hyperkeratotic.

The incubation period is from 7 to 20 days.

Bacteriology

The infective agent is *Treponema carateum*, a spirochaete which is morphologically indistinguishable from *T. pallidum*.

Epidemiology

Pinta occurs predominantly in the dark-skinned people of Mexico, Central and South America, North Africa, Middle East, India, the Philippines and some areas in the Pacific.

Reservoir

The reservoir of infection is in human beings; the patients with early active lesions are the sources of infection.

Transmission

Transmission is mainly from direct non-sexually transmitted contact, or through indirect contact. It has been suggested that certain biting insects play a role but this is not proven.

Host factors

Infection is commoner in children than in adults. There is some cross-immunity with syphilis and other treponemal infections but protection is partial and syphilis may coexist with pinta.

Control

■ As for yaws.

ENDEMIC (NON-VENEREAL) SYPHILIS

Distribution:	Tropical Africa, Middle and Near East, southern Europe
Organism:	Treponema pallidum
Reservoir:	Humans
Transmission:	Direct and indirect contact
Control:	Mass survey and chemotherapy with penicillin
	Improvement in personal hygiene

This refers to a manifestation of infection with *Treponema pallidum* in an epidemiological situation in which the infection is highly endemic with non-sexually transmitted transmission occurring predominantly in young persons.

A primary chancre is not commonly encountered and it is mainly extragenital. In the secondary stage, mucosal lesions (mucous patches) occur in the mouth, tongue, larynx and nostrils. Condylomata lata are also found in the moist areas: anogenital area, groins, axillae, below the breasts and the angles of the mouth. A variety of other skin lesions may also be present at this stage. Late lesions include skin gummata, nasopharyngeal ulceration, and bone lesions (osteitis, gummata). Cardiovascular and neurological involvement may occur but are apparently rare. Congenital infection is also rare.

The incubation period is 2 weeks to 3 months.

Bacteriology

The causative organism, *T. pallidum*, is indistinguishable from the aetiological agent of sexually transmitted syphilis.

Epidemiology

The infection is found in remote rural areas in parts of tropical Africa, the Middle and Near East, and southern Europe. It has virtually been eliminated from most of these areas where it was formerly endemic.

Reservoir and transmission

The reservoir of infection is in humans. Transmission is by close person to person contact; indirect transmission may occur through sharing pipes, cups and other utensils.

Host factors

The distribution of the disease is associated with poverty, overcrowding and poor personal hygiene. Early infections occur predominantly in childhood. With improvement in social conditions, the endemic syphilis recedes, few children become infected but adults acquire venereally transmitted syphilis.

Laboratory diagnosis

The organism can be seen under dark-field microscopy from wet lesions such as mucous patches and condylomata. Serology becomes positive by the time that secondary lesions occur.

Control

■ As for yaws.

Chlamydial infections

The spectrum of clinically distinct diseases produced by infection with the different serotypes of *Chlamydia trachomatis* is summarized in Table 5.8. They include lymphogranuloma venereum (LGV – see p. 115), trachoma and inclusion conjunctivitis (TRIC) agents and also the strains involved in various genital tract infections. With the exception of lymphogranuloma venereum strains which have a predilection for lymph nodes, *Chlamydia trachomatis* only grows in the columnar epithelial cells found in the conjunctiva, cervix, urethra, the respiratory and gastrointestinal tracts and the rectal mucosa. This is reflected in the spectrum of diseases that they cause.

The members of this species are natural parasites of man only in contrast to the other species of chlamydia, *Chl. psittacii*, which is primarily a pathogen of birds, only occasionally infecting man.

Table 5.8: Serotypes and diseases of *Chlamydia trachomatis*

Serotypes	Diseases
A, B, C	Trachoma*
D-K	Inclusion conjunctivitis*
	Non-gonococcal urethritis
	Post-gonococcal urethritis
	Epididymitis in adults
	Proctitis
	Cervicitis
	Salpingitis
	Perihepatitis
	Inclusion conjunctivitis
	Pneumonia in neonates
	Otitis media
L1, L2, L3	Lymphogranuloma venereum*

*Described in this chapter.

TRACHOMA

Occurrence:	Worldwide, uneven distribution, mainly tropical and subtropical
Organism:	*Chlamydia trachomatis* (serotypes A, B, C)
Reservoir:	Humans
Transmission:	Contact, fomites, mechanically by flies
Control:	'SAFE' strategy: **S**urgery, **A**ntibiotics, **F**ace Washing and **E**nvironmental measures

Trachoma is a major cause of blindness in the tropics and is characterized by a mucopurulent discharge initially progressing to a chronic keratoconjunctivitis, with the formation of follicles, with hyperplasia, vascular invasion of the cornea and, in the late stage, gross scarring with deformity of the eyelids. Vision may be impaired, and in severe cases it may lead to blindness.

According to WHO's estimates, trachoma is responsible for at least 15% of the world's blindness, 6 million people irreversibly blinded by the disease and about 150 million active cases in need of treatment to prevent blindness.

The incubation period is from 4 to 12 days.

Bacteriology

The organism responsible for trachoma *Chlamydia trachomatis* is also termed the TRIC agent (trachoma inclusion conjunctivitis agent). It was first isolated with certainty in Peking and confirmed in the Gambia. Trachoma is caused by serotypes A, B and C.

Epidemiology

The occurrence of the infection is worldwide, including tropical, subtropical, temperate and cold climates, but the distribution of disease is uneven, being mostly in the Middle East, Mediterranean coast, parts of tropical Africa, Asia and South America (Plate 38). In the USA, it selectively affects certain groups such as American Indians and Mexican immigrants. It is estimated that throughout the world 300 million persons are infected with trachoma and 20 million are blind.

Reservoir and transmission

The reservoir of infection is in human beings. The common mode of transmission is mechanical from eye to eye by contaminated fingers, cloths, towels, bed clothes and flies (particularly *Musca sorbers*). Infected nasal discharge and tears can also be agents of transmission. The more severe the infection the greater is the degree of virus shedding.

Host factors

In most areas of the world infection occurs in children under 10 years of age. It is particularly common where there is poor personal hygiene; exposure to sun, wind and sand may aggravate the clinical manifestations.

Immunity to trachoma is only partial and non-protective. Cell-mediated immunity develops eventually, leading to hypersensitivity which is responsible for the blinding complications of trachoma. The disease traces a variable course with spontaneous healing in some cases or progressive damage in others. In countries with a high incidence of bacterial conjunctivitis, particularly of the seasonal epidemic variety, the severity of the trachoma is increased and disabling complications are more frequent. In other areas the disease is mild, and serious sequelae are uncommon.

Laboratory diagnosis

Intracytoplasmic inclusion bodies 0.25–0.04 μm in diameter, staining purple with Giemsa or reddish brown by iodine, may be seen in conjunctival scrapings. These elementary particles have been termed Halberstaedter–Prowazek bodies and are the principal microscopic diagnostic feature in trachoma but are also seen in inclusion conjunctivitis of the newborn. The number of inclusions tends to be proportional to the intensity of the infection and are most numerous in scrapings from the upper lid.

In early lesions neutrophils may be abundant. In later lesions plasma cells, lymphoblasts and macrophages containing necrotic debris (Leber cells) may be seen.

The agent may be cultured in the yolk sac of the embryonated egg.

Control

International agencies have adopted a common strategy summarized under the acronym 'SAFE':

- *Surgery* to correct advanced disease; this is a simple procedure that can be safely and effectively carried out by specially trained field staff.
- *Antibiotics* to treat active infection – the drug of choice is azithromycin, a 1-day treatment by mouth; where it is not available and for young children, the alternative treatment is a course of tetracyline ointment instilled into the eyes.
- *Face washing* to reduce disease transmission; it requires no more than three handfuls of water per person.
- *Environmental change* to increase access to clean water, improve sanitation, and promote health education to eliminate disease altogether. Hygienic measures include improvement in personal cleanliness, and avoiding the sharing of handkerchiefs, towels and eye cosmetics. It involves health education and the provision of adequate water supply. Home-made fly traps using old plastic bottles and faeces have been shown to reduce the fly population by 40% and the number of trachoma cases by 36% in the Masai area of Kenya.

Active research on vaccination is making slow progress. It only provides partial protection, and on the whole, has so far proved disappointing.

WHO is leading a global alliance aimed at eliminating trachoma as a blinding disease by the year 2020.

INCLUSION CONJUNCTIVITIS

Occurrence:	Worldwide
Organism:	*Chlamydia trachomatis*, (serotypes D–K)
Reservoir:	Humans
Transmission:	Intrapartum, contact, swimming
Control:	Early treatment
	Chlorination of swimming pools

Inclusion conjunctivitis is a condition similar to but milder than trachoma. It produces an acute purulent conjunctivitis in neonates (ophthalmia neonatorum) and a follicular conjunctivitis in adults.

The incubation period is 5–12 days.

Virology

The causative agent is *Chlamydia trachomatis*, serotypes D–K, which differ from those producing trachoma in that their primary habitat is the human genital tract rather than the eye.

Epidemiology

The distribution of infection is probably worldwide but the frequency is not fully appreciated except in places where interested clinicians have adequate laboratory facilities.

Reservoir

The reservoir of infection is in human beings, the usual habitat of the organism being the genital tract: the cervix in females, the urethra in males. The genital infection is often asymptomatic in women, but an important cause of non-gonococcal (NGU) and postgonococcal (PGU) urethritis in men.

Transmission

The newborn baby is infected from its mother's genital tract during delivery, which may lead to pneumonia or otitis media in addition to inclusion conjunctivitis. The infection may also be transmitted mechanically from eye to eye, but adults often acquire the infection in the swimming pool.

Control

Topical treatment with tetracycline ointment is usually effective but sulphonamides may also be administered by the oral route. Routine eye toilet of newborn babies is of no apparent value. Systemic treatment with erythromycin is effective against all forms of neonatal disease.

Chlorination of swimming pools is useful in preventing adult infections.

Leprosy

Occurrence:	Indian subcontinent, tropical Africa, South East Asia, South America
Organisms:	Mycobacterium leprae
Reservoir:	Humans
Transmission:	Close contact
Control:	Multidrug therapy
	Leprosy elimination campaigns
	Community participation
	Self-administration
	Education
	BCG

This is an infection due to the specific microorganism, *Mycobacterium leprae*, which is of low invasive power and pathogenicity. The four main clinical forms described are: indeterminate leprosy (I), tuberculoid leprosy (TT) borderline (BB) (probably the most common form), and lepromatous leprosy (LL) (Fig. 5.1). The incubation period is long. Studies on patients born and resident in non-endemic areas but who spent periods in endemic areas indicate incubation periods of 2–5 years for tuberculoid leprosy and 8–12 years for lepromatous leprosy.

BACTERIOLOGY

Mycobacterium leprae is a slender rod-like organism which is both acid and alcohol fast and Gram-positive. It is found singly or in masses (globi). The viable organism stains deeply and uniformly; irregular staining or beading indicates non-viability. The bacilli are scanty in some clinical separate forms of leprosy (indeterminate and tuberculoid), while they are very numerous in the lesions of lepromatous leprosy. The organism has never been consistently cultured on artificial media. *M. leprae* has been successfully inoculated into the footpads of mice; it thrives in the armadillo and the hedgehog.

EPIDEMIOLOGY

This disease is common in the Indian subcontinent, tropical Africa, South East Asia and South America (Fig. 5.2). Small foci of infection exist in southern Europe and in the countries bordering the Mediterranean. Leprosy has been introduced by immigrants into countries that have been free of indigenous cases for many years, for example the UK. It was estimated that the total number of cases throughout the world exceeded 12 million. The introduction of multidrug therapy regimens has led to a dramatic decline in the prevalence of the disease (Plate 39).

Reservoir

Humans are the only source of infection. There is no positive evidence for the existence of an extrahuman reservoir of leprosy bacilli, nor for different strains.

Transmission

The infectiousness of leprosy is not high, and repeated skin to skin contact seems to be necessary. The mechanism of contagion probably consists of the transfer of living *M. leprae* from skin to skin, and the introduction of the bacilli into the corium by some slight and unremembered trauma. The discovery of the viability of the large numbers of bacilli emerging from the nasal mucosa of patients with lepromatous leprosy is very important, pointing to inhalation as a mode of transmission. *M. leprae* may also be shed by such patients from lepromatous skin ulcers, in the milk of lactating mothers, in much smaller numbers from the skin appendages. The role of fomites, contaminated by skin squames or by nasal secretions is not clear. Conjugal infections are usually 5% or less.

While prolonged and intimate contact is still classically considered to be necessary for infection

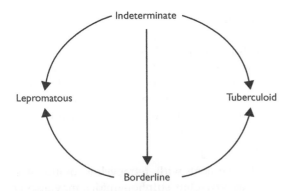

Figure 5.1: Natural history of leprosy.

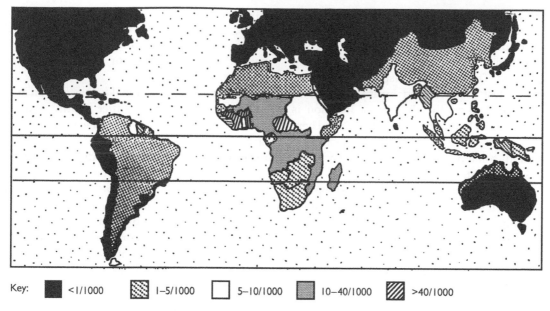

Key: ◼ <1/1000   ▨ 1–5/1000   ☐ 5–10/1000   ▦ 10–40/1000   ▨ >40/1000

Figure 5.2: Distribution of leprosy per 1000 population (1973).

to develop, there are well-authenticated cases of patients acquiring the infection after a brief passing contact with a person suffering from leprosy. Studies have shown that immunological conversion has taken place in a large proportion of leprosy contacts. These observations provide a firmer basis for placing leprosy in the group of infectious diseases (e.g. tuberculosis and poliomyelitis) in which the rate of transmission of the infecting agent is very significantly higher than the disease attack rate. It is quite rare, for example, for workers in leprosaria to contract leprosy. Although leprosy is commonest in moist and humid lands, climatic factors *per se* are probably not important.

Host factors

Even those exposed to repeated contact with open cases of leprosy may not contract the disease. Children and adolescents are commonly held to be more susceptible than adults, as are males more than females, but these generalizations are not as definite as they are sometimes made out to be. Hormonal influences may play a part, since there seems to be an increased incidence at puberty in both sexes, and clinical exacerbation of the disease may occur during pregnancy and particularly after parturition. Racial and genetic susceptibility affect the pattern of the disease from Central Africa since,

as one moves eastwards or westwards from this central point, the ratio of lepromatous to tuberculoid patients increases.

The diverse clinical manifestations of *M. leprae* infection result from differences in immunological response: in *lepromatous leprosy*, the host offers little resistance to the infection, which is severe and progressive. *Tuberculoid leprosy*, at the other end of the spectrum, is characterized by cell-mediated immunity and a type IV hypersensitivity response to the lepromin test (see below). Despite much tissue and nerve destruction there is a strong tendency towards spontaneous healing.

Recent work has emphasized the complex nature of the immune response in leprosy. Both immunoglobulins and lymphocyte-mediated immune mechanisms are involved. Patients whose resistance is impaired lack cell-mediated immunity. Studies from Surinam, India and China have shown that HLA-DR2 and DR3 alleles are associated with TT, whereas the HLA-DQwl is expressed more frequently in LL and lepromin-negative individuals.

THE LEPROMIN TEST

The antigens used for the lepromin test are prepared by the maceration of tissue containing great numbers of bacilli, such as a nodule obtained from a patient suffering from active lepromatous leprosy. The organisms are killed by heat or by other means. A refined lepromin is obtained by treating the tissue with chloroform and ether, and then centrifuging at high speed. The deposit is suspended in carbol-saline. The test is performed by injecting 0.1 ml of antigen intradermally; the site of injection is inspected after 24 hours, and daily thereafter. There are other methods of preparing a suitable antigen from bacillus containing material and sundry modifications of the test.

There are two types of cutaneous response to the lepromin test. The early reaction of Fernandez consists of an erythematous infiltrated area which appears 24–72 hours after injection, while the Mitsuda reaction is nodular in form and most intense 21–30 days after injection. The early reaction is now interpreted as a response to soluble substances of the bacillus, and the late reaction as resistance to the bacillus excited by insoluble substances. Variation of the intensity of the lepromin test occurs among leprosy patients as well as among contacts. The best site for the inoculation is the anterior aspect of the forearm.

The Mitsuda reaction is negative in pure lepromatous leprosy, strongly positive in major tuberculoid leprosy, and variably positive in intermediate forms. BCG vaccination may result in conversion of a negative lepromin reaction to positive, this conversion occurring in a variable proportion of subjects to a variable degree.

Neither an early nor late lepromin reaction proves immunity. The lepromin test is essentially an allergic reaction, though many leprologists believe that the reaction tests both allergy and immunity to leprosy bacilli. The proportion of persons in endemic areas giving positive Mitsuda reactions increases with age from nil at birth up to 80% in adults. It has been speculated that an intrinsic natural factor (N) exists that gives an individual the capacity to react specifically to *M. leprae*. Thus about 20% of the population, for no apparent reason, will not become lepromin positive however strong the natural or artificial extrinsic stimuli may be, this minor group probably lacks intrinsic factor N.

SOCIAL AND PSYCHOLOGICAL FACTORS

In no other disease do social and psychological factors loom so large as in leprosy. Since no specific psychological changes can be attributed to leprosy *per se*, the factors determining the psychological changes that occur are rather the outcome of the patient's attitude to his or her disease and the attitude of society.

In the patient, traditional beliefs as well as guilt feelings may result in either apathy and resignation or a resentful aggressiveness towards society. Leprosy in the present 'incarnation' may be regarded as retribution for misdeeds in a previous one, so that nothing can or should be done to ameliorate it. When seen as punishment for a sexual misdemeanour, leprosy may lead to such intense feelings of remorse and recrimination that suicide is contemplated or even committed. On the other hand, the person with leprosy may be led to believe that their only hope of cure is to deflower a virgin and thus pass on their disease to someone else.

Tolerance by society is the exception rather than the rule. As a result the patient tries to conceal his or her trouble for as long as possible, for the consequences may be compulsory segregation or shunning of the whole family by the community. Apparently healthy relatives are regarded as 'tainted' and may find it impossible to secure marriage partners, or those already married may be forced to divorce. Concealment of early (and treatable) leprosy lesions not only allows the disease to progress to irreversible deformity but also perpetuates an endemic situation. As the curability of leprosy becomes more widely recognized, social attitudes will change for the better and the social stigma leprosy has carried for centuries will disappear.

LABORATORY DIAGNOSIS

The cardinal point in diagnosis is the demonstration of *M. leprae* in a smear of a clinical lesion stained by the Ziehl–Neelson method. The best sites for taking smears are: the active edge of the most active lesion, the ear lobes, and the mucosa of the nasal septum.

Biopsy of typical macules, nodules infiltrations or enlarged nerves is often used. Bacterial assessment of patients with leprosy is made by counts on skin smears or biopsy specimens, from which two indices, the morphological index (MI) and the bacteriological index (BI) can be derived. The morphological index is the average percentage of morphologically normal and viable (i.e. solid staining or deeply staining) bacilli in smears from the various sites. The bacteriological index, expressed by various notations (0–4 or 5/6), is a measure of the average concentration of recognizable bacillary forms in smears from various sites on the skin (and possibly nasal mucosa).

CONTROL

Where determined and sustained efforts can be made, leprosy can be cured in the individual and controlled in the community (Plate 39).

Multidrug therapy (MDT)

This is the cornerstone for the control of leprosy. The following clinical classification for control programmes has been formulated: (a) paucibacillary (PB) single-lesion leprosy (one skin lesion); (b) paucibacillary leprosy (2–5 skin lesions); and (c) multibacillary (MB) leprosy – (more than 5 skin lesions) or smear-positive patients:

(a) *paucibacillary (PB) single-lesion leprosy*: a *single* dose of Rifampicin 600 mg + Ofloxacin 400 mg + Minocycline 100 mg;
(b) *paucibacillary (PB) leprosy*: self-administration of 100 mg Dapsone *daily* + 600 mg Rifampicin *monthly* for 6 months;
(c) *multibacillary (MB) leprosy*: self-administration of 100 mg Dapsone *daily* + 50 mg Clofazimine daily for 12 months as well as *supervised* administration of 600 mg Rifampicin + 300 mg Clofazimine *monthly* for 12 months.

MDT is produced in blister packs for WHO and the cost varies between $3.00 and $16.00, for a curative course for PB and MB respectively, which is covered by governments, WHO and donor agencies. MDT is free of charge to all patients.

The provision of an uninterrupted supply of MDT is mandatory for the conduct of a successful programme.

Strategies for high prevalence areas and special population groups

In most endemic countries patients can get MDT from the primary health dispensaries and supervision can be provided by the primary health workers.

However, in certain countries access to healthcare facilities is limited and in such areas leprosy elimination campaigns (LEC) are used to clear up undetected cases which have accumulated over time in the community. Three major activities are envisaged under LEC: (i) capacity building in local health workers to improve MDT services; (ii) increasing community participation; and (iii) diagnosing and curing patients.

In order to reach patients living in difficult-to-access areas or where the health infrastructure does not exist special action projects for the elimination of leprosy (SAPEL) can be embarked upon. This involves: (i) diagnosing and curing all cases found; (ii) promotion of self reliance; and (iii) community involvement.

Community involvement

Communities and their leaders will play a key role in the elimination of leprosy. In some situations they are the only ones capable of delivering MDT drugs, supervising the monthly administration, retrieving defaulters and rehabilitating affected patients.

Prevention of disability depends on the patient, who must be suitably instructed and each procedure demonstrated several times. Ideally, a community or family member should also be trained in the procedure to avoid disability.

BCG

BCG has been shown to provide valuable protection in a series of field trials ranging from 20 to 80%. Chemoprophylaxis is not currently recommended by WHO in leprosy endemic areas.

LEPROSY ELIMINATION

This must not be confused with 'eradication', which refers to complete interruption of transmission. In leprosy, the elimination goal is defined as reaching a prevalence of less than one case per 10 000 population, by the year AD 2000. Some countries did not achieve this objective by the specified date, but there is little doubt that MDT is being increasingly and widely applied.

Monitoring leprosy elimination in endemic countries will require special activities such as independent leprosy elimination monitoring (LEM) and the use of geographic information systems (GIS).

FUNGAL INFECTIONS

Superficial fungal infections

Occurrence:	Worldwide, but certain manifestations, e.g. clefts, are more severe in the tropics
Organisms:	Various species of *Epidermophyton*, *Trichophyton* and *Microsporon*; also *Mallassezia furfur* (now *Pityrsporum orbiculare*)
Reservoir:	Humans, animals and soil
Transmission:	Direct contact, indirect contact with contaminated articles
Control:	Personal hygiene Sanitation in baths and pools

A wide variety of fungi infect skin, hair and nails, without deeper penetration of the host tissues. The infective agents include species of *Epidermophyton*, *Trichophyton*, *Microsporon* and *Mallassezia furfur* (causative agent of tinea versicolor).

The various clinical manifestations include favus, ringworm of the scalp, body, feet (athlete's foot) and nails; some produce dyspigmentation, for example tinea versicolor. The lesions are mostly disfiguring but apart from the aesthetic aspect some are disabling, for example athlete's foot could lead to splitting of the skin and secondary bacterial infection.

EPIDEMIOLOGY

These infections have a worldwide distribution but some of the clinical manifestations such as ringworm of the feet tend to be more severe in the moist tropics. There are geographical variations in the incidence of various species, for example the predominant cause of tinea capitis in North America is *Microsporon audouinii* but it is *Trichophyton tonsurans* in South America.

Reservoir

Humans and animals represent the main reservoir of many of these infections but some of the fungi are also found in the soil. Domestic pets play an important role for some infections, for example *Microsporon canis*, which is transmitted from dogs and cats.

Transmission

Transmission may be from direct contact but also indirectly through contact with contaminated floors, barbers' instruments, clothing, combs and other personal articles.

Host factors

All age and racial groups are susceptible to these infections but some of the infections show variation with age and sex, for example ringworm of the scalp due to *Microsporon audouinii* is most prevalent in prepubertal children. Subclinical infections occur: some of these organisms can be cultured from persons who do not show clinical signs.

LABORATORY DIAGNOSIS

Specimens for examination include scrapings from the skin and nails, and also infected hairs. The organisms may be demonstrated on microscopy of skin scrapings which can be cleared with a solution of 10% potassium hydroxide. Some of the organisms can be cultured on selective media such as Sabouraud's glucose agar at 20°C. Some of the fungal lesions in hairy areas display fluorescence when examined under ultraviolet light ('Wood's light') and this serves as a useful screening test.

CONTROL

Prompt identification and treatment of infected persons will help to reduce the reservoir of infection, but the existence of subclinical infections may limit the value of this measure. General hygienic measures in homes, schools and public places such as baths and swimming pools can help reduce the hazard of infection. The sharing of towels and other personal toilet articles should be discouraged. The handling of animals including domestic pets is also an avoidable risk.

Candidiasis

Occurrence:	Worldwide
Organism:	*Candida albicans*
Reservoir:	Humans
Transmission:	Contact, parturition
Control:	Careful use of broad-spectrum antibiotics

> Elimination of local predisposing factors
> Treatment of pregnant women

This is a mycotic infection which usually affects the following sites:

- oral cavity (thrush);
- female genitalia (vulvovaginitis);
- moist skin folds (dermatitis);
- nails (chronic paronychia).

Rarely, the organism becomes disseminated systemically in immunocompromised persons, for example HIV/AIDS, leukaemia and other neoplasms, especially when under treatment with corticosteroids and broad-spectrum antibiotics.

The incubation period varies widely, but in children, it may be of the order of 2–6 days.

MYCOLOGY

Candida albicans is the main pathogenic organism producing these lesions; rarely, other organisms such as *Saccharomyces* may produce a similar oral lesion.

EPIDEMIOLOGY

Candidiasis has a worldwide distribution.

Reservoir

The reservoir of infection is in human beings. The carrier state is very common, the organism being found as part of the normal oral and intestinal flora. The occurrence of disease is therefore largely determined by host susceptibility.

Transmission

Transmission is by contact with infected persons, both patients and carriers. The newborn infant may be infected by the mother during childbirth.

Host factors

Susceptible groups include:

- newborn babies and infants;
- immunocompromised and debilitated patients (e.g. HIV/AIDS patiens, diabetics, cachectic patients, advanced tuberculosis).

Local factors may predispose to candidiasis lesions:

- ill-fitting dentures;
- tuberculous cavities;
- alterations is the normal gut flora – following treatment with broad-spectrum antibiotics;
- prolonged soaking, e.g. housewives, cleaners, bar tenders, may develop paronychia.

CONTROL

This includes prompt treatment of infections using mycostatin, in severe cases. Genital infections should be treated in late pregnancy. Prolonged use of broad-spectrum antibiotics should be avoided.

ARTHROPOD INFECTIONS

Scabies

Occurrence:	Worldwide, in overcrowded poor areas
Organism:	Sarcoptes scabiei
Reservoir:	Humans
Transmission:	Direct contact, or indirectly through contaminated clothing
Control:	Improvement in personal hygiene Treatment of affected persons

This is an infection of the skin by the mite, *Sarcoptes scabiei*. The skin rash typically consists of small papules, vesicles and pustules, characterized by intense pruritus. Another typical feature is the presence of burrows, which are superficial tunnels made by the adult mite. Secondary bacterial infection is common. Lesions occur most frequently in the moist areas of skin, for example the web of the fingers.

The incubation period ranges from a few days to several weeks.

CAUSATIVE AGENT

The infective agent is the mite *S. scabiei*. The female mite which is larger than the male, measures 0.3–0.4 mm. The gravid female lays its eggs in superficial tunnels. Within 3–5 days, the eggs hatch to produce larvae and nymphs which pass through four stages and finally moult after 3 weeks to become sexually mature adults. The adults pair and mate on the skin surface.

EPIDEMIOLOGY

The distribution of the disease is widespread in the tropics with particular concentration in poor overcrowded areas; it is also found in the temperate zones, especially in slums and where disasters such as wars have led to crowding and insanitary conditions.

Reservoir

The reservoir of infection is in human beings. There is a related species of mite in animals – *S. mange*; humans may acquire this infection on contact with infected dogs, but this mite cannot reproduce on human skin.

Transmission

Transmission of scabies is by direct contact with an infected person or indirectly through contaminated clothing. Infection may be acquired during sexual intercourse.

Host factors

All persons are apparently susceptible but infection is particularly common in children; several cases are commonly found within the same household.

LABORATORY DIAGNOSIS

The adult mite can be seen using a hand lens, and identified under the microscope; the female mite can be brought to the surface by teasing the burrows with a sharp pointed needle.

CONTROL

A high standard of personal hygiene must be maintained. Regular baths with soap and water, frequent laundering of clothes, and the avoidance of overcrowding help to prevent the spread of infection.

Infected persons should be treated by the application of benzyl benzoate emulsion or tetraethylthiuram monosulphide following a thorough bath. Other affected members of the family should be treated at the same time to prevent reinfection. Mass treatment may be useful in large institutions such as work camps.

INFECTIONS ACQUIRED FROM NON-HUMAN SOURCES

Non-human sources of infection through skin and mucous membranes include:

- soil (tetanus, hookworm);
- water (schistosomiasis, leptospirosis);
- contact with animals or their products (anthrax);
- animal bites (rabies).

The causative agents include viruses, bacteria and helminths.

VIRAL INFECTIONS

Rabies

Occurrence:	Endemic in most parts of the world except Great Britain, Australia, New Zealand, Scandinavia, parts of the West Indies and the Pacific Islands
Organism:	Rabies virus
Reservoir:	Wild animals, strays and pets
Transmission:	Bite of infected animals Air-borne in restricted circumstances
Control:	Immunization of pet dogs, control of stray dogs Passive and active immunization after exposure Prophylactic immunization of high-risk groups

Rabies is a viral infection which produces fatal encephalitis in man. The clinical features include convulsions, dysphagia, nervousness and anxiety, muscular paralysis and a progressive coma. The painful spasms of the throat muscles make the patient apprehensive of swallowing fluids (hydrophobia), even his or her own saliva. Once clinical signs are established the infection is invariably fatal.

The incubation period is usually 4–6 weeks but it may be much longer, 6 months or more.

VIROLOGY

Rabies virus is a myxovirus which can be isolated and propagated in chick embryo or tissue culture from mouse and chick embryos. The freshly isolated virus ('street virus') in experimental infections has a long incubation period (1–12 weeks) and it invades both the central nervous system and the salivary glands. After serial passage in rabbit brain, the virus ('fixed virus') multiplies rapidly solely in brain with a short incubation period of 4–6 days after experimental inoculation.

EPIDEMIOLOGY

The infection is endemic in most parts of the world with the exception of Great Britain, Australia, New Zealand, Scandinavia, areas of the West Indies and the Pacific Islands. The disease is most commonly encountered in parts of South East Asia, Africa and Europe.

Reservoir

Rabies is a zoonotic infection of mammals, especially wild carnivores in the forest (foxes, wolves, jackals). The urban reservoir includes stray and pet dogs, cats and other domestic mammals, and in a part of South America, vampire bats play an important role in spreading infection to fruit bats, cattle and other animals, including man.

Clinical features

With the exception of the vampire bat which tolerates chronic rabies infection with little disturbance, other mammals rapidly succumb to this infection once clinical signs develop. At first, there may be a change in the behaviour of the animal: restlessness, excitability, unusual aggressiveness or friendliness. Later, there are signs of difficulty in swallowing fluids and food. Paralysis of the lower jaw gives the 'dropped jaw' appearance in dogs. Even at the terminal stage the animal may be running around, attacking indiscriminately ('furious rabies'). Finally, it becomes comatose and paralysed ('dumb rabies').

Transmission

The transmission of the infection is by the bite of the infected animal, the virus being present in the saliva. It can also presumably be transmitted by the infected animal licking open sores and wounds. Air-borne infection has been demonstrated in some special circumstances, notably in caves heavily populated by bats.

LABORATORY DIAGNOSIS

Various laboratory tests are used to establish the diagnosis in suspected animals or in human cases. The rabies virus may be demonstrated in the brain tissue, saliva, spinal fluid and urine, but brain tissue is most commonly examined. Microscopic examination of the brain may show characteristic cytoplasmic inclusion bodies (Negri bodies) in the nerve cells, especially those of the hippocampal gyrus. These may be demonstrated on microscopic sections of the brain or by staining smear impressions from fresh brain tissue. The organism can be demonstrated by inoculation of suspected material into mice (intracerebral) or into hamsters (intramuscular), infection being identified by the presence of Negri bodies in the brains of the animals which die, by the fluorescent antibody technique or by neutralization tests using specific antibody.

CONTROL

Animal reservoir

In urban areas, the problem is best tackled by the control of dogs; stray dogs should be impounded and destroyed if unclaimed. Pet dogs, and preferably also cats, should be vaccinated every 3 years. In rabies-free areas, the importing of dogs, cats and other mammalian pets should be strictly controlled, such animals being kept in quarantine for at least 6 months. Whenever a dog is found to be rabid, other animals that have been exposed to it should be traced so that they can be vaccinated, kept under observation or destroyed. Some western European countries have used oral vaccination campaigns to eliminate rabies in wildlife. This technique could eventually eliminate rabies from its terrestrial reservoirs in western Europe. Improved postexposure treatment of humans and the vaccination of dogs have resulted in dramatic decreases in human cases of rabies during recent years in China, Thailand, Sri Lanka and Latin America.

POSTEXPOSURE TREATMENT

Local treatment

The wound should be cleaned thoroughly with soap or detergent; an antiseptic such as chlorine bleach should be applied.

IMMUNIZATION

Rabies can be prevented in persons who have been exposed to risk by the use of active immunization alone (rabies vaccine) or in combination with passive immunization (rabies immunoglobulin). Immunoglobulin confers immediate protection while the patient responds to vaccination. The preparations available are listed in Table 5.9. The decision to use immunization should be based on a careful consideration of the risk in each case. Three points need to be carefully considered (see Table 5.9):

Prevalence of rabies in the area

Vaccine may not be indicated in areas which are consistently free of animal rabies.

Biting animal: its species and state of health

Carnivores are particularly important in the spread of rabies.

In the case of a dog bite, the animal should be captured alive if possible, and kept under observation for 10 days. If the animal has been killed or if it dies during the period of observation, steps should be taken to find out if it was rabid; the animal should be decapitated and the head sent to the laboratory. A dog which has been adequately vaccinated is unlikely to be rabid.

In the case of a wild animal, it should be killed and the brain examined for rabies. It must be assumed that there has been exposure to rabies in cases of unprovoked bites by wild animals, or if the biting animal has escaped or been destroyed without examination.

Severity of the bite: site and extent

This may be classified into severe or mild exposure. Severe exposure includes cases of multiple or deep puncture wounds; bites on the head, neck, face, hands or fingers. After such a severe exposure, the incubation period tends to be very short. Mild exposure includes single bites, scratches and lacerations away from the dangerous areas listed under severe exposure; also the licking of open wounds.

PRE-EXPOSURE TREATMENT

Certain groups, such as veterinarians, dog catchers and hunters, who run a high risk of rabies can be protected by using HDCV (see Table 5.9). Three 1-ml injections are given intramuscularly on days 0, 7 and 21. If HDCV is not available, DEV is also effective (e.g. two doses of 1 ml given subcutaneously 1 month apart, followed by a booster dose 6–7 months later).

BACTERIAL INFECTIONS

Tetanus

Occurrence:	Worldwide, but very low incidence in developed countries as a result of immunization programme
Organism:	*Clostridium tetani*
Reservoir:	Humans
Transmission:	Through wounds including the umbilicus in newborn babies
Control:	Toilet of wounds
	Clean delivery and management of the umbilical cord
	Penicillin prophylaxis
	Passive immunization (antitetanus serum)
	Active immunization (tetanus toxoid)

This is an acute disease characterized by an increase in muscle tone, with spasms, fever and a high fatality rate in untreated cases. Usually the hypertonia and the spasms are generalized, but in some mild cases the muscle rigidity may be confined to a local area (e.g. a limb) and spasms may also be localized to the laryngeal muscles. Trismus is usually an early symptom. A peculiar grimace

Table 5.9: Guide for postexposure treatment for prevention of rabies

Category	Type of contact with a suspect or confirmed rabid domestic or wild* animal, or animal unavailable for observation	Recommended treatment
I	Touching or feeding of animals Licks on intact skin	None, if reliable case history is available
II	Nibbling of uncovered skin Minor scratches or abrasions without bleeding Licks on broken skin	Administer vaccine immediately** Stop treatment if animal remains healthy throughout an observation period*** of 10 days or if animal is euthanized and found to be negative for rabies by appropriate laboratory techniques
III	Single or multiple transdermal bites or scratches Contamination of mucous membrane with saliva (i.e. licks)	Administer rabies immunoglobulin and vaccine immediately** Stop treatment if animal remains healthy throughout an observation period*** of 10 days or if animal is killed humanely and found to be negative for rabies by appropriate laboratory techniques

*Exposure to rodents, rabbits and hares seldom, if ever, requires specific antirabies treatment.
**If an apparently healthy dog or cat in or from a low-risk area is placed under observation, it may be justified to delay specific treatment.
***This observation period applies only to dogs and cats. Except in the case of threatened or endangered species, other domestic and wild animals suspected as rabid should be euthanized and their tissues examined using appropriate laboratory techniques.

'risus sardonicus' is often noted in these patients. In tetanus neonatorum, the first symptom is failure to suck in a baby who had sucked normally for the first few days after delivery.

The incubation period is usually between 3 days and 3 weeks. The interval between the first symptom of stiffness and the appearance of spasms is known as the period of onset.

BACTERIOLOGY

Clostridium tetani is a Gram-positive rod, an obligate anaerobe, which forms terminal spores giving it a characteristic drumstick shape. The spores are highly resistant to drying and to high temperatures: they may withstand boiling for short periods.

EPIDEMIOLOGY

Tetanus is found worldwide with a high concentration in some parts of the tropics. Farmers and others living in rural areas are usually more frequently affected than urban dwellers. With routine immunization of children and prophylactic care of wounds, the disease is now rare in the developed countries.

Reservoir and transmission

The reservoir of infection is the soil and the faeces of various animals, including man. The organism gains entry into the host through wounds; any wound may serve as the portal of entry for tetanus:

- *Post-traumatic.* Deep penetrating wounds especially when associated with tissue necrosis, and particularly when contaminated with earth, dung or foreign organic material. Superficial wounds including burns may also cause tetanus. The umbilical wound is the usual portal of neonatal tetanus.
- *Postpuerperal and postabortal.* These arise from the use of contaminated instruments and dressings.
- *Neonatal tetanus* is usually acquired through contamination of the umbilical wound in the newborn baby.

- *Postsurgical.* These may also be from instruments and dressings, but the infection may be endogenous, from the presence of the organism in the host's bowel or wounds.
- *Chronic ulcers and discharging sinuses.* Chronic ulcers, guinea-worm infections, chronic otitis media, and infected tuberculous sinuses may serve as portals of entry.
- *Cryptogenic.* In a high proportion of cases, no focus is found, presumably some of these are due to minor injuries which have healed. All non-immune persons in all age groups are susceptible. Infection does not confer immunity: repeated attacks occur.

LABORATORY DIAGNOSIS

A firm clinical diagnosis can be made without laboratory tests. The isolation of the organism from the wound is of little value since it may be recovered from the wounds of persons who show no sign of tetanus.

CONTROL

There are three main lines of prevention:

Antibacterial measures

These include the protection of wounds from contamination, adequate cleansing of wounds and careful debridement. Antibiotics especially long-acting penicillin can also be given to suppress the multiplication of *Clostridium tetani.* If the wound is old (i.e. more than 12 hours), tetanus may occur despite an adequate dose of penicillin.

Doctors, midwives and traditional birth attendants should use clean instruments for cutting the umbilical cord and sterile dressings to protect it until it heals.

Passive immunization

Tetanus immune globulin (TIG) from human blood is now used in place of tetanus antitoxin (ATS), which was derived from horse serum; the latter carried a serious risk of severe allergic reactions including anaphylactic shock. TIG is used to protect individuals with dirty wounds who have no clear history of active immunization with tetanus toxoid.

Active immunization

Active immunization with tetanus toxoid is the most satisfactory method of preventing tetanus. Ideally, everyone should be given a course of active immunization. This is given in combination with diphtheria toxoid and pertussis vaccine in a triple vaccine formulation (DPT). Three doses, at monthly intervals starting at 2 months, are recommended. Booster doses of tetanus toxoid can then be given periodically, for example every 5 years or whenever the person is injured. Active immunization of the pregnant woman will protect the infant from neonatal tetanus.

WHO estimates that in 1999, there were 270 000 deaths from neonatal tetanus; these could have been prevented cheaply with the administration of two doses of tetanus toxoid to pregnant women. The persistence of clinical cases of tetanus in any community is a direct indictment of the health authorities of the country concerned because tetanus toxoid is simple to administer, safe, effective and cheap.

Mycobacterium ulcerans infection (Buruli ulcer)

Occurrence:	Major foci in Uganda, New Guinea
Organism:	*Mycobacterium ulcerans*
Reservoir:	Probably grass
Transmission:	Skin, by abrasion or insect bite
Control:	Possible benefit from BCG vaccination

Mycobacterium ulcerans causes chronic necrotizing ulcers of the skin and subcutaneous tissues. The predominance of lesions occur in the extremities. The usual incubation period is about 4–10 weeks.

BACTERIOLOGY

M. ulcerans grows preferentially at a temperature of 32–33°C. It belongs to the group of slow-growing mycobacteria requiring 4–18 weeks to grow from initial isolation.

EPIDEMIOLOGY

The infection has been recognized in at least 31 countries in Africa, Australasia and in other regions. The prevalence of Buruli disease varies considerably in the various reported areas. In an epidemiological study in Uganda, the outstanding geographic feature was the distribution of Buruli lesions near the Nile. Thus, the section of the Kinyara refugee settlement closest to the Nile had the highest incidence of the disease. In these parts, more than 25% of refugee children under 1 year of age developed Buruli lesions.

Reservoir and transmission

Both the reservoir and the mode of transmission are still uncertain. The reservoir is probably grasses and transmission is probably through abrasions or insect bites.

Host factors

Buruli disease occurs from infancy to old age, but the highest incidence is in children from 5 to 14 years. Among adults, it is more common among women than men. Two factors are mainly responsible for the age and sex distribution: immunity to the disease and exposure to the agent. People with a naturally positive tuberculin reaction are partially protected from Buruli disease. The most important reasons for the age, sex distribution and differences in anatomical sites are probably attributable to differential exposure.

LABORATORY DIAGNOSIS

Classically, histological examination of the lesions reveals complete necrosis of subcutaneous tissue with numerous organisms in subcutaneous fibrous septa. There is a notable absence of inflammatory cells.

CONTROL

The individual

The first principle of surgical treatment is excision of all involved tissue; the second is early covering of the denuded area with skin.

The community

BCG vaccination has given promising results. Health education emphasizing to the communities the significance of the early lesion – a small nodule – has resulted, in Uganda, in an overall reduction in

total hospitalization and theatre time, as well as the elimination of crippling deformities.

Leptospirosis

Occurrence:	Worldwide
Organisms:	Leptospira spp. (various serotypes)
Reservoir:	Domestic and wild animals
Transmission:	Contact with polluted water, ingestion of water or food
Control:	Limit animal contact with human sources of water
	Avoid contact with contaminated water
	Immunization

This is an acute febrile illness usually accompanied by malaise, vomiting, conjunctival infection and meningeal irritation; in severe cases, jaundice, renal involvement and haemorrhage may occur. The incubation period is from 3 days to 3 weeks.

BACTERIOLOGY

Leptospira are thin spirochaetal organisms, which can remain viable in water for several weeks. Many different serotypes have been identified, some of the common ones being *Leptospira icterohaemorrhagica* (the agent of Weil's disease), *L. canicola* (canicola fever), *L. pomona* and *L. bovis*.

EPIDEMIOLOGY

Various pathogenic species of leptospira are present in most parts of the world. The occurrence of human disease is determined by the distribution of the organisms in animal reservoirs.

Reservoir

The reservoir of infection is in various vertebrates; both wild and domestic animals are involved – cattle, dogs, pigs, rats and other rodents, and reptiles. Urine is the source of infection.

Transmission

The infection may be acquired by contact with infected water, the organism penetrating the skin, or by ingestion of contaminated water or food.

Host factors

Certain occupations carry the risk of exposure to leptospirosis, for example fish workers, persons working in sewers, rice paddies, or other collections of surface water, and soldiers who may have to wade across streams.

LABORATORY DIAGNOSIS

The organisms may be seen on microscopy of blood or a centrifuged specimen of urine using dark-ground illumination, or of a thick blood film stained with Giesma's technique. The organism can be isolated on culture or by inoculation of blood intraperitoneally into hamsters or guinea-pigs. The serotype is identified by serological tests. Agglutination and complement fixing antibodies can be detected in infected patients.

CONTROL

Domestic animals should be segregated as far as possible from water sources for human use. The reservoir in wild animals should also be eliminated, for example by the control of rodents.

Human contact with potentially contaminated water should be avoided, and where such contact is unavoidable, protective clothing should be worn.

Immunization for persons at high risk has been suggested using the local strain of leptospira as antigen; similarly pet dogs can be vaccinated.

Anthrax

Occurrence:	Widespread in agricultural areas
Organism:	*Bacillus anthracis*
Reservoir:	Farm animals
Transmission:	Contact with infected animals or their products; inhalation; ingestion
Control:	Isolation of sick animals
	Careful disposal of infected carcasses
	Disinfection of hides, skins and hair
	Protective clothing (e.g. gloves)

This is an acute infection which may present as a localized necrotic lesion of the skin (malignant pustule) with regional lymphadenopathy; further dissemination will cause septicaemia. Pulmonary and gastrointestinal forms of infection occur from inhalation or ingestion of the infected material.

The incubation period is usually less than 1 week.

BACTERIOLOGY

The causative agent, *Bacillus anthracis*, is an anaerobic, Gram-positive spore-bearing rod. The resistant spore survives drying, routine disinfection and other adverse environmental conditions; it remains viable for long periods on hides, skins and hair.

EPIDEMIOLOGY

The infection is endemic in most agricultural areas, both tropical and temperate.

Reservoir

Anthrax is a zoonosis, the reservoir of infection being farm animals: cattle, sheep, goats, horses and pigs. The animal products such as hides, skins and hair (e.g. brushes) are potential sources of infection.

Transmission

Transmission may be by contact with these infected materials or animals. The organism may also be inhaled (wool sorter's disease) or swallowed, for example in contaminated milk.

LABORATORY DIAGNOSIS

A smear of the skin lesion may show typical organisms as chains of large, Gram-positive rods. The organism can be isolated from skin, sputum or blood, by culture on blood agar. Virulence is tested by intraperitoneal injection into mice.

CONTROL

Sick animals should be isolated. The carcasses of animals that die should be burnt or buried in lime, avoiding any contamination of soil. Animals and human beings at high risk can be immunized using a live attenuated vaccine. Animal products such as hides, bone meal, and brushes, should be disinfected usually by autoclaving where feasible. Protective clothing especially gloves should be worn when handling potentially infected material.

HELMINTHIC INFECTIONS

Hookworm

Occurrence:	Tropics and subtropical areas of Africa, South America and Asia
Organisms:	*Necator americanus, Ankylostoma duodenale*
Reservoir:	Humans
Transmission:	Contact with contaminated soil Oral (*A. duodenale*)
Control:	Chemotherapy Correction of anaemia Sanitary disposal of faeces

This is an important intestinal parasite which occurs commonly in warm climates, especially in communities with poor environmental sanitation. Anaemia secondary to blood loss is the most important clinical feature of hookworm infection. Although light to moderate loads of infection may be tolerated in well-nourished persons who have an adequate intake of iron, heavy infection usually leads to iron-deficiency anaemia and occasionally to severe protein depletion. Thus, the occurrence of disease in hookworm infection depends on the interaction of the load of infection, the state of the iron stores and the diet of the host.

PARASITOLOGY

The two main species which infect humans are *Ankylostoma duodenale* and *Necator americanus*. (Fig. 5.3) illustrates their life cycle.

Ankylostoma duodenale (unlike *Necator americanus*) may also be contracted by the faeco-oral route. The hookworms of cats and dogs, *Ankylostoma braziliense* and *A. caninum*, fail to achieve full maturity in humans but may cause a serpiginous skin rash – cutaneous larva migrans.

LABORATORY DIAGNOSIS

Hookworm infection is diagnosed by the identification of the eggs in the stool; concentration methods are used for detecting light infections. Quantitative assessment of the load can be made by using the Kato–Katz method, or other quantitative techniques. The larvae can be cultured from the stool on moist filter paper at room temperature (25°C). The species of worm can be identified from the larval stage or from expelled adults.

EPIDEMIOLOGY

Hookworm is endemic in the tropics and subtropics; it is receding from the more developed areas being most prevalent in the rural areas of the moist tropics. It occurs in various parts of tropical Africa, southeastern USA, Mediterranean countries, Asia and the Caribbean (Fig. 5.4). In parts of West Africa, Central and South America, and elsewhere, mixed infections of both species occur. *A. ceylanicum* has occasionally also been reported to cause disease in humans.

Reservoir

Humans are the only important source of human hookworm infection. The epidemiology of the disease is dependent upon the interaction of three factors:

- suitability of the environment for eggs or larvae;
- mode and extent of faecal pollution of the soil;
- mode and extent of contact between infected soil and skin.

Survival of hookworm larvae is favoured in a damp, sandy or friable soil with decaying vegetation, and a temperature of 24–32°C. *A. duodenale* eggs resist desiccation more than those of *Necator*. The development of hookworm larvae in the eggs and subsequent hatching can be retarded in the absence of oxygen.

Transmission

Insanitary disposal of faeces or the use of human faeces as fertilizer are the chief sources of human infection in countries where individuals are barefooted. Thus, it is to be expected that hookworm infection will have a higher prevalence in agricultural than in town workers and that in many tropical countries it is an occupational disease of the farming community.

Oral route

It has been shown that although *Necator* infection is acquired almost exclusively by the percutaneous route, *Ankylostoma* infection may be contracted either percutaneously or orally. The latter mode of entry gives special significance to the reports of contamination of vegetables by these larvae and

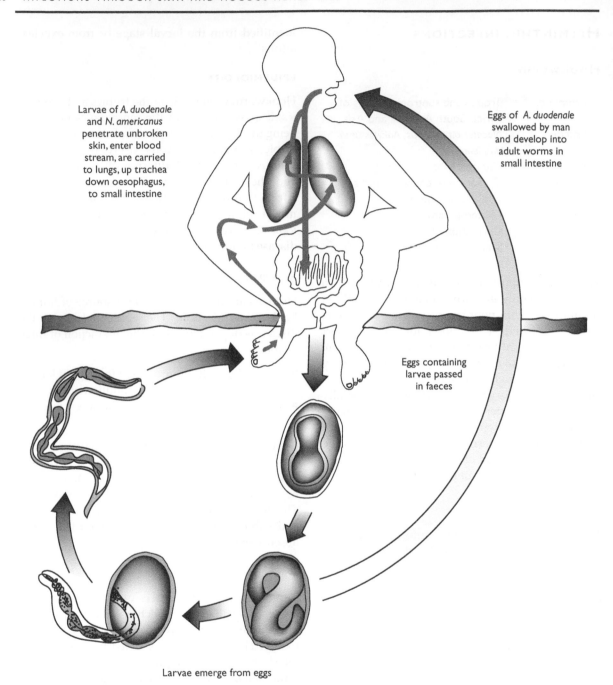

Larvae of *A. duodenale* and *N. americanus* penetrate unbroken skin, enter blood stream, are carried to lungs, up trachea down oesophagus, to small intestine

Eggs of *A. duodenale* swallowed by man and develop into adult worms in small intestine

Eggs containing larvae passed in faeces

Larvae emerge from eggs

Figure 5.3: Life cycles of *Ankylostoma duodenale* and *Necator americanus*.

underlines the biological differences between the two species.

Transplacental transmission
Transplacental transmission of *A. duodenale* probably also occurs.

Seasonal shedding
Contrary to the general belief, it has been shown that larvae of *A. duodenale* do not always develop directly to adulthood upon invasion of humans. Thus, in West Bengal, India, arrested development (hypobiosis) appears to be a seasonal

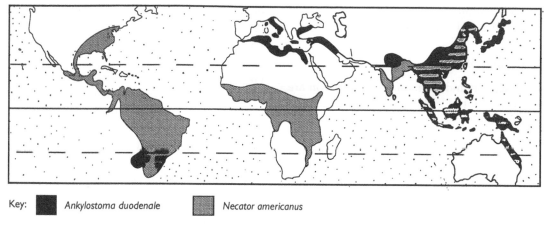

Key: ▉ *Ankylostoma duodenale*   ▨ *Necator americanus*

Figure 5.4: Distribution of hookworm infection.

phenomenon which results in:

- reduction of egg output wasted in seeding an inhospitable environment;
- a marked increase in eggs entering the environment just before the monsoon begins.

Host factors

Provided people are equally exposed to hookworm infection, both sexes and all ages are susceptible. In communities in which the parasite has long been endemic, the inhabitants develop a host/parasite balance in which the worm load is limited, thus although the infection rate in some rural areas of the tropics may be 100% only a small proportion develop hookworm anaemia. It is not known whether these heavy infections resulting in anaemia are dependent upon repeated exposure to a high intensity of infection, or whether they are due to other factors. Even low infections with hookworm may adversely influence growth of older children and reduce appetite, physical fitness and cognition.

Other factors

Although the basic epidemiology of hookworms infection is relatively simple, its quantitative epidemiology is much more complex. Some of the important features based on studies by Anderson, Schad and others can be summarized as follows:

- Distribution of worm numbers per person tends to be highly aggregated in form, where most individuals harbour few parasites and a few harbour heavy burdens.
- Worm fecundity appears to decline as the worm burden within an individual increases.
- Changes with age. The average *intensity* of infection tends to be convex in form. Changes in *prevalence* with age are less convex in form than those observed for average intensity of infection.
- Predisposition of heavily infected individuals within a community due to a variety of yet undetermined factors (behavioural, social, nutritional or genetic).
- Reinfection following chemotherapy tends to be common, the rate of return depending on a variety of circumstances. Longitudinal studies suggest that parasites are regularly lost and subsequently reacquired in the following transmission season and there is some evidence for herd immunity. However, if hookworms do elicit protective immunity in humans, the concept remains to be conclusively proven.
- In agricultural exposure to infection, rural sociological factors, such as the work done, determine the groups at greatest risk e.g. adult women in the tea plantations or men ploughing contaminated fields.

CONTROL

Control of hookworm infection involves the following approaches:

- chemotherapy;
- correction of anaemia;

- health education;
- sanitary disposal of faeces.

Sanitation and education

Health education and promotion of sanitation are crucial to the control of hookworm infections. In most of the least developed countries improved sanitation is a long-term objective but none the less one worth achieving for its all-round beneficial use. The use of fresh human faeces as a fertilizer should be discouraged.

Chemotherapy

There is a consensus that the morbidity caused by hookworm and other helminthic infections can be reduced by the proper use of anthelminthic drugs.

Even though re-infection is likely following chemotherapy until environmental hygiene is considerably improved, the short-term relief from the burden of disease is thought to be well worth the cost and effort of delivery. A Cochrane review has recently challenged this conclusion.

Mass treatment, selective chemotherapy or targeted chemotherapy or combinations of these strategies can be used.

Regimen

The recommended anthelminthics are relatively non-toxic and in most instances can be given straight away, even to debilitated patients. When the anaemia is very severe (less than 5 g/100 ml) some practitioners prefer to raise the haemoglobin level to about 7–8 g/100 ml before dealing with the worm infection specifically. Patients with severe hypoalbuminaemia should be adequately and quickly dewormed.

Repeated treatments are usually necessary except in light infection. In the past, laxatives were routinely given before and after treatment; they are now considered unnecessary except in the presence of constipation.

The timing of chemotherapy is important. In countries where transmission is seasonal, two treatments are advocated: one at the beginning of the wet season will reduce the number of infective eggs in the environment, while a second treatment 4–6 weeks after the end of the rains, when overall prevalence is generally high, will reduce the chances of re-infection during the subsequent dry season. In areas of perennial transmission such a strategy will produce less impressive results.

Drugs

Several drugs are available for treating hookworm infections. Their efficacy varies according to the species in question. Broad-spectrum anthelminthics, effective against more than one parasite, are useful in the treatment of multiple intestinal helminth infections, common in the rural tropics:

- Albendazole;
- Mebendazole;
- Pyrantel;
- Levamisole.
- Nitazoxanide.

When infection is light, the convenience, range and economic advantages of such drugs make them well worth considering. In heavy infections, however, selective treatment for the appropriate species of helminthic infection is preferable.

In many countries of the tropics economic considerations must determine the choice of drug. In addition, ease of administration, number of doses, treatment time, side-effects, palatability, shelf-life and storage requirements are all factors that have to be taken into consideration when comparing different drugs. Albendazole is now the most widely used anthelminthic. In some school programmes Albendazole has been combined simultaneously with administration of vitamin A.

Anaemia

The response to iron therapy is usually rapid. A cheap and very effective treatment is ferrous sulphate, 200 mg thrice daily given by mouth and continued for 3 months after the haemoglobin concentration has risen to 12 g/100 ml. Even without deworming, this regime will rectify the anaemia and a rise in haemoglobin of 1 g/100 ml per week occurs; unless the worms have been removed, however, the haemoglobin will drop as soon as iron therapy is discontinued and anthelminthics are therefore mandatory in heavy infections. When indicated, for example if regular oral administration cannot be guaranteed, intramuscular or intravenous iron preparations are given.

Strongyloidiasis

Occurrence:	Worldwide
Organism:	Strongyloides stercoralis
Reservoir:	Humans
Transmission:	Contact with contaminated soil
	Auto-infection/faeco-oral
	transmission
Control:	Sanitary disposal of faeces
	Personal hygiene

Strongyloidiasis is caused by the nematode *Strongyloides stercoralis*. The clinical picture varies from an asymptomatic infection to a creeping linear erythematous eruption ('larva currens') malabsorption and disseminated fatal strongyloidiasis usually seen in the immunocompromised host including AIDS patients.

PARASITOLOGY

The life cycle of *S. stercoralis* is illustrated in Figure 5.5.

EPIDEMIOLOGY

The global distribution of *S. stercoralis* varies widely. It is commonly found in South East Asia, Africa and Latin America. In Europe, pockets of strongyloidiasis have been identified in Yugoslavia, Romania and elsewhere. One of the areas of highest endemicity is Brazil: in some parts of the northeast a prevalence rate of 60% has been reported.

Reservoir and transmission

Humans are the reservoir of infection. Strongyloidiasis is transmitted most commonly through contact with soil contaminated with infective larvae. The free-living stages develop well in hot, wet climates and in rich soil in organic matter. Studies of infection in former prisoners of war from Thailand and Burma have shown that some may remain infected for more than 35 years after leaving the endemic area (auto-infection). A few cases of strongyloidiasis acquired from dogs have occurred.

LABORATORY DIAGNOSIS

Special techniques for isolation of larvae are usually required, for example Baerman or Harada-Mori.

Scanty larvae can sometimes be seen on direct examination of stools. Serological tests are also available.

CONTROL

This is basically similar to that of hookworm infection (see p. 140). The most satisfactory drug for the treatment of strongyloidiasis is ivermectin, whether at the individual or community level.

Schistosomiasis

Occurrence:	Schistosoma haematobium –
	tropical Africa, Middle East
	S. mansoni – tropical Africa and
	South America
	S. japonicum – China and other
	areas in Far East
Organisms:	Schistosoma haematobium,
	S. mansoni, S. japonicum,
	S. intercalatum, S. mekongi
Reservoir:	S. haematobium – humans
	S. mansoni – humans
	S. japonicum – humans, various
	domestic and wild animals
Vector:	Snails
Transmission:	Contact with infected fresh water
Control:	Many methods (in particular
	chemotherapy and moluscicides)
	Integrated wherever possible

This remains one of the most important parasitic infections in the tropics. Human infection, due mainly to *Schistosoma haematobium*, *S. mansoni* and *S. japonicum*, causes chronic inflammatory changes with progressive damage to various organs. The localization of the worms varies from species to species. At first the lesions are granulomatous with damage to parenchymatous host cells; later fibrotic changes take place. Even after the worms have been eliminated, residual sequelae may persist. Three clinical stages are identified: (i) the stage of invasion (cercarial dermatitis); (ii) the stage of migration (toxaemia); and (iii) the stage of established infection (urinary, intestinal tract and liver).

PARASITOLOGY

These worms are trematodes with the peculiar morphological feature that the body of the male is

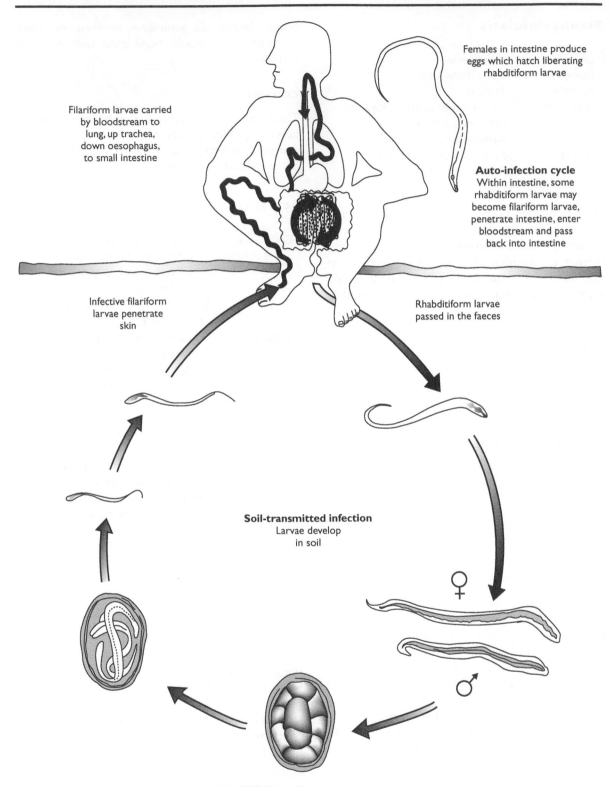

Females in intestine produce
eggs which hatch liberating
rhabditiform larvae

Filariform larvae carried
by bloodstream to
lung, up trachea,
down oesophagus,
to small intestine

Auto-infection cycle
Within intestine, some
rhabditiform larvae may
become filariform larvae,
penetrate intestine, enter
bloodstream and pass
back into intestine

Infective filariform
larvae penetrate
skin

Rhabditiform larvae
passed in the faeces

Soil-transmitted infection
Larvae develop
in soil

♀

♂

Figure 5.5: Life cycle of *Strongyloides stercoralis*.

folded to form a gynaecophoric canal in which the female is carried. The adult worms are found in the veins; *S. haematobium* are predominantly in the vesical plexus, *S. mansoni* in the inferior mesenteric veins and *S. japonicum* predominantly in the superior mesenteric veins.

Other schistosomes which infect man include *S. intercalatum*, *S. mekongi* and occasionally *S. bovis* and *S. matthei*.

LIFE CYCLE (FIGS 5.6 AND 5.7)

Intermediate hosts

All the intermediate hosts of schistosomes are freshwater snails of the Gastropoda class in the orders Pulmonata and Prosobronchiata. Various species of *Bulinus* snails are the vectors of *S. haematobium*, whilst species of *Biomphalaria*, are the intermediate hosts of *S. mansoni*. Both *Bulinus* and *Biomphalaria* are aquatic snails that breed in ponds, lakes, streams, marshes, swamps, drains, dams and irrigation canals. *Oncomelania* species, the intermediate host of *S. japonicum*, are amphibious snails, living in moist vegetation. These snail hosts are affected by physical factors such as temperature; and by chemical factors, pH and oxygen tension. The snails are hermaphrodite but not self-fertilizing; they lay eggs usually on vegetation; these hatch and grow to mature adult forms. During the dry season, the aquatic snails aestivate in the drying mud, with the openings of the shells covered with dried mucus. Although snails with immature infections may survive the dry season, those with mature infections usually die. *Oncomelania*, being an operculated snail, survives drying much better than the non-operculated snails.

EPIDEMIOLOGY

It has been estimated that a total of about 200 million persons are affected in various parts of the world. *S. haematobium* occurs in many parts of Africa (North, West, Central and East Africa) and parts of the Middle East; *S. japonicum* occurs in China, the Philippines and other foci in the Far East; while *S. mekongi* is found in the countries around the Mekong river in South East Asia (Fig. 5.8).

S. mansoni is found in the Nile delta, West, East and Central Africa, South America and the Caribbean; *S. intercalatum* occurs in Central Africa (Fig. 5.9).

Reservoir

Humans are the main reservoir of *S. haematobium* and *S. mansoni* but naturally acquired infection with *S. mansoni* has also been found in various mammals (cats, dogs, cattle, pigs and rats) and they may constitute a part of the reservoir. In contrast, animal reservoirs both wild and domestic, contribute significantly to human *S. japonicum* infection. Other schistosomes, for example *S. bovis* and *S. mathei*, are basically infections of animals with occasional infection to man.

Transmission

Humans acquire the infection by wading, swimming, bathing or washing clothes and utensils in the polluted streams. Certain occupational groups, for example farmers and fishermen, may be exposed to a high risk (Plates 40–48). Considerable interest exists in mathematical models of schistosome transmission and their relevance to control strategy.

Host factors

The age and sex distribution of schistosomiasis varies from area to area.

Age
One fairly common pattern is of high prevalence rates of active infection in children, who excrete relatively large quantities of eggs, and a lower prevalence rate of active infection among adults; the latter show late manifestations and sequelae. In general, age-prevalence–intensity data for *S. haematobium* infection conform to Figure 5.10(a) while the typical age-prevalence–intensity curve for *S. mansoni* infection is shown in Figure 5.10(b). The curve for *S. japonicum* is less well defined. These age-related trends in prevalence and intensity often parallel age-related water contact patterns.

Load of infection
In general, the form of age-prevalence curves remains the same whether the mean intensity of infection is high or low. Epidemiological studies indicate that the load of infection is an important factor in determining the severity of pathological lesions and clinical manifestations.

Immunity
Epidemiological evidence also suggests that some degree of immunity to all schistosomal infections also occurs in humans.

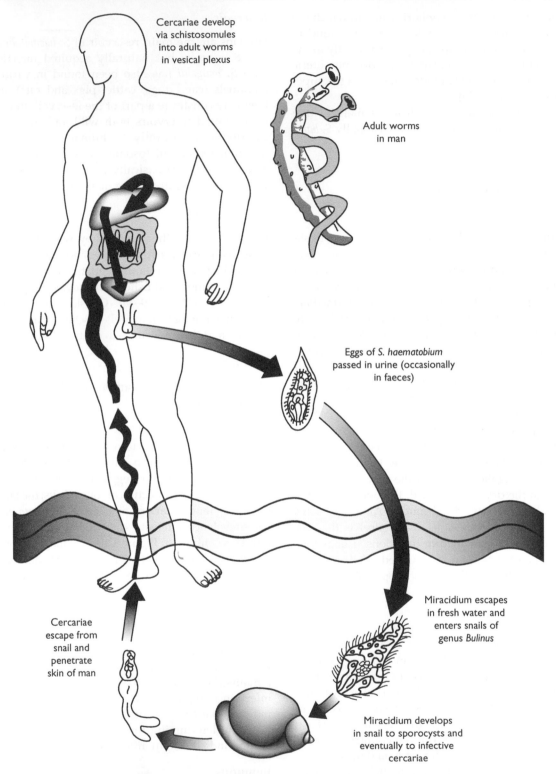

Cercariae develop
via schistosomules
into adult worms
in vesical plexus

Adult worms
in man

Eggs of *S. haematobium*
passed in urine (occasionally
in faeces)

Miracidium escapes
in fresh water and
enters snails of
genus *Bulinus*

Cercariae
escape from
snail and
penetrate
skin of man

Miracidium develops
in snail to sporocysts and
eventually to infective
cercariae

Figure 5.6: Life cycle of *Schistosoma haematobium*.

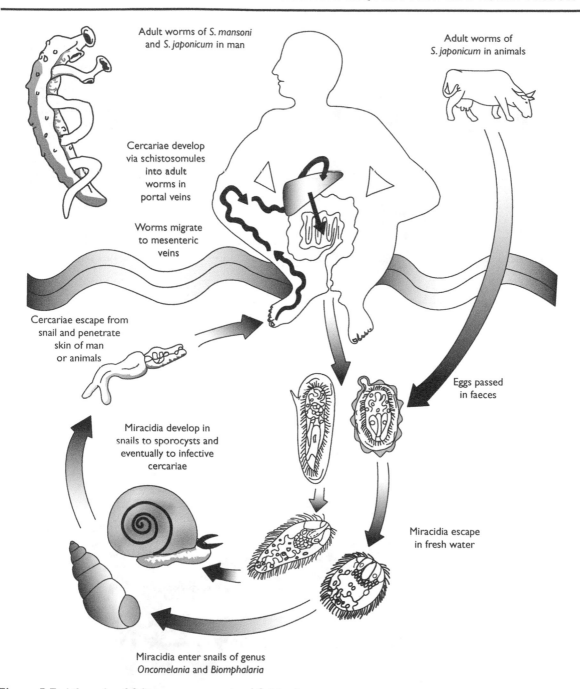

Adult worms of S. mansoni and S. japonicum in man

Adult worms of S. japonicum in animals

Cercariae develop via schistosomules into adult worms in portal veins

Worms migrate to mesenteric veins

Cercariae escape from snail and penetrate skin of man or animals

Eggs passed in faeces

Miracidia develop in snails to sporocysts and eventually to infective cercariae

Miracidia escape in fresh water

Miracidia enter snails of genus Oncomelania and Biomphalaria

Figure 5.7: Life cycle of Schistosoma mansoni and S. japonicum.

Development: man-made water resources

In the past two decades water resource development programmes were undertaken in endemic areas of the world and during this period an increase has been observed in the transmission of schistosomiasis in the areas around man-made lakes and irrigation schemes. Real economic returns could well be seriously jeopardized unless provision for human welfare is made at the planning stage. The basis for our current understanding of the epidemiology of schistosomiasis is summarized in Table 5.10.

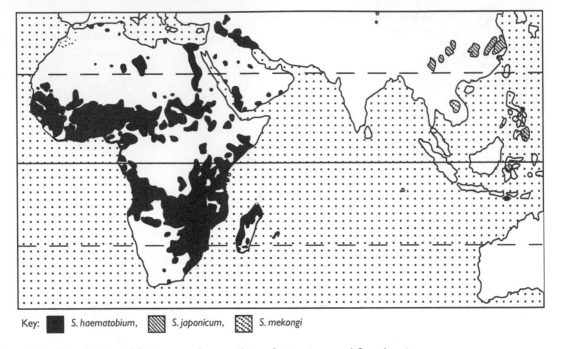

Key: ▓ S. haematobium,   ▨ S. japonicum,   ▨ S. mekongi

Figure 5.8: Distribution of *Schistosoma haematobium*, *S. japonicum* and *S. mekongi*.

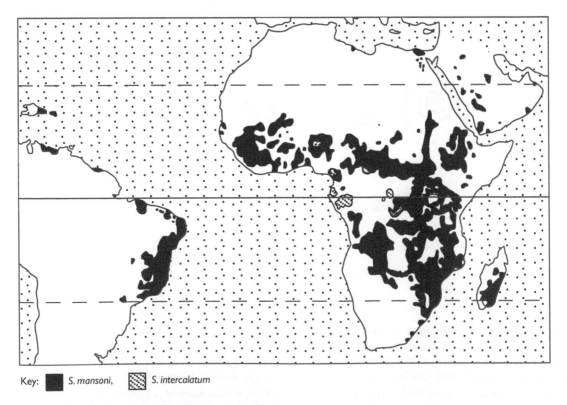

Key: ■ S. mansoni,   ▨ S. intercalatum

Figure 5.9: Distribution of *S. mansoni* and *S. intercalatum*.

DIAGNOSIS

Parasitological and immunological methods are used in the diagnosis of schistosomiasis. Visible haematuria is a reliable indicator of heavy infection. In

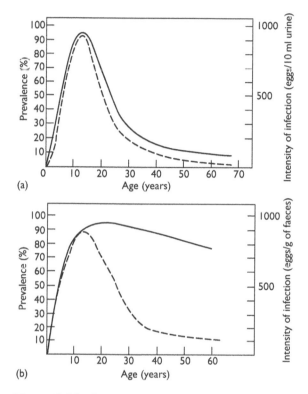

Figure 5.10: Generalized distributions of prevalence (——) and intensity (–––) for (a) *Schistosoma haematobium* infection; (b) *S. mansoni* infection. Source: Sleight & Mott (1986).

endemic areas it is tantamount to a positive diagnosis of *S. haematobium*. Reagent strips for haematuria are simple to use and widely available. A simple questionnaire can give a good indication of how frequent schistosomiasis is present in a community in *S. haematobium* endemic areas. The vernacular for schistosomiasis and haematuria are well understood in such areas. 'Blood in stool', 'grow', 'toto' and 'gloujen' have been found reliable symptoms in rapid and low cost identification of *S. mansoni* in the Ivory Coast.

PARASITOLOGY

Urine

Eggs of *S. haematobium* are usually found in urine and occasionally in faeces. For a quantitative assessment of the load of infection, a 24-hour collection of urine can be examined, or timed collection around midday (e.g. 10 am–2 pm) when egg count is highest, may be used. Eggs of *S. mansoni* are occasionally found in urine.

Faeces

For *S. mansoni* and *S. japonicum* infection, examination of faeces may reveal the eggs; concentration techniques may be required for light infections; quantitative techniques are available and are useful in determining both pathogenicity as well as the effects of intervention. The Kato–Katz quantitative method is generally used for intestinal schistosomiasis while for *S. haematobium* the quantitative filtration technique is employed.

Table 5.10: Summary of the epidemiological knowledge in schistosomiasis

Detection and grading	Schistosoma infections can be detected and graded by urine or faecal egg counts
Distribution	The prevalence and intensity of infection varies greatly from one focus to another. Within a zone of endemic infection, transmission is frequently focal. Population growth, migration and socio-economic development schemes (e.g. water resources) aggravate and expand transmission
Intensity	The mean intensity of infection tends to increase in parallel with the prevalence. Only a small proportion of an infected population carry heavy infections. The risk of fibro-obstructive disease is proportional to the intensity of infection. However, at each stratum of intensity of load there is variation in the pathological effects and clinical manifestations
Age	In endemic areas, the prevalence and intensity of infection usually peaks between 10 and 17 years of age. The age-related rise and fall in the prevalence and intensity of infection often (but not invariably) parallels the age-related water contact pattern
Immunity	Some individuals seem to develop immunity to superinfection

Rectal biopsy

Rectal biopsy ('rectal snip') is useful in diagnosing infections, particularly those due to *S. mansoni* and *S. japonicum* but it is also positive in some cases of *S. haematobium*; the specimen is easily obtained by curetting the superficial layers of the rectal mucosa and examining the material fresh between two glass slides; it can later be fixed and stained.

IMMUNOLOGY

Immunological tests, for example circumoval precipitin (COP), Cercariahfillen, and fluorescent antibody tests (ELISA), are used for the diagnosis of schistosomiasis; the tests are group specific and so cannot identify the particular infecting species. Some of the tests (e.g. COP) become negative after treatment or spontaneous cure, but others (e.g. the skin test) remain positive for indefinitely long periods. False-positive results may occur in persons who have been exposed to avian and other non-human schistosomes. ELISAs for the detection of circulating anodic antigen (CAA) and circulating cathodid antigen (CCA) are sensitive newer methods.

Other techniques for diagnosis and assessment

Other diagnostic techniques include cystoscopy, ultrasonography, pyelography, liver biopsy, and biochemical tests of hepatic and renal function. These are mainly used for the detailed assessment of individual patients but some, especially ultrasonography, have been adapted for field surveys. The frequency of gross haematuria, and the degree of haematuria and proteinuria detectable by chemical reagent strips, correlate with the intensity of infection.

CONTROL

The control of schistosomiasis depends on a profound understanding of the epidemiology of the disease complex, and in particular of the biology, ecology and distribution of the parasites, their snail intermediate hosts and mammalian reservoir hosts. A sound knowledge of the role of humans and their behaviour in maintaining the infection is crucial. Moreover, the ultimate success of any control programme is dependent upon a full understanding of the local socio-economic conditions, upon the appreciation by the health authorities as well as by the community of the benefits of the proposed measures.

There are six basic approaches to the control of schistosomiasis:

- elimination of the reservoir: chemotherapy;
- avoidance of pollution of surface water;
- elimination of the vector;
- prevention of human contact with infected water;
- health education;
- community participation.

Ideally, control should involve an integrated approach, using as many as possible of these methods, as described below.

Elimination of the reservoir: chemotherapy

The use of chemotherapy in control requires a clear definition of aims, selection of the appropriate chemotherapeutic agent, and decisions on the dosage and frequency of administration to be followed as well as on the organization of the delivery system.

Primary and secondary control

While other approaches to schistosome control merely reduce transmission without any direct effects on human worm load, chemotherapy reduces the output of live eggs from the patient's body and, in doing so, diminishes transmission.

Moreover, killing worms in the treated individual not only reduces the risk of morbidity and mortality due to the disease, but also enables the patient to recover from reversible lesions. It is important to distinguish between these two beneficial effects. The second, a fall in disease risk, benefits only those who are treated, while the first, a reduction in transmission, helps the whole community. Even when the reduction in transmission is incomplete, the fall in disease risk may still be considerable. Chemotherapy is thus a tool for both primary and secondary control of schistosomiasis.

Primary control   The object of primary control is clearly to end output, especially in those most likely to pollute transmission sites. In situations where egg output cannot be reduced to zero, it is not known at what level persisting egg excretion ceases to be a public health problem. Some epidemiological models suggest that egg production is so great, relative to what is needed for continued transmission, that even a small residual percentage of egg output will be sufficient to maintain transmission at a considerable level; however, enough data are not yet available to test this hypothesis. Nor is it possible to say whether a few people with high egg excretion rates are epidemiologically more or less of a problem than a large number of people with a low egg output. It follows that the goal of primary control should be to reduce the egg output of as large a part of the population as possible to as near zero as can be obtained within the constraints of drug toxicity, cost, and possible effects on immunity.

Secondary control   This is aimed at minimizing the pathological effects of the infection. The severity of schistosomiasis increases with rising egg output and intensity of infection. An appreciable proportion of patients with low egg excretion rates also show severe lesions, though it is not clear whether these lesions are due to a previous heavy infection or greater susceptibility to pathological consequences. Again, as with primary control, it is desirable to treat all infected individuals.

Praziquantel – the broad-spectrum antischistosomal drug – is now the most effective and widely used drug for the control of schistosomiasis. The price is now affordable by most endemic-country governments and successful campaigns have been carried out in Brazil, Egypt, China, several countries in Africa and elsewhere, resulting in a significant reduction of clinical disease. Integration with primary health services is increasingly occurring.

Strategies

The choice between mass chemotherapy, selective chemotherapy and targeted chemotherapy depends upon balancing maximum control with safety and economic consideration. The frequency of treatment will depend on a variety of factors which can only be determined by individual health and national control programmes and are likely to vary from country to country.

Avoidance of pollution of surface water

This can be achieved by providing suitable sanitary facilities for the disposal of excreta and teaching people how to use them appropriately. It is important for the programme to include children since

they usually have relatively high outputs of viable eggs. Unless the programme is highly successful, little benefit will be derived from these measures because infected communities usually produce more eggs than are required to maintain infection in the snails.

Elimination of the vector

Physical

Alteration of the habitat (e.g. drainage of swamps) may solve the problem by eliminating the breeding sites of the snails. Where such a radical cure is not feasible, the situation can be improved by rendering the environment hostile to the snails, for example removal of acquatic vegetation, altering the flow rate of the streams, or building concrete linings to the walls of drains.

Chemical

Only one molluscicide – Baylucide – is predominantly used in control programmes (Plate 49). Endod (*Phytolaca dodecandra)* and *Swartzia madagascariensis* remain the most thoroughly studied field examples of a molluscicide of plant origin.

Molluscicide can be applied focally or area-wide depending on specific situations. Administration must be carried out under the direction of those who have expert knowledge and experience to assure effective action against the snails and minimal risk to humans and other living things. Selective focal mollusciciding is generally preferred to area-wide.

Biological

Experience has shown that predatory snails and fishes are successful only in very specific habitats and biological control is not a practical option at present.

Prevention of human contact with infected water

This requires the provision of alternative supplies of safe water, coupled with health education. Where contact with infected water is unavoidable, protective clothing such as rubber boots should be worn; this may prove impractical for peasant farmers or subsistence fishermen. It has recently been shown that artemether can be used prophylactically to prevent the development of infection.

Health education

Human attitudes towards water and water-borne disease transmission frequently need to be modified, particularly in areas with endemic schistosomiasis.

Health education should be the responsibility of all health workers and should be based on a clear understanding of the people's perception of disease and its relation to the environment. Efforts should be directed towards those groups that are at greatest risk and most involved in transmission – usually young children. It is recommended that, whenever possible, efforts be positive rather than negative in orientation. In other words, it is better to encourage children to refrain from initially polluting water sources than to try to prevent water contact. Infection is likely to be associated with certain types of water-contact behaviour, which will vary in different transmission situations. If a link is established between specific activities and schistosomiasis transmission, then these activities should be discouraged.

An effective health-education programme should promote active community participation (see below). Such participation may range from a community installing its own water supply to a community simply co-operating with the health authorities in reducing contact with unsafe water bodies.

Community participation

Community participation must be considered as an essential element of any schistosomiasis control programme.

National interest should be promoted once the schistosomiasis problem is considered to be a serious public health problem. Governments or communities implementing schistosomiasis control programmes have the responsibility of organizing national or local efforts through mechanisms acceptable to the communities concerned.

Recognition of the problem by the local population and its awareness of the risks and possible consequences of infection must be the basis of its co-operation. To this end the advice should be prepared in a clear, simple and convincing form, and presented in the most suitable style. Simple, inexpensive and appropriate technology must be carefully selected and transmitted to those members of the community most involved in schistosomiasis control.

Community participation must be organized as an integral part of the basic health-care activities and the primary health workers must be prepared to assume their responsibilities at the local level.

REFERENCES AND FURTHER READING

Genta R.M. (1987) Strongyloidiasis. In: Pawloski Z. (Ed.) *Intestinal Helminthic Infections.* Baillière Tindall, London, pp. 645–667.

Lucas A., *et al.* (1966) Radiological changes after medical treatment of vesical schistosomiasis. *Lancet* 1: 631–634.

Niamey Working Group (1999) Ultrasound in schistosomiasis. WHO document. TDR/Sch/Ultrason/99.

Pawlowski Z.S., Schad G.A. & Stott G.J. (1991) *Hookworm Infection and Anaemia.* WHO, Geneva.

Sleight A.C. and Mott K.E. (1986) Schistosomiasis. In: Gilles H.M. (Ed.) *Epidemiology and Control of Tropical Diseases.* W.B. Saunders, Philadelphia, pp. 643–670.

Srini Vasan H. (1993) *Prevention of Disabilities in Patients with Leprosy; A Practical Guide.* WHO, Geneva.

UNDP/World Bank/WHO (1998) TDR's contribution to the development of multidrug therapy for leprosy. TDR/ER/RD/98.4.

UNDP/World Bank/WHO (1995) *The Schistosomiasis Manual.* TDR/SER/MSR/95.2.

WHO (1977) *Social and Health Aspects of Sexually Transmitted Diseases.* Public Health Papers No. 65. WHO, Geneva.

WHO (1978) *7th WHO Expert Committee on Leprosy.* Technical Report Series No. 874. WHO, Geneva.

WHO (1980) *Epidemiology and Control of Schistosomiasis.* Technical Report Series No. 643. WHO, Geneva.

WHO (1982) *Chemotherapy of Leprosy for Control Programmes.* Technical Report Series No. 675. WHO, Geneva.

WHO (1984) *Expert Committee on Rabies, Seventh Report.* Technical Report Series No. 709. WHO, Geneva.

WHO (1985) *Epidemiology of Leprosy in Relation to Control.* Technical Report Series No. 716. WHO, Geneva.

WHO (1985) *The Control of Schistosomiasis.* Technical Report Series No. 728. WHO, Geneva.

WHO (1985) *Viral Haemorrhagic Fevers.* Technical Report Series No. 721. WHO, Geneva.

WHO (1986) *WHO Expert Committee on Sexually Transmitted Diseases and Treponematoses.* Technical Report Series No. 736. WHO, Geneva.

WHO (1987) *Community-Based Education for Health Personnel.* Technical Report Series No. 746. WHO, Geneva.

WHO (1987) *Prevention and Control of Intestinal Parasitic Infections.* Technical Report Series No. 749. WHO, Geneva.

WHO (1992) *Epidemiological Modelling for Schistosomiasis Control.* TDR/IDE/Sch-Mod/92.1.

WHO (1992) *WHO Expert Committee on Rabies.* Technical Report Series No. 824. WHO, Geneva.

WHO (1993) *The Control of Schistosomiasis.* Technical Report Series No. 830. WHO, Geneva.

WHO (1996) Report of the WHO informal consultation on hookworm infection and anaemia in girls and women. WHO/CTD/SIP/06.1. WHO, Geneva.

WHO (1998) *Guidelines for the Evaluation of Soil Transmitted Helminthiasis and Schistosomiasis at Community Level.* WHO/CDS/SIP/98.1. WHO, Geneva.

WHO (1998) *WHO Expert Committee on Leprosy.* Technical Report Series No. 874. WHO, Geneva.

WHO (1999) Report of the WHO informal consultation on monitoring the drug efficacy in the control of schistosomiasis and intestinal nematodes. WHO, Geneva.

WHO (2002) Prevention and control of schistosomiasis and soil-transmitted helminthiasis. WHO Technical Report Series No. 912. WHO, Geneva.

LATE ADDENDUM

Leprosy – A genetic basis for susceptibility of an individual to leprosy has been established, it is in Locus 6q25 of the chromosome region. Locus 10p13 determines the development of paucibacillary leprosy.

CHAPTER SIX

INFECTIONS THROUGH THE RESPIRATORY TRACT

- Infective agents
- Transmission
- Host
- Control of air-borne infections

- Viral infections
- Bacterial infections
- Fungal infections
- References and further reading

Infections of the respiratory tract are acquired mainly by the inhalation of pathogenic organisms. Lower acute respiratory infections (ARI) are an important cause of death of children in the tropics (Plate 50).

INFECTIVE AGENTS

The infective agents that cause respiratory infections include viruses, bacteria, rickettsiae and fungi (Table 6.1). The spread of infection from the respiratory tract may lead to the invasion of other organs of the body. Bacterial meningitis is often secondary to a primary focus in the respiratory tract, for example infections due to *Streptococcus pneumoniae*, *Haemophilus influenzae* or *Mycobacterium tuberculosis*. In the case of meningococcal infection, there are usually no local symptoms from the primary focus of infection in the nasopharynx.

These pathogens vary in their ability to survive in the environment. Some are capable of surviving for long periods in dust, especially in a dark, warm, moist environment, protected from the lethal effects of ultraviolet rays of sunshine. For example, *M. tuberculosis* can survive for long periods in dried sputum.

Table 6.1: The infective agents

Viral infections
Measles (measles virus)
Rubella (rubella virus)
Mumps (mumps virus)
Influenza (influenza viruses)
Acute upper respiratory tract infection
   (rhinoviruses, reoviruses, enteroviruses)
Infectious mononucleosis (Epstein–Barr virus)
Chickenpox* (varicella-zoster virus)

Rickettsial infections
Q fever* (*Coxiella burnetii*)

Bacterial infections
Tuberculosis (*Mycobacterium tuberculosis*)
Pneumococcal pneumonia (*Streptococcus pneumoniae*)
Other pneumonias (*Streptococcus pyogenes*,
   Staphylococcus aureus, *Klebsiella pneumoniae*,
   Haemophilus influenzae)
Psittacosis (*Chlamydia psittaci*)
Atypical pneumonia (*Mycoplasma pneumoniae*)
Meningococcal infection (*Neisseria meningitidis*)
Streptococcal infection, rheumatic fever
   (*Streptococcus pyogenes*)
Whooping cough (*Bordatella pertussis*)
Diphtheria (*Corynebacterium diphtheriae*)
Pneumonic plague** (*Yersinia pestis*)

Fungal infections
Histoplasmosis (*Histoplasma capsulatum*)

*See Chapter 5.
**See Chapter 7.

Humans are the reservoir of most of these infections but some have a reservoir in lower animals, for example plague in rodents. Carriers play an important role in the epidemiology of some of these infections, for example in meningococcal infection carriers represent the major part of the reservoir.

TRANSMISSION

There are three main mechanisms for the transmission of air-borne infections – droplets, droplet nuclei and dust.

Droplets

These are particles that are ejected by coughing, talking, sneezing, laughing and spitting. They may contain food debris and micro-organisms enveloped in saliva or secretions of the upper respiratory tract. Being heavy, droplets tend to settle rapidly. The transmission of infection by this route can only take place over a very short distance. Because of their relatively large size, droplets are not readily inhaled into the lower respiratory tract.

Droplet nuclei

These are produced by the evaporation of droplets before they settle. The small dried nuclei are buoyant and are rapidly dispersed. The droplet nuclei are also usually small enough to pass through the bronchioles into the alveoli of the lungs.

Dust

Dust-borne infections are important in relation to organisms that persist in dust for long periods and dust can act as the reservoir for some of them. The organisms may be derived from sputum, or from settled droplets.

Other mechanisms

Streptococci or staphylococci may also be derived from skin and infected wounds.

HOST

Non-specific defences

A number of non-specific factors protect the respiratory tract of man. These include mechanical factors such as the mucous membrane, which traps small particles on its sticky secretions and cleans them out by the action of its ciliated epithelium. In addition, the respiratory tract is also guarded by various reflex acts such as coughing and sneezing which are provoked by foreign bodies or accumulated secretions. Mucoid secretions which contain lysozyme and some biochemical constituents of tissues have antimicrobial action.

Immunity

Specific immunity may be acquired by previous spontaneous infection or by artificial immunization. For some of the infections, a single attack confers life-long immunity (e.g. measles) but in other cases, because there are many different antigenic strains of the pathogen, repeated attacks may occur (e.g. influenza).

CONTROL OF AIR-BORNE INFECTIONS

The main principles involved in the control of respiratory infections are outlined under three headings – infective agent, the mode of transmission and host factors.

Infective agent

- Elimination of human and animal reservoirs.
- Disinfection of floors and the elimination of dust.

Mode of transmission

- Air hygiene: good ventilation; air disinfection with ultraviolet light (in special cases).
- Avoid overcrowding. Bedrooms of dwelling-houses and public halls.
- Personal hygiene. Avoid coughing, sneezing, spitting or talking directly at the face of other

persons. Face masks should be worn by persons with respiratory infections to limit contamination of the environment.

Host

- Specific immunization: active immunization (e.g. measles, whooping cough, influenza); passive immunization in special cases (e.g. gamma globulin for the prevention of measles).
- Chemoprophylaxis (e.g. isoniazid in selected cases for the prevention of tuberculosis).

VIRAL INFECTIONS

MEASLES

Occurrence:	Worldwide
Organism:	Measles virus
Reservoir:	Humans
Transmission:	Droplets, air-borne, contact
Control:	Active immunization with live attenuated virus
	Improvement in the nutrition of the children
	Vitamin A supplementation

Measles is an acute communicable disease which presents with fever, signs of inflammation of the respiratory tract (coryza, cough), and a characteristic skin rash. The presence of punctate lesions (Koplik's spots) on the buccal mucosa may assist diagnosis in the early prodromal phase. Deaths occur mainly from complications such as secondary bacterial infection, with bronchopneumonia and skin sepsis. Post-measles encephalitis occurs in a few cases.

The incubation period is usually about 10 days, at which stage the patient presents with the prodromal features of fever and coryza. The skin rash usually appears 3–4 days after the onset of symptoms. The aetiological agent is the measles virus.

Epidemiology

Measles is a familiar childhood infection in most parts of the world. Until recent years there were a few isolated communities in which the infection was unknown, but the disease is endemic in virtually all parts of the world.

RESERVOIR AND TRANSMISSION

Humans are the reservoir of infection. Transmission is by droplets or by contact with sick children or with freshly contaminated articles such as toys or handkerchiefs.

HOST FACTORS

The outcome of measles infection is largely determined by host factors, in particular the state of nutrition of the child. Measles tends to be a severe killing disease in malnourished children; the infection not infrequently precipitates severe protein-calorie malnutrition ('kwashiorkor'). It has been shown that measles has an immunosuppressive effect. One attack confers lifelong immunity. Babies are usually immune during the first few months of life through the transplacental transmission of passive immunity from immune mothers.

The disease tends to occur in epidemic waves; in some areas, large epidemics occur on alternate years in densely populated urban areas but at longer intervals in sparsely populated rural areas: the explosive outbreaks seem to occur only when there has been a sufficient accumulation of susceptible children.

Laboratory diagnosis

Serological tests show a four-fold rise in antibody titres of haemagglutination-inhibiting (HI) and neutralizing (N) antibodies, between acute and convalescent sera. A capture antibody assay for measles IgM antibodies has a high sensitivity and specificity. Polymerase chain reaction (PCR) assays can detect virus from urine specimens.

Control

Isolation of children who have measles is of limited value in the control of the infection because the disease is highly infectious in the prodromal coryzal phase before the characteristic rash appears. Thus, often by the time a diagnosis of measles is made or even suspected, a number of contacts would have been exposed to infection.

ACTIVE IMMUNIZATION

The best means of reducing the incidence of measles is by having an immune population. Children should be vaccinated at 8 months, with one dose of live attenuated measles virus vaccine. The protection conferred appears to be durable (12 years).

During shipment and storage, prior to reconstitution, freeze-dried measles vaccine must be kept at a temperature between 2 and 8°C and must be protected from light. Using revised immunization strategies, some WHO regions have set goals for the elimination of measles by 2010.

PASSIVE IMMUNIZATION

Measles infection may be prevented or modified by artificial passive immunization using immune gamma globulin. If the gamma globulin (0.25 ml/kg) is given early, within 3 days of exposure, the infection will be prevented; if a smaller dose (0.05 ml/kg) is given 4–6 days after exposure, the infection may be modified, the child presenting with a mild infection which confers lasting immunity. Since passive immunity by itself gives only transient protection, it is more desirable to achieve a modified attack rather than complete suppression of the infection unless the presence of some other serious condition in the child absolutely contraindicates even a mild attack. (For the new strategy on vaccination see p. 174.)

RUBELLA ('GERMAN MEASLES')

Occurrence:	Worldwide
Organism:	Rubella virus
Reservoir:	Humans
Transmission:	Droplets, contact (direct, indirect)
Control:	Active immunization
	Passive immunization if exposed during pregnancy

Rubella or German measles is an acute viral infection which presents with fever, mild upper respiratory symptoms, a morbiliform or scarlatiniform rash and lymphadenopathy usually affecting postauricular, postcervical and suboccipital lymph nodes. The illness is almost always mild, but infection with rubella during the first trimester of pregnancy is associated with a high risk (up to 20%) of congenital abnormalities in the baby.

The incubation period is 2–3 weeks. The aetiological agent is the rubella virus.

Epidemiology

Rubella has a worldwide distribution. Humans are the reservoir of infection which is spread from person to person by droplets or by contact, direct or through contamination of fomites. Infection results in lifelong immunity. Infection during early pregnancy may cause such abnormalities as cataract, deaf mutism and congenital heart disease in the baby.

Laboratory diagnosis

Clinical differentiation from other mild exanthematous fever may be difficult or impossible. Serological methods will detect a rise in antibody concentration. Specific IgM antibodies and M-antibody capture assays are preferred.

Control

The main interest is to prevent the infection of women who are in the early stages of pregnancy, and thus avoid the risk of rubella-induced foetal injury. One practical approach is the deliberate exposure of prepubertal girls to infection with rubella or vaccinating them with a single dose of vaccine. Pregnant women should avoid exposure to rubella, especially during the first 4 months of pregnancy; those who have been in contact with the disease should be protected with human immunoglobulin.

MUMPS

Occurrence:	Worldwide
Organism:	Mumps virus
Reservoir:	Humans
Transmission:	Droplets and contact
Control:	Isolation of cases
	Active immunization of susceptible groups

This is an acute viral infection which typically affects salivary glands, especially the parotids, but may also involve the submandibular or the sublingual salivary glands. Pancreatitis, orchitis, inflammation of the ovaries or meningo-encephalitis may complicate the infection; some of the complications occasionally occur in the absence of obvious clinical symptoms or signs of salivary gland infection.

The incubation period varies from 2 to 4 weeks; usually it is about 21 weeks. The infectious agent is the mumps virus.

Epidemiology

Mumps has a worldwide distribution.

RESERVOIR

Humans are the reservoir of infection. The virus is present in the saliva of infected persons; it may be isolated as early as 1 week before clinical signs occur, and it may persist for 9 days after the onset of signs. Healthy carriers, who remain asymptomatic throughout the infection, may also transmit the infection. The source of infection therefore, includes sick patients, incubatory ('precocious') carriers and healthy carriers.

TRANSMISSION

The infection is transmitted by droplets or by contact, directly or indirectly, through fomites.

HOST FACTORS

One infection, whether clinical or subclinical, confers lifelong immunity. Artificial active immunization with live or inactivated vaccine provides protection for a limited period of a few years.

Laboratory diagnosis

The typical case can be identified clinically but confirmation of diagnosis may be required in atypical cases. Serological tests (haemagglutination, neutralization and complement-fixation) are available; the organism may be cultured from saliva, blood or cerebrospinal fluid.

Control

INDIVIDUAL

The sick patient should be isolated, if possible, during the infectious phase; strict hygienic measures should be observed in the cleansing of spoons, cups and other utensils handled by the patient, and also in the disposal of his or her soiled handkerchiefs and other linen.

VACCINATION

A live mumps virus vaccine is available. Vaccination is of value in protecting susceptible young persons in residential institutions in which epidemics occur frequently. It has proved very effective in controlling mumps in the USA. A combined vaccine for measles, mumps and rubella is available (MMR). Fears for the use of this vaccine seem unjustified on present evidence.

INFLUENZA

Occurrence:	Worldwide local endemic/epidemic picture; massive pandemics
Organism:	Influenza viruses (A, B, C)
Reservoir:	Humans
Transmission:	Air-borne, contact
Control:	Killed vaccine (identical antigenic strain)

This is an acute respiratory infection that is characterized by systemic manifestations – fever, rigors, headache, malaise and muscle pains, and by local manifestations of coryza, sore throat and cough. Secondary bacterial pneumonia is an important complication. The case fatality rate is low but deaths tend to occur in debilitated persons, those with underlying cardiac, respiratory or renal disease, and in the elderly.

The incubation period is usually 1–3 days.

Virology

There are three main types of the influenza virus – influenza A, B and C; A and B types consist of several serological strains. An important feature of the epidemiology of influenza is the periodic emergence of new antigenically distinct strains which account for massive pandemics. Most epidemic strains belong to type A. They have been recovered from various types of animals and birds which may well act as important sources of new strains showing major antigenic changes (antigenic shift). Pandemics may originate where there is close contact between humans and animals. Sporadic cases and limited outbreaks occur annually throughout the world and are the result of progressive, minor antigenic change (antigenic drift).

Laboratory diagnosis

The virus can be isolated on culture of throat washings. Serological tests include complement-fixation and haemagglutination tests; these can be performed on sera of acute and convalescent patients to show the rising titre of antibodies. Enzyme immunoassays (EIAs) rapidly diagnose type A influenza while PCR can detect influenza virus RNA in clinical specimens.

Epidemiology

Massive epidemics of influenza periodically sweep throughout the world with attack rates as high as 50% in some countries. The pandemic may first appear in a specific focus (Asiatic 'flu, Hong Kong 'flu) from which it spreads from continent to continent. Rapid air travel has facilitated the global dissemination of this infection.

RESERVOIR AND TRANSMISSION

Humans are the reservoir of infection of human strains of the influenza virus. The infection is transmitted by droplets, and also by contact, both direct and indirect, through the handling of contaminated articles.

HOST FACTORS

All age groups are susceptible, but if the particular strain causing an epidemic is antigenically related to the cause of an earlier epidemic, the older age group with persisting antibodies may be less susceptible.

Deaths occur mostly in cases with some underlying debilitating disease.

Control

Active immunization with inactivated influenza virus protects against infection with that specific strain. Polyvalent vaccines are also available but they are only effective if they contain the antigens of the particular strain causing the epidemic. Sometimes, it may be possible to prepare vaccine from strains that are isolated early in the epidemic for use in other areas or countries which have not been affected. Based on serological surveys and antigenic analysis WHO recommends vaccine formulations on a year to year basis. WHO collaborating centres are strategically placed in various countries in the world. The vaccine is especially recommended for the elderly and other vulnerable groups, for example, chronic lung disease.

ACUTE UPPER RESPIRATORY TRACT INFECTION

Occurrence:	Worldwide
Organisms:	Rhinoviruses, reoviruses, some enteroviruses, etc.
Reservoir:	Humans
Transmission:	Air-borne, contact
Control:	Avoid exposure of young children to infected persons

Acute infection of the upper respiratory tract is a common but mainly benign disease. The most typical manifestation, 'the common cold', presents with coryza, irritation of the throat, lacrimation and mild constitutional upset. Local complications may occur with secondary bacterial infection and involvement of the paranasal sinuses and the middle ear. Infection may spread to the larynx, trachea and bronchi.

The incubation period is from 1 to 3 days.

Microbiology

These symptoms can be induced by infection with various viral agents, including the rhinoviruses, certain enteroviruses, influenza, para-influenza, adenoviruses, reoviruses and the respiratory syncitial virus. Superinfection with various bacteria may determine the clinical picture in the later stages of the illness.

Laboratory diagnosis

Some of the viruses can be isolated from the throat washings or stool but this diagnostic test is not routinely done.

Epidemiology

Humans are the reservoir of these infections. Transmission is by air-borne spread, or by contact both direct and indirect (contaminated toys, handkerchiefs, etc.). All age groups are susceptible but the manifestations and complications tend to be severe in young children. Repeated attacks are very common. Epidemics occur commonly in households, offices, schools and in other groups having close contact.

Control

No specific control measures are available. Infected persons should avoid contact with others. The exposure of young persons to infected persons should be avoided if possible.

INFECTIOUS MONONUCLEOSIS

Occurrence:	Worldwide
Organism:	Epstein–Barr virus
Reservoir:	Humans
Transmission:	Air-borne, contact
Control:	No effective measures

This is an acute febrile illness which is characterized by lymphadenopathy ('glandular fever'), splenomegaly, sore throat and lymphocytosis. A skin rash and small mucosal lesions may be present. Occasionally, jaundice and rarely meningoencephalitis may occur.

The incubation period is from about 4 days to 2 weeks.

The causative agent is the Epstein–Barr virus, which is also associated with Burkitt's lymphoma.

Laboratory diagnosis

In the acute phase, there is marked leucocytosis mainly due to an increase in monocytes and large lymphocytes. The presence of IgM antibodies to viral capsid antigen provides the most reliable diagnostic test. The rapid screening Monospot test is also reliable.

Epidemiology

Isolated cases and epidemics of the disease have been reported from most parts of the world.

Humans are presumed to be the reservoir of infection, with saliva being regarded as the most likely source of infection. Transmission may be air-borne or by person to person occurring in closed institutions for young adults; there is some suggestion that kissing may be an important route. Infection occurs mostly in children and young adults. It is uncommon in developing countries.

Control

No satisfactory control measures are available. For SARS see page 174.

BACTERIAL INFECTIONS

TUBERCULOSIS

Occurrence:	Worldwide
Organism:	*Mycobacterium tuberculosis* (human and bovine strains)
Reservoir:	Humans, cattle
Transmission:	Air-borne droplets, droplets nuclei and dust
	Milk and infected meat
Control:	General improvement in housing
	Nutrition and personal hygiene
	Immunization with BCG
	Chemoprophylaxis
	Case finding and treatment, DOTS

Tuberculosis remains one of the major health problems in many tropical countries; in some countries the situation is being aggravated by dense overcrowding in urban slums. An estimated 8–10 million people develop overt tuberculosis annually as a result of primary infection, endogenous reactivation or exogenous reinfection. The worst affected country is India which is estimated to have 30% of the world's cases of TB and 37% of the deaths from TB (Plate 51).

The coexistence of HIV infection and tuberculosis has been hailed as one of the most serious threats to human health since the Black Death and has been labelled 'the cursed duet' (Plate 52). Drug-resistant tuberculosis is on the increase in many countries of the world.

Tuberculosis presents a wide variety of clinical forms, but pulmonary involvement is common and is most important epidemiologically as it is primarily responsible for the transmission of the infection.

Primary complex

On first infection, the patient develops the primary complex which consists of a small parenchymal lesion and involvement of the regional lymph node; in the lungs, this constitutes the classical Ghon focus, with a small lung lesion and invasion of the mediastinal lymph node. In most cases the primary complex heals spontaneously, with fibrosis and calcification of the lesions, but the organisms may persist for many years within this focus.

Early complications

In a small proportion of cases the primary complex progresses to produce more severe manifestations locally (e.g. caseous pneumonia) or there may be haematogenous dissemination to other parts of the body. Thus within a few years of the primary infection, especially during the first 6 months, there is the danger of haematogenous spread either focal (e.g. bone and joint lesions) or disseminated (in the form of miliary tuberculosis and tuberculosis meningitis).

Secondary infection

Apart from the primary complex and its early complications, the 'adult' pulmonary form of tuberculosis may occur either as a result of the reactivation of an existing lesion or by exogenous re-infection. Destruction of the lung parenchyma, with fibrosis and cavitation are important features of this adult form. Clinically, it may present with cough, haemoptysis and chest pain, with general constitutional symptoms – fever, loss of weight and malaise; often it remains virtually asymptomatic especially in the early stages.

The incubation period is from 4 to 6 weeks.

Bacteriology

The causative agent is *Mycobacterium tuberculosis*, the tubercle bacillus. The human type produces most of the pulmonary lesions, also some extra-pulmonary lesions; the bovine strain of the organism mainly accounts for extrapulmonary lesions. Other types of *M. tuberculosis* (avian and atypical strains) rarely cause disease in humans, but infection may produce immunological changes, with a non-specific tuberculin skin reaction.

Tubercle bacilli survive for long periods in dried sputum and dust.

Laboratory diagnosis

The organism may be identified on examination of sputum and other pathological specimens (cerebrospinal fluid, urine, pleural fluid or gastric washings). The tubercle bacillus is Gram-positive, but because of its waxy coat it does not stain with the standard procedure. It is usually demonstrated by the Ziehl–Neelsen method, using hot carbolfuchsin stain; the tubercle bacillus like other mycobacteria resists decolorization with acid ('acid fast bacilli') but unlike the others it is also not decolorized by alcohol ('acid and alcohol fast').

The organism can be isolated on culture using special media, or by inoculation into guinea pigs. Radiometric and DNA amplification by PCR are available in special centres.

Tuberculin test

With the first infection with *M. tuberculosis,* the host develops hypersensitivity to the organism; this hypersensitivity is the basis of various tuberculin skin tests. The material used may be a concentrated filtrate of broth in which tubercle bacilli have been grown for 6 weeks ('old tuberculin') or a chemical fraction, the purified protein derivative (PPD). The skin reaction to tuberculin is of the delayed hypersensitivity type, and the tuberculin test result is usually read in 48 or 72 hours. In the Mantoux test, the material is injected intradermally, a positive reaction being denoted by an induration of 10 mm diameter or larger in response to five tuberculin units. The tuberculin test can also be performed using the Heaf gun.

The tuberculin test usually becomes positive 4–6 weeks after primary infection with tubercle bacilli; and after BCG immunization other mycobacteria may produce cross-sensitivity. A negative reaction usually indicates that the patient has had no previous exposure to tubercle bacilli but occasionally the test is negative in patients with overwhelming infection or in certain conditions which suppress the allergic response, for example measles, sarcoidosis.

The tuberculin test can be used in various ways:

- *Clinical diagnosis* – the tuberculin test is usually positive in infected persons, and tends to be strongly positive in cases of active disease. In previously unexposed health workers seroconversion from negative to positive may be used as an indication of disease.
- *Identifying susceptible groups* – a negative reaction usually indicates that the person has had no previous exposure to tuberculous infection and therefore, no acquired immunity.
- *Epidemiological surveys* – to determine the pattern of infection and immunity in the community.

Epidemiology

Tuberculosis has a worldwide distribution. Until recently, it was absent from a few isolated communities where the local populations are now showing widespread infections with severe manifestations on first contact with tuberculosis.

RESERVOIR

Humans are the reservoir of the human strain and patients with pulmonary infection constitute the main source of infection.

The reservoir of the bovine strain is cattle, with infected milk and meat being the main sources of infection.

TRANSMISSION

Transmission of infection is mainly air-borne by droplets, droplet nuclei and dust; thus it is enhanced by overcrowding in poorly ventilated accommodation. Infection may also occur by ingestion, especially of contaminated milk and infected meat.

HOST FACTORS

The host response is an important factor in the epidemiology of tuberculosis. A primary infection may heal, the host acquiring immunity in the process. In some cases the primary lesion progresses to produce extensive disease locally, or infection may disseminate to produce metastatic or miliary lesions. Lesions that are apparently healed may subsequently break down with reactivation of disease. Certain factors such as malnutrition, measles infection and HIV infection, use of corticosteriods and other debilitating conditions predispose to progression and reactivation of the disease.

Control

In planning a programme for the control of tuberculosis, the entire population can be conveniently considered as falling into four groups:

- *No previous exposure to tubercle bacilli* – they would require protection from infection.
- *Healed primary infection* – they have some immunity but must be protected from reactivation of disease and reinfection.
- *Diagnosed active disease* – they must have effective treatment and remain under supervision until they have recovered fully.
- *Undiagnosed active disease* – without treatment the disease may progress with further irreversible damage. As potential sources of infection, they constitute a danger to the community.

The control of tuberculosis can be considered at the following levels of prevention:

- general health promotion;
- specific protection – active immunization, chemoprophylaxis, control of animal reservoir;
- early diagnosis and treatment;
- limitation of disability;
- rehabilitation;
- surveillance.

GENERAL HEALTH PROMOTION

Improvement in housing (good ventilation, avoidance of overcrowding) will reduce the chances of air-borne infections. Health education should be directed at producing better personal habits with regard to spitting and coughing. Good nutrition enhances host immunity.

SPECIFIC PROTECTION

Three measures are available: (i) active immunization with BCG (Bacille Calmette Guerin);

(ii) chemoprophylaxis; and (iii) control of animal tuberculosis.

BCG vaccination

This vaccine contains live attenuated tubercle bacilli of the bovine strain. It may be administered intradermally by syringe and needle or by the multiple-puncture technique. It confers significant but not absolute immunity; in particular, it protects against the disseminated miliary lesions of tuberculosis and tuberculous meningitis.

Immunization strategy

BCG vaccination may be used selectively in tuberculin-negative persons who are at high risk, for example close contacts, doctors, nurses and hospital ward attendants. A strain of BCG that is resistant to isoniazid has been developed; this can be used in vaccinating tuberculosis contacts who require immediate protection with isoniazid. BCG may also be used more widely in immunizing tuberculin-negative persons, especially children, in the community. In some developing countries where preliminary tuberculin testing may significantly reduce coverage, BCG may be administered in mass campaigns without tuberculin tests. The disadvantage of this method of 'direct BCG vaccination' is that those who are tuberculin-positive are likely to show more severe local reactions at the site of vaccination.

BCG vaccination of the new-born is widely practised in the tropics. Overall, the evidence suggests that it confers considerable protection against tuberculosis in infants and young children. The strategy introduced recently in expanded immunization programmes, is to give BCG vaccination a few months after birth. The implications of this different timing have yet to be assessed.

Disadvantages

Various complications have been encountered in the use of BCG. These may be:

- *local* – chronic ulceration, discharge, abscess formation and keloids;
- *regional* – adenitis which may or may not suppurate or form sinuses;
- *disseminated* – a rare complication.

The protective efficacy of BCG vaccine has varied considerably in different countries.

Chemoprophylaxis

Isoniazid has proved an effective prophylactic agent in preventing infection and progression of infection to severe disease.

Treatment with isoniazid for 1 year is recommended for the following groups:

- close contacts of patients;
- persons who have converted from tuberculin-negative to tuberculin-positive in the previous year;
- children under 3 years who are tuberculin-positive from naturally acquired infection.

The tuberculin-negative person may be protected by BCG or isoniazid, the decision as to which method to use would depend on local factors, the acceptability of regular drug therapy, and the availability of effective supervision.

Control of bovine tuberculosis

The ideal is to maintain herds that are free of tuberculosis. Infected animals can be identified by the tuberculin skin test and eliminated. Milk, especially from herds that are not certified tuberculosis free, should be pasteurized. After slaughter, carcasses of cattle should be examined for signs of tuberculosis. Such infected meat should be condemned.

EARLY DIAGNOSIS AND TREATMENT

Case-finding operations should aim at identifying active cases at an early stage of the disease. This would depend on maintaining a high index of suspicion in clinical practice and carrying out routine screening, especially of high-risk groups.

Screening

Screening methods include tuberculin testing, sputum and chest X-ray examination.

- *Tuberculin test*. The interpretation of the tuberculin test would depend on local epidemiological factors.
- *Sputum*. Microscopic examination of Ziehl–Neelsen stained smears of sputum is a simple cheap screening technique which is particularly useful in rural areas of developing countries where resources are limited.
- *Chest X-ray*. Mass miniature radiography (MMR) has been widely applied and has been particularly valuable in detecting presymptomatic

disease, but it is: (i) relatively expensive to establish and run; (ii) it requires highly trained personnel; and (iii) it has little specificity, showing many lesions that are definitely non-tuberculous or of doubtful origin. WHO no longer recommends its routine use for screening.

High-risk and special groups that should be screened include:

- contacts of tuberculous patients (both household contacts and workmates);
- persons who have cough persisting for 3 weeks or more;
- workers in hospitals and sanatoria;
- teachers, food handlers and other persons who come into contact with the public;
- immigrants from high-incidence regions;
- residents in common lodging houses.

DRUG TREATMENT

WHO recommends the short course directly observed therapy (DOTS). This consists of 2 months of isoniazid, rifampicin, pyrazanimide and ethambutol given daily, followed by 4 months of isoniazid and rifampicin given thrice weekly.

As part of the DOTS strategy, health workers counsel and observe their patients swallowing each dose, and the health service monitors the patients' progress until each is cured. Political and financial commitments and a dependable drug supply are essential parts of the DOTS strategy.

Despite the fact that DOTS is very cost-effective ($20 for 6 months of medicines), not all endemic countries have adopted it yet. In terms of disability-adjusted life years (DALYs), treatment of smear-positive cases of TB with DOTS works out at $3 per DALY saved – a very effective intervention. The DOTS strategy is being reviewed and may be modified in the future. An urgent need for new effective anti-tuberculous drugs exists.

LIMITATION OF DISABILITY

Apart from early diagnosis and effective drug treatment, steps should be taken to limit the physical, mental and social disability associated with the disease. The physical aspect may require active physiotherapy, for example breathing exercises, appropriate body exercises and support for diseased bones and joints. The mental disability may be limited by suitable diversional or occupational therapy and by simple reassurance or more expert psychotherapy.

REHABILITATION

This should, as always, commence from the beginning of the treatment of the patient. Most patients recover sufficiently well to return to their former occupation. Where chronic physical disability is unavoidable, the patient can be retrained for alternative employment.

Careful health education of relatives and the community by breaking down prejudices will assist the rehabilitation of patients.

SURVEILLANCE OF TUBERCULOSIS

For effective control of tuberculosis, there should be a surveillance system to collect, evaluate and analyse all pertinent data, and use such knowledge to plan and evaluate the control programme. The sources of data will include:

- notification of cases;
- investigation of contacts, post-mortem reports;
- special surveys – tuberculin, sputum, chest X-ray;
- laboratory reports on isolation of organisms including the pattern of drug sensitivity;
- records of BCG immunization – routine and mass programmes;
- housing, especially data about overcrowding;
- data about tuberculosis in cattle;
- utilization of antituberculous drugs.

Stop TB Initiative

Recognizing that TB was one of the most neglected health problems and that the TB epidemic was out of control in many of the developing countries of the world, TB was declared by WHO to be a global emergency in April 1993.

The STOP TB Initiative is based at WHO, and is a partnership of countries where TB is a serious problem, including UN and other international organizations, bilateral donors, scientific and public health institutions and NGOs.

Its main thrust is to promote the use of the cost effective Directly Observed Treatment, Short Course (DOTS); increase political commitment, guarantee adequate financing and human resources; improve organization and management capacity and ensure uninterrupted supplies of high-quality anti-TB drugs. A ministerial conference for 20 of the world's highest TB burden countries was held in Amsterdam in March 2000 and all signed a declaration to stop TB.

WHO TB CONTROL POLICY PACKAGE

This includes the following four elements: (i) government commitment; (ii) case detection through predominantly positive case finding; (iii) administration of DOTS to at least all confirmed sputum smear positive cases of TB; and (iv) establishment and maintenance of a monitoring system to be used for programme supervision and evaluation.

Key operations of a national TB programme (NTP)

All countries where TB is a public health problem should establish a national TB programme, the key specifics of which are:

- establishment of a central unit to guarantee the political and operational support for the various levels of the programme;
- prepare a programme manual;
- establish a seconding and reporting system;
- initiate a training programme;
- establish microscopy services;
- establish treatment services;
- secure a regular supply of drugs and diagnostic material;
- design a plan of supervision;
- prepare a project development plan.

The overall objective is to reduce mortality, morbidity and transmission of TB until it is no longer a threat to public health as speedily as possible.

Constraints in meeting targets are: (i) lack of political will and commitment; (ii) inadequate financial resources; (iii) insufficient skilled human resources; (iv) interruption of drug supplies; and (v) prevalence of HIV and emergence of multidrug resistance.

PNEUMONIAS

A variety of organisms may cause acute infection of the lungs. The non-tuberculous pneumonias are usually classified into three groups:

- pneumococcal;
- other bacterial;
- atypical.

Pneumococcal pneumonia

Occurrence:	Worldwide; epidemics occur in work camps, prisons
Organism:	*Streptococcus pneumoniae*
Reservoir:	Humans
Transmission:	Droplets, dust, air-borne contact, fomites
Control:	Avoid overcrowding
	Good ventilation
	Improve personal hygiene (spitting, coughing)
	Chemoprophylaxis to control institutional outbreaks
	Vaccination

Pneumococcal infection of the lungs characteristically produces lobar consolidation but bronchopneumonia may occur in susceptible groups. Typically, the untreated case resolves by crisis, but with antibiotic treatment there is usually a rapid response. Metastatic lesions may occur in the meninges, brain, heart valves, pericardium or joints. Pneumonia and bronchopneumonia are two of the major causes of death in the tropics, especially in children.

The incubation period is 1–3 days. The disease is usually notifiable.

BACTERIOLOGY

The aetiological agent is *Streptococcus pneumoniae*, a Gram-positive, lancet-shaped diplococcal organism. It is enveloped in a polysaccharide capsule. There are 83 serotypes of pneumococcus, the lower-numbered serotypes are most frequently responsible for disease. In Papua New Guinea, which has a high rate of pneumococcal disease, serotypes 2, 3, 5, 8 and 14 are most commonly identified.

EPIDEMIOLOGY

The disease has a worldwide distribution.

Reservoir

Humans are the reservoir of infection; this includes sick patients as well as carriers.

Transmission

Transmission is by air-borne infection and droplets, by direct contact or through contaminated articles. Pneumococcus may persist in the dust for some time.

Host factors

All ages are susceptible, but the clinical manifestations are most severe at the extremes of age. Negroes seem to be more susceptible than Caucasians.

Pneumonia may complicate viral infection of the respiratory tract. Exposure, fatigue, alcohol and pregnancy apparently lower resistance to this infection. On recovery, there is some immunity to the homologous type.

Epidemics of pneumococcal pneumonia occur in prisons, barracks and work camps, for example South African gold miners.

LABORATORY DIAGNOSIS

The organism may be recovered on culture of the sputum, material from a throat swab and, less commonly, the blood. The specific type can be identified by direct serological testing of the sputum or, later, the organisms isolated on culture. Countercurrent immunoelectrophaesis (CIE), latex agglutination and ELISA are all reliable tests.

CONTROL

S. pneumoniae generally responds well to penicillin but strains with intermediate resistance occur and strains with high resistance have been isolated (Plate 53).

The general measures for the prevention of respiratory infections apply – avoidance of overcrowding, good ventilation and improved personal hygiene with regard to coughing and spitting. Prompt treatment of cases with antibiotics penicillin, cephalosporins, vancomycin would prevent complications. Chemoprophylaxis with penicillin is indicated in cases of outbreaks in institutions. A polyvalent polysaccharide vaccine is available and has been successfully used in children with sickle cell disease. It is not effective in children under 2 years.

Other bacterial pneumonias

Occurrence:	Worldwide
Organisms:	*Mycoplasma pneumoniae,*
	Staphylococcus aureus,
	Legionella pneumophila,
	Chlamydia pneumoniae,
	Haemophilus influenzae

Reservoir:	Humans
Transmission:	Air-borne, contact
Control:	Prevention and treatment of respiratory disease
	Improvement in housing conditions

The other bacteria which can cause pneumonia include: *Staphylococcus aureus, Chlamydia pneumoniae, Haemophilus influenzae, Legionella pneumophila, Mycoplasma pneumoniae* and *Chlamydia psittaci* (a zoonotic infection – see below).

Although in some cases one particular organism predominates, it is not unusual to encounter mixed infections, especially in persons with chronic lung disorders. The organisms can be isolated on culture of the sputum or occasionally from blood.

EPIDEMIOLOGY

These infections have a worldwide distribution and the organisms are commonly found in humans and their environment. Transmission is by droplets, air-borne infection and contact.

Host factors

The occurrence of infection is largely determined by host factors such as the presence of viral infection of the respiratory tract (e.g. influenza, measles) or debilitating illness (e.g. diabetes, chronic renal failure). Patients suffering from chronic bronchitis are particularly susceptible.

CONTROL

The frequency of these bacterial pneumonias can be diminished by:

1 The prevention or prompt treatment of respiratory disease:
   - viral infection (e.g. measles and influenza vaccination);
   - upper respiratory infection (especially in children and the elderly);
   - chronic lung disease (especially chronic bronchitis).
2 Improvement in housing conditions.

Psittacosis

Occurrence:	Worldwide
Organism:	*Chlamydia psittaci*
Reservoir:	Birds (e.g. parrots)
Transmission:	Air-borne; person to person contact
Control:	Quarantine of imported birds Antibiotic therapy to eliminate carriers Destruction of infected birds

This may present as an acute severe pneumonia that may prove fatal, but mild, subclinical infections do occur. The incubation period is about 4–14 days. The causative agent is *Chlamydia psittaci*.

The organism may be isolated on culture of sputum, blood or vomitus, on yolk sacs of embryonated eggs or by inoculation into mice.

Serological tests on paired sera may show rising titres in complement fixing, neutralization or agglutination tests.

EPIDEMIOLOGY

The distribution of the disease in humans is determined by infection in parrots, budgerigars and other psittacine birds. These birds are found in Australia, Africa and South America, but may be imported as pets to other parts of the world.

Reservoir

Psittacosis is basically a zoonotic infection of birds. The affected birds excrete the organisms in their faeces, and through the respiratory tract.

Transmission

Humans acquire the infection by inhalation of the infective agent from bird faeces; those who own and handle such birds are at high risk. Person to person spread may occur in close contacts.

CONTROL

The importation of these birds should be strictly controlled. They can be held in quarantine to ensure that they are free from infection; infected birds can also be detected by serological tests. Broad-spectrum antibiotics, for example tetracycline, can be used to eliminate the carrier state. In case of human infection, the source of infection should be traced and the bird destroyed.

Mycoplasma pneumoniae

Occurrence:	Worldwide
Organism:	*Mycoplasma pneumoniae*
Reservoir:	Humans
Transmission:	Droplets, contact
Control:	General measures for controlling respiratory infection Treatment of patients with tetracycline

This is an acute febrile illness usually starting with signs of an upper respiratory infection, later spreading to the bronchi and lungs.

Radiological examination of the lungs shows hazy patchy infiltration.

The incubation period is usually about 12 days, ranging from 7 to 21 days. The infective agent is *Mycoplasma pneumoniae* (pleuro-pneumonia-like organism).

EPIDEMIOLOGY

The geographical distribution is worldwide. Humans are the reservoir of infection. It is transmitted from sick patients as well as from persons with subclinical infection. Transmission is by droplet infection and by contact. Only a small proportion of infected persons (1 in 30) show signs of illness. After recovery, the patient is immune for an undefined period. *M. pneumoniae* spreads easily in institutions such as schools, and military units, the highest incidence is in under 20-year-olds.

LABORATORY DIAGNOSIS

The diagnosis can be established by showing a rising complement fixation titre of antibodies to *M. pneumoniae*. The organism can also be identified by collecting sputum or throat washings at an early stage of the infection, using antigen capture enzyme immunoassay, PCR or detection of ribosomal RNA genes. A useful bedside test is the presence of cold agglutinins which first appear 7–9 days after infection with a peak after 4–6 weeks.

CONTROL

General measures for the control of respiratory diseases apply (see p. 154). Treatment with tetracycline is advocated in cases of pneumonia.

Legionella pneumophila

This organism was named after an epidemic occurred in legionnaires attending a conference in Philadelphia and resulted in a pneumonia-like disease – Legionnaires' disease.

Legionella survive in water for long periods – air-conditioning equipment, shower heads and hot water taps spread the disease. The most important preventative measure is to render water sources safe, for example hospital cooling towers and water supplies by hyperchlorination or heating. Pneumonia is the second most common nosocomial infection after urinary tract infection.

MENINGOCOCCAL INFECTION

Occurrence:	Worldwide; epidemics: 'meningitis belt' of tropical Africa, recruits in military barracks
Organism:	Neisseria meningitidis
Reservoir:	Humans
Transmission:	Air-borne, droplets, direct contact
Control:	Treatment of patients and contacts
	Avoid overcrowding
	Mass immunization
	Surveillance

A variety of clinical manifestations may be produced when human beings are infected with Neisseria meningitidis: the typical clinical picture is of acute pyogenic meningitis with fever, headache, nausea and vomiting, neck stiffness, loss of consciousness and a characteristic petechial rash is often present. The wide spectrum of clinical manifestations ranges from fulminating disease with shock and circulatory collapse to relatively mild meningococcaemia without meningitis presenting as a febrile illness with a rash. The carrier state is common.

The incubation period is usually 3–4 days, but may be 2–10 days.

Bacteriology

N. meningitidis (meningococcus) is a Gram-negative, bean-shaped, diplococcal organism. It is differentiated from other neisserial organisms, including the commensal N. catarrhalis, by fermentation reactions. Several major antigenic strains (A, B, C, W-135, X and Y) have been identified on serological testing. In the 'meningitis belt' of Africa, type A is the major causative agent of most epidemics but outbreaks due to type C have also occurred.

Epidemiology (Plate 54)

There is a worldwide distribution of this infection. Sporadic cases and epidemics occur in most parts of the world, in particular South America and the Middle East, but also in the developed countries of the temperate zone. Massive epidemics occur periodically in the so-called 'meningitis belt' of tropical Africa, a zone lying 5–15′N of the equator and characterized by annual rainfall between 300 and 1100 mm. In this zone, the epidemic comes in waves: the outbreaks usually begin in the dry season, reaching a peak at the end of the dry season, and end sharply at the onset of the rains. However, in 1989 an epidemic of meningitis due to N. meningitis type A occurred during the rainy season in Tanzania (which is outside the meningitis belt). A major outbreak was anticipated in Ethiopia in 2000 and 1 million people were vaccinated, thus aborting the epidemic (Plate 55).

RESERVOIR

Humans are the reservoir of infection. Nasopharyngeal carriage ranges from 1 to 50% and is responsible for infection to persist in a community.

TRANSMISSION

Transmission is by air-borne droplets or from a nasopharyngeal carrier or less commonly from a patient through contact with respiratory droplets or oral secretions. It is a delicate organism, dying rapidly on cooling or drying, and thus indirect transmission is not an important route. Travel and migration, large population movements (e.g. pilgrimages – Plate 56), and overcrowding (e.g. slums), facilitate the circulation of virulent strains inside a country or from country to country.

HOST FACTORS

In countries within the meningitis belt the maximum incidence is found in the age group 5–10 years; but in epidemics all age groups may be affected. In institutions such as military barracks, new entrants and recruits usually have higher attack rates than those who have been in long residence.

The genetically determined inability to secrete the water-soluble glycoprotein form of the ABO blood group antigens into saliva and other body fluids, is a recognized risk factor for meningococcal disease. The relative risk of non-secretors developing meningococcal infection was found to be 2.9 in a Nigerian study. The reasons why non-secretors are more susceptible are not known.

Laboratory diagnosis

The organism can be recovered from bacteriological examination of nasopharyngeal swabs, blood and cerebrospinal fluid; Gram stain will reveal the meningococci. The cerebrospinal fluid will, in addition, show the typical changes of pyogenic meningitis: cloudy fluid, numerous pus cells, raised protein content, low or absent glucose. Latex agglutination permits rapid detection of meningococcal antigen while PCR is specific and sensitive.

Control

There are four basic approaches to the control of meningococcal infections:

- the management of sick patients and their contacts;
- environmental control designed to reduce air-borne infections;
- immunization;
- surveillance.

SICK PATIENTS AND THEIR CONTACTS

The most effective and simplest treatment for the individual case is a single injection of 3 g of long-acting chloramphenicol (Tifomycin); long-acting penicillin or, if affordable, ceftriaxone can be used.

To prevent disease among close household contacts rifampicin can be used coupled with immunization (see below), or immunization alone if rifampicin is ruled out because of economic considerations.

Sulphonamide resistance is now so widespread that it is inadvisable to use these drugs either for treatment or prophylactically.

MANAGEMENT OF EPIDEMICS

A number of practical problems have to be solved in dealing with outbreaks of meningitis in rural Africa. The cases tend to overwhelm the local health services and they are usually supplemented by mobile teams which can be organized and rapidly deployed to deal with the emergency. A 'cold chain' must be maintained for storage of the vaccine. In the most peripheral units, the management of cases may have to rely mainly on auxiliary personnel.

COMMUNITY: ENVIRONMENTAL CONTROL

Overcrowding should be avoided in institutions such as schools, boarding-houses and military barracks; the dormitories should be spacious and well-ventilated. In areas where people tend to live in cramped, overcrowded accommodation, they should be advised to sleep out of doors to limit the risk of transmission.

IMMUNIZATION

Groups A, C, W-135 and Y capsular polysaccharide vaccines are available and controlled field trials have demonstrated their effectiveness in many areas. The new meningococcal group C conjugated vaccine is immunogenic in children from 2 months of age, and appears to induce immunological memory so that further boosting is likely not to be needed. The recommended schedule is three doses for children aged 2, 3 and 4 months, two doses for children over 4 months and under 1 year and one dose for all others. Vaccination of large numbers of persons can be accomplished using jet injection guns appropriately. In malarious areas the concomitant use of antimalarial drugs (e.g. single oral dose of four tablets of chloroquine) may enhance the antibody response to the vaccines. Immunization provides the most effective means of controlling an epidemic.

SURVEILLANCE

For the effective control of this disease, a system of epidemiological surveillance must be established. Data derived from treatment centres, hospitals, laboratories and special surveys must be collated, evaluated, analysed and disseminated to those who have to take action in the field. National data on epidemics should be made available to neighbouring states and co-ordinated through the World Health Organization.

In countries where meningitis epidemics are common, an established committee responsible for meningococcal disease should be established and meet at regular intervals to plan control strategies.

The community must be accurately informed about an epidemic in order to avoid panic. For countries in the meningitis belt, a rate of 15 cases per 100 000 per week in a given area, averaged over two consecutive weeks, is indicative of an impending epidemic. Once an epidemic is detected in a given area, 5 cases/100 000 per week is the threshold that can be used for a contiguous area.

STREPTOCOCCAL INFECTIONS

Occurrence:	Worldwide; varying pattern from area to area
Organism:	Streptococcus pyogenes, group A
Reservoir:	Humans
Transmission:	Air-borne, contact or milk-borne
Control:	As for other air-borne infections
	Pasteurization of milk
	Penicillin or sulphonamide prophylaxis

Streptococcus pyogenes, group A haemolytic streptococci can invade various tissues of human skin and subcutaneous tissues, mucous membranes, blood and some deep tissues. The common clinical manifestations of streptococcal infection include streptococcal sore throat, erysipelas, scarlet fever and puerperal fever. Some strains produce an erythrogenic toxin which is responsible for the characteristic erythematous rash of scarlet fever. Rheumatic fever (see below) and acute glomerulonephritis result from allergic reactions to streptococcal infections.

Bacteriology

There are at least 40 serologically distinct types of group A streptococci; some of these specific serological types tend to be associated with particular forms of streptococcal disease, for example type 12, group A is frequently associated with glomerulonephritis. Apart from group A, other groups of streptococci, B, C, D, F and G, have been identified.

Epidemiology

Streptococcal infections have a worldwide occurrence, but the pattern of the distribution of streptococcal disease varies from area to area.

RESERVOIR

Humans are the reservoir of infection; this includes acutely ill and convalescent patients, as well as carriers, especially nasal carriers.

TRANSMISSION

The sources of infection are the infected discharges of sick patients, droplets, dust and fomites. The infection may be air-borne, through droplets, droplet nuclei or dust. It may be spread by contact or through contaminated milk.

HOST FACTORS

Although all age groups are liable to infection, children are particularly susceptible. Repeated attacks of tonsillitis and streptococcal sore throat are common but immunity is acquired to the erythrogenic toxin and thus it is rare to have a second attack of scarlet fever with the scarlatinous rash.

Laboratory diagnosis

The organism can be isolated by culture of bacteriological swabs taken from the throat, nose or pus. The particular group and serological type can be identified from cultures grown on blood agar. Organisms can also be isolated from blood culture. Sera that are elevated above the 'upper limit of normal' are useful in establishing previous streptococcal infection in cases of suspected rheumatic fever or glomerulonephritis. This value varies in different populations. Antigen detection methods are also available.

Control

The general measures for the control of air-borne infections are applicable. In addition, such measures as the pasteurization of milk and aseptic obsteric techniques are of value.

Specific chemoprophylaxis with penicillin is indicated for persons who have had rheumatic fever and for those who are liable to recurrent strepto-coccal skin infections. The penicillin can be given orally in the form of daily doses of penicillin V.

RHEUMATIC FEVER

Occurrence:	Worldwide: declining in developed countries but increasing in some tropical developing countries
Aetiology:	Complication of group A streptococcal throat infection
Reservoir:	Humans
Transmission:	See 'Streptococcal infections'
Control:	Control of streptococcal infections Long-term chemoprophylaxis to prevent recurrences

Rheumatic fever is a complication of infection with group A haemolytic streptococci. The initial infection may present as a sore throat or may be sub-clinical; the onset of rheumatic fever is usually 2–3 weeks after the beginning of the throat infection. Apart from fever, the patient may develop pancar-ditis, arthritis, chorea, subcutaneous nodules and erythema marginatum. Residual damage in the form of chronic valvular heart disease may com-plicate clinical or subclinical cases of rheumatic fever; the complication is more liable to occur after repeated attacks.

Bacteriology and laboratory diagnosis

Group A haemolytic streptococci may be isolated from the bacteriological swab of the throats of some of these patients but not from the heart or the joints, which are not directly invaded by the organism.

Antistreptolysin 0 titres are revised above the 'upper limit of normal'; this figure varies in popu-lations of different ages, in different locations and with different frequencies of streptococcal infec-tion. Nucleic acid probe methods for both group A and B streptococci are now available.

Epidemiology

The disease has a worldwide occurrence. Although there is a falling incidence in the developed countries of the temperate zone, it is becoming a more prominent problem in the overcrowded urban areas of some tropical and subtropical coun-tries, for example in South East Asia and the Middle East.

Rheumatic fever represents an allergic response in a small proportion of persons who have strepto-coccal sore throat. The factors that determine this sensitivity reaction are not known.

Control

The control of rheumatic fever involves the control of streptococcal infections in the community generally and the prevention of recurrences by chemoprophylaxis after recovery from an attack of rheumatic fever.

PERTUSSIS (WHOOPING COUGH)

Occurrence:	Worldwide
Organism:	Bordetella pertussis
Reservoir:	Humans
Transmission:	Air-borne, contact
Control:	Active immunization with killed vaccine

Infection with Bordetella pertussis leads to inflam-mation of the lower respiratory tract from the trachea to the bronchioles. Clinically, the infection is characterized by paroxysmal attacks of violent cough; a rapid succession of coughs typically ends with a characteristic loud, high-pitched inspira-tory crowing sound – the so-called 'whoop'.

The incubation period is usually 7–10 days but may be as long as 3 weeks. The pertussis organism is a Gram-negative rod which can be cultured on blood-enriched media. It can be differentiated by immunological tests from *B. parapertussis,* which produces a similar but milder disease.

Epidemiology

The disease has a worldwide distribution but there is falling morbidity and mortality following immunization programmes. Humans are the reservoir of infection. Transmission of infection may be air-borne or by contact with freshly soiled articles.

Children under 1 year old are highly susceptible and most deaths occur in young infants.

Laboratory diagnosis

The organism can be recovered from infected patients during the early stages of the infection, from nasopharyngeal swabs or from cough plates, followed by culture on special media.

Control

INDIVIDUAL

Sick children should be kept away from susceptible children during the catarrhal phase of the whooping cough; isolation need not be continued beyond 3 weeks because the patient is no longer highly infectious even though the whoop persists.

VACCINATION

Routine active immunization with killed vaccine is highly recommended for all infants. The pertussis vaccine is usually incorporated as a constituent of the triple antigen DPT (diphtheria–pertussis–tetanus), which is used for the immunization of children starting from 2 to 3 months. It provides immunity for about 12 years.

DIPHTHERIA

Occurrence:	Worldwide, but now largely controlled in developed countries except some states of former USSR (Plate 57)
Organism:	*Corynebacterium diphtheriae*
Reservoir:	Humans
Transmission:	Air-borne, contact (direct, indirect), contaminated milk
Control:	Active immunization with toxoid

This disease is caused by infection with *Corynebacterium diphtheriae* (Klebs–Loeffler bacillus). There may be acute infection of the mucous membranes of the tonsils, pharynx, larynx or nose; skin infections may also occur and are of particular importance in tropical countries. Much faucial swelling may be produced by the local inflammatory reaction and the membranous exudate in the larynx may cause respiratory obstruction. The exotoxin which is produced by the organism may cause nerve palsies or myocarditis.

The incubation period is 2–5 days. Diphtheria is usually included in the list of diseases that are notifiable nationally.

Bacteriology

C. diphtheriae is a Gram-positive rod, with a characteristic bipolar metachromatic staining. Virulent strains produce a soluble exotoxin which is responsible for the systemic manifestations and the sequelae of the disease. Three major types, gravis, intermedius and mitis, have been differentiated, as associated with severe, moderately severe and mild clinical manifestations respectively.

Epidemiology

Although there is a worldwide occurrence of the disease, this once common epidemic disease of childhood is now well controlled in most developed countries by routine immunization of infants. There is evidence to suggest that in some parts of the tropics a high proportion of the community acquires immunity through subclinical infections, mainly in the form of cutaneous lesions. Since the acceptance of the expanded programme of immunization by most of the developing countries, the incidence of diphtheria has dropped dramatically.

RESERVOIR

Humans are the reservoir of infection; this includes clinical cases and also carriers.

TRANSMISSION

The infective agents may be discharged from the nose and throat or from skin lesions. The transmission of the infection may be by:

- air-borne infection;
- direct contact;
- indirect contact through fomites;
- ingestion of contaminated raw milk.

HOST FACTORS

All persons are liable to infection but susceptibility to infection may be modified by previous natural exposure to infection and immunization. The newborn baby may be protected for up to 6 months through the transplacental transmission of antibodies from an immune mother.

The most severe illness is associated with faucial or laryngeal infection in children; nasal infections tend to be more chronic and less severe; and the cutaneous lesions which are often not recognized produce immunization of the host with low morbidity.

Susceptibility to infection may be tested by means of the Schick test: a test dose of 0.2 ml of diluted toxin is injected intradermally into one forearm, with a similar injection of toxin, destroyed by heat, into the other forearm to serve as a control. A positive Schick test, consists of an area of redness 1–2 cm diameter at the site of the test dose, reaching its maximum size in 3–4 days, later fading into a brown stain. This positive reaction is confirmed by the absence of reaction at the site of the control injection. Redness at both sides is recorded as a pseudoreaction, and probably represents non-specific sensitivity to some of the protein substances in the injection. A negative Schick test is recorded when there is no redness at either injection site. Both the pseudoreaction and the negative Schick test are accepted as indicating resistance to diphtheria infection. Currently, there are several methods available for assessing levels of circulating diphtheria antibody. Clinical diagnosis can be confirmed by bacteriological examination of swabs of the nose and throat or of skin lesions.

Control

THE INDIVIDUAL

Antitoxin should be given promptly on making the clinical diagnosis and without awaiting laboratory confirmation. Treatment with penicillin or other antibiotics may be given in addition to, but not instead of, serum. The patient should be isolated until throat cultures cease to yield toxigenic strains. However, a patient is expected to be non-contagious within 48 hours of antibiotic administration. Isolation should be maintained until elimination of the organisms is demonstrated by two negative cultures obtained at least 24 hours apart after completion of antimicrobial therapy.

CONTACTS

Non-immune young children who have been in direct contact with the patient should be protected by passive immunization with antitoxic serum and at the same time, active immunization with toxoid is commenced. Susceptible (Schick-positive) adult contacts should be protected with active immunization and a booster dose can be given to immune (Schick-negative) persons. It is now recommended that all close contacts should receive antibiotic prophylaxis to be maintained for a week.

THE COMMUNITY

The search for carriers and their treatment with antibiotics may be indicated in the special circumstances of an outbreak in a closed community such as a boarding school, but the major approach to the control of this infection is routine active immunization of the susceptible population.

ACTIVE IMMUNIZATION

Active immunization with diphtheria toxoid has proved a reliable measure for the control of this infection. It is usually administered in combination with pertussis vaccine and tetanus toxoid (DPT or triple antigen) from the age of 2 to 3 months. A booster dose of diphtheria toxoid is recommended at school entry and this may be given in combination with typhoid vaccine.

The following are the internationally accepted interpretations of the levels of circulating diphtheria toxin antibodies expressed in IU/ml:

<0.01: Susceptible
0.01–0.09: Basic protection
0.1: Full protection
>1.0: Long-term protection

FUNGAL INFECTIONS

HISTOPLASMOSIS

Occurrence:	Parts of America, Africa, Asia and the Pacific
Organism:	*Histoplasma capsulatum*
Reservoir:	Soil, especially those contaminated with bird droppings
Transmission:	Air-borne from spores in soil
Control:	Avoid exposure to infected areas

The classical form of histoplasmosis due to *Histoplasma capsulatum* presents a variety of clinical manifestations. Infection is mostly asymptomatic, being detected only on immunological tests. On first exposure there may be an acute benign respiratory illness, which tends to be self-limiting, healing with or without calcification. Progressive disseminated lesions may occur with widespread involvement of the reticulo-endothelial system; without treatment this form may have a fatal outcome. The incubation period is from 1 to 21 weeks.

H. duboisii, a variant confined to tropical Africa produces distinct clinical and pathological features. Little is known about its reservoir, mode of transmission or other epidemiological factors.

Mycology

The causative agent is *H. capsulatum*, a dimorphic organism (both yeast phase and mycelial phase occur). In the host tissues only the yeast phase is found. Spores can survive in the soil for long periods. They flourish particularly well in soil that is manured by bird or bat droppings, especially in caves.

Laboratory diagnosis

The organism can be isolated on culture of pathological specimens – sputum, or biopsy material – by culture on selective media (e.g. enriched Sabouraud's medium). The skin test with histoplasmin is useful epidemiologically to detect inapparent infections, including old infections. Serological tests (e.g. complement fixation) are also positive on infection: a rising titre may indicate recent exposure or current disease.

Epidemiology

The infection is endemic in certain parts of North, Central and South America, Africa and parts of the Far East.

RESERVOIR

The reservoir is in soil, especially chicken coops, bat caves and areas polluted with pigeon droppings.

TRANSMISSION

The infection is acquired by inhalation of the spores. Person to person transmission is rare.

HOST FACTORS

It is not clear why in some patients the infection progresses to severe disease.

Control

The main measure is to avoid exposure to contaminated soil and caves. Infected patients with significant disease can be treated with Amphotericin B.

REFERENCES AND FURTHER READING

Foundation Marcel Merieux (1995) *Control of Epidemic Meningococcal Disease*. WHO. *Practical Guidelines*.

WHO (1994) *Acute Respiratory Infections in Children: Case Management in Small Hospitals in Developing Countries. A manual for Doctors and other Senior Health Workers*. WHO/AR/94.5. WHO, Geneva.

WHO (1994) *Framework for Effective Tuberculosis Control*. WHO/TB/94. 17.9. WHO, Geneva.

WHO (1997) *Packaged Treatment for First Line Case in Cerebral Malaria and Meningitis*. WHO/MaI/97. 1083. WHO, Geneva.

WHO (1998) *Report of the AD HOC Committee on the Tuberculosis Epidemic*. WHO/TB/98. 245. WHO, Geneva.

WHO (1999) *Global Tuberculosis Control*. WHO/TB/99. 259. WHO, Geneva.

WHO (1999) *The Evolution of Diarrhoeal and Acute Respiratory Disease Control at WHO*. WHO/CHS/CAH/99. 12. WHO, Geneva.

WHO (2001) *Management of the Child with a Serious Infection or Severe Malnutrition*. WHO/FCH/CAH/OO. 1. WHO, Geneva.

LATE ADDENDA

The new strategy for measles vaccination

PAHO has pioneered a three-pronged strategy of:

- "Catch-up" one-time only mass measles vaccination of all children 1–14 years,
- "Keep-up" routine vaccination of 95% of children in each subsequent birth cohort (using Measles-Mumps-Rubella vaccine), and
- "Follow-up" periodic measles vaccination of all children age 1–4 years every four years.

The PAHO strategy also includes intensive surveillance of rash illnesses, including active case searches in problem areas and laboratory confirmation of all sporadic cases and of a sample of cases in each outbreak, as well as aggressive investigation of all suspected cases. With this strategy, measles cases in the Americas have been reduced from 246,612 cases reported in 1990 to 2,109 cases in 1996 and a provisional total of only 533 cases, many of which were imported from other regions, in 2001.

Tuberculosis

Dots-plus is the strategy used when *M. tuberculosis* is resistant to first line drugs. The second line drugs are more expensive, more difficult to administer and poorly tolerated.

Severe Acquired Respiratory Syndrome (SARS)

The SARS epidemic started in Guangdong, China in November 2002 and by June 2003 had affected over 8,000 patients and caused 800 deaths. China, Hong Kong, Taiwan, Singapore and Canada were the countries worst affected. The clinical features include influenza-like prodromal symptoms, cough, dyspnoea and large volume watery diarrhoea. Bacterial sepsis and pneumonia occur, particularly in the elderly.

Virology

The disease is caused by a novel coronavirus (SARS-COV).

Epidemiology

The mean incubation period is 5 days with a range of 2–10 days. The disease is most likely transmitted by droplet infection. Nosocomial transmission has been a striking feature of SARS ranging from 16–53% among health workers. Children are rarely affected. The role of animals in transmission is being investigated.

An unusual outbreak occurred in a block of flats complex in Hong Kong resulting from a breakdown of the sewage treatment plant in the complex and contaminated sewage being drawn through the bath drains into the bathrooms.

Laboratory diagnosis

The diagnosis can be confirmed by PCR positive for SARS-COV; Seroconversion by ELISA or IFA and by virus isolation.

Control

1 Isolation of all suspected cases in a single room with an extractor fan. Where single rooms are not available, the space between beds should be at least 2 metres and very strict droplet and contact precautions observed at all times.
2 No visits or very restricted visits by family members.
3 All health workers should be protected using N95 masks with tight fitting seals or three-ply surgical masks and disposable second layer of protective clothing to be discarded before leaving room.
4 Hand washing, barrier precautions, gowns, gloves, mask eye protection.
5 Active surveillance of exposed health workers and contacts of patients with temperature monitored several times a day. No treatment is available for SARS. WHO has produced guidelines for Alert, verification and public health management of SARS and provided a list of focal points (http://www.who.int/CSR/SARS/postoutbreak/en/).

Avian flu

See page 361.

CHAPTER SEVEN

ARTHROPOD-BORNE INFECTIONS

- The infective agents
- Transmission
- Host factors
- Control of arthropod infections
- Insecticides in public health
- Biological control

- Arbovirus infections
- Rickettsial infections
- Bacterial infections
- Protozoal infections
- Helminthic infections
- References and further reading

Arthropods play an important, and in some cases a determinant role, in the transmission of some infections. The epidemiology of these infections is closely related to the ecology of the arthropod vector, and hence the most effective measures for the control of these infections often relate to the control of the vector. The arthropod vector introduces a further dimension to the complex host-parasite interrelationship, and for some of these infections, a fourth factor is added when there is a non-vertebrate animal reservoir. Arthropod vectors of importance include various species of flies, mosquitoes, fleas, ticks and mites.

THE INFECTIVE AGENTS

These include a wide variety of organisms ranging from viruses to helminths, as listed in Table 7.1. The viral infections are known under the collective term 'arboviruses', a contraction of 'arthropod-borne viruses'.

TRANSMISSION

VECTOR–PARASITE RELATIONSHIP

The role of the vector in transmission may be either biological or mechanical.

BIOLOGICAL

The vector may be specifically involved in the biological transmission of the infective agent, in which case, this is an essential phase in the life cycle of the agent. The phase within the vector, which is often referred to as the extrinsic incubation period, may involve:

- morphological development without multiplication, e.g. filarial worms;
- asexual multiplication, e.g. arboviruses, plague;
- sexual multiplication, e.g. malaria.

The extrinsic incubation is important epidemiologically, for only after its completion is the infection transmissible. Usually, the arthropod acquires the infection on biting an infected host but in a few specific instances the vector may acquire the infection congenitally by transovarian passage, for example mites in scrub typhus.

MECHANICAL

The vector may bring about a simple mechanical transfer of the agent from the source to the susceptible host. The vector may carry the infective agent on its body or limbs, or the infective agents may be ingested by the vector passing through its body

Table 7.1: The infective agents

Arbovirus infections
Yellow fever
Dengue fever
Japanese B encephalitis
Kyasanur Forest disease
Other arboviruses: Sandfly fever, Rift Valley fever,
West Nile

Rickettsial infections
Epidemic, louse-borne typhus (*Rickettsia prowazekii*)
Murine typhus (*Rickettsia typhi*)
Scrub typhus (*Rickettsia orientalis*)
African tick typhus (*Rickettsia conorii*)
Q fever (*Coxiella burnetii*)

Bacterial infections
Plague (*Yersinia pestis*)
Tick-borne relapsing fever (*Borrelia duttoni*)
Louse-borne relapsing fever (*Borrelia recurrentis*)
Bartonellosis (*Bartonella bacilliformis*)

Protozoal infections
Malaria (*Plasmodium* spp.)
African trypanosomiasis (*Trypanosoma brucei
gambiense, T.b. rhodesiense*)
South American trypanosomiasis (*Trypanosoma cruzi*)
The leishmaniases (*Leishmania* spp.)

Helminthic infections
Filariases (*Wuchereria bancrofti, Brugia malayi*)
Loaiasis (*Loa loa*)
Onchocerciasis (*Onchocerca volvulus*)
Other filarial infections (*Detrapetalonema perstans,
Tetrapetalonema streptocerca, Mansonella ozzardi,
Dirofilaria* spp.)

unmodified and excreted in faeces. The housefly and other filth flies are important mechanical vectors of various infections especially gastrointestinal infections (e.g. shigellosis), which rely on the faeco-oral route of transmission. These are dealt with in Chapter 4.

TRANSMISSION FROM VECTOR TO HOST

The infected vector may inoculate the infective agents from its salivary secretions into a new host, for example malaria. In other cases, the host becomes infected through contamination of his or her mucous membranes or skin by the infective faeces of the vector, for example Chagas' disease;

or by the infective tissue fluids which are released when the vector is crushed, for example louse-borne relapsing fever. The host may acquire infection by ingesting the vector: the transmission of guinea-worm occurs by this unusual route, when man ingests the infected cyclops, the crustacean intermediate host of this worm (see p. 81).

HOST FACTORS

HOST PREFERENCE

Many of the arthropod vectors which bite mammals show marked host preferences. Some of them bite man preferentially, and these are said to be anthropophilic; whereas others which bite animals preferentially are zoophilic. There is some evidence that mosquitoes are attracted to and bite some persons more often than others, but the basis for this preference is not, as yet, clearly understood.

IMMUNITY

Acquired immunity plays an important role in the epidemiology of some of the arthropod-borne infections. For example, previous exposure to the yellow fever virus may confer lifelong immunity; some protection from yellow fever may also be derived from exposure to related viruses of the B group (see p. 180). In other cases, immunity is of short duration and is not absolute, for example plague.

CONTROL OF ARTHROPOD INFECTIONS

INFECTIVE AGENT

- *Destruction of animal reservoir*, e.g. rats in the control of plague.
- *Isolation and treatment of cases*, e.g. yellow fever patient is nursed in a mosquito-proof room or bed.

TRANSMISSION

Prevention of vector–host contact

- *Physical barriers*, e.g. clearing an area to free it of breeding and resting places for the vectors; siting houses away from known breeding places of mosquitoes.
- *Mechanical barriers*, e.g. protective clothing, screening of houses, impregnated mosquito nets.

Destruction of vectors

TRAPPING, COLLECTION AND DESTRUCTION

Various mechanical devices are in use, e.g. sticky strips to which flies adhere.

INSECTICIDES

Some of these are active against the larval aquatic forms, others are directed against the adult vectors. For a full account of the various types, methods of application and effects of insecticides, see below.

PHYSICAL AND BIOLOGICAL METHODS

These include the alteration of the physical environment, alteration of the flora and fauna, and use of bacteria, for example *Bacillus thuringiensis israeliensis*.

HOST

- *Immunization*, e.g. yellow fever prophylaxis with a live attenuated virus.
- *Chemoprophylaxis*, e.g. antimalarials.

INSECTICIDES IN PUBLIC HEALTH

Most of the insecticides manufactured are used in agriculture, many of them affect insects of importance in public health and may cause poisoning in humans. In general, the use of insecticides is discouraged for environmental reasons. However, a balanced risk and benefit analysis is required before final decisions are made, especially in countries where they may be essential for endemic and epidemic control of important prevalent diseases.

MODE OF ACTION

Insecticides in public health are used either for a quick knock down or for a residual effect.

Knock-down insecticides

Most knock-down insecticides contain pyrethrum (sometimes with addition of DDT to improve their efficacy). They are used, usually as a fine spray, to get rid of adult insects quickly, but the effect lasts for only a short time. They can be used when rapid control is required, as in an epidemic of an insect-borne disease, or to kill insects in aircraft. This quick knock-down can be achieved with insecticidal fogs, smoke and aerial spraying, also by impregnating mosquito nets.

Residual insecticides

For long-continued effect (e.g. 6 months duration) residual insecticides are used: DDT for example, applied to wall surfaces at a dose of $2\,g/m^2$, will kill mosquitoes that rest indoors, providing they are still susceptible.

DDT the oldest, is still the best and cheapest, for malaria control. It is relatively non-toxic. Only India and China now produce DDT. Until alternatives to DDT affordable to many of the malaria endemic countries become available, it is unethical to ban it in those countries that truly need it. A properly constructed phase-out of DDT is required, rather than an outright immediate ban. Benzene hexachloride (BHC), is less long-lasting; Dieldrin is too toxic for general use without strict precautions.

Various organic phosphorus insecticides have been used in situations where DDT is not effective. These vary enormously in their toxicity, from parathion which is very dangerous indeed (it is used in agriculture but seldom in public health) to malathion which is only slightly more toxic than DDT. They are less long-lasting and more expensive than DDT.

METHODS OF APPLICATION

The insecticides can be applied in many ways, depending on the objective to be achieved. Some of these formulations are:

- aerosols;
- fogs;
- vapours;
- smokes;
- paints.

These are used where penetration is required but does not give a long-lasting residual effect. Recently ultra-low volume (ULV) aerosols have been popular, dispensing about 0.1 l/min of concentrated insecticide.

Aerial spraying

Spraying from low levels (up to 100 m) by slow-flying (250–320 km/h) aeroplanes, or by helicopters, may be useful for treating large or inaccessible breeding grounds of some pests, such as mosquito larvae in large swamps, or tsetse flies in extensive bush. Air spraying can be done only during still air conditions. In tropical countries ground heating during the day produces violent air convection, which restricts spraying to about an hour either just after sunrise or just before sunset. Aerial spraying is very useful in epidemic situations.

Larvicides

These have been successfully used in the control of mosquitoes (see p. 207) especially when breeding sites are restricted or close to houses, for example *Aedes aegypti* (see p. 184). They have also been successful in controlling *Simulium* (see p. 231). The decision of which insecticide and formulation should be used depends on the circumstances of the particular problem.

Water-dispersible powders (WDP)

These are used for applying insecticides to wall surfaces. They are cheap but messy, leaving a white deposit of inert powder on the wall. Most malaria eradication campaigns use 5% DDT (WDP).

Solutions, emulsions

These have the same effect as water-dispersible powders. The solvent evaporates, leaving the insecticide on the wall. On some surfaces, however, for example mud, soakage takes place and the insecticidal effect is markedly lessened. Impregnation of nets with deltamethrin is now widely being used. Cheap commercial kits for home use are now available.

RESISTANCE

Insects of public health importance have developed resistance to insecticides. House flies rapidly become resistant (therefore good sanitation is the control method of choice); anopheline mosquitoes are less liable to become resistant to DDT, than to dieldrin or BHC. The only measure to overcome resistance is to change the insecticide or limit its use. The mechanisms of resistance are complex and beyond the scope of this book.

TOXICITY

All the residual insecticides are toxic to humans, but the degree varies enormously: DDT and BHC are only slightly toxic; parathion is extremely toxic.

Common-sense precautions, for example not eating when using insecticides, washing and changing clothes at the end of the day's work, avoiding contact with concentrated insecticides especially when in solution or emulsion, must be taken by everyone involved in spraying operations. Special precautions must be taken when anything more toxic than DDT or BHC is being applied.

OTHER EFFECTS OF INSECTICIDES

There is a worldwide controversy about the relative damage caused by residual insecticides to wild-life and the benefits they give by increasing food production. It is important to appreciate in this context that indoor spraying does not contribute materially to the pollution of the environment and that pesticides widely used for agricultural purposes are a far greater hazard in this respect. The decision as to the choice of insecticides, timing of application, dosage and formulation demands a careful study of each situation. Unless this is done, money may be wasted and the desired result may not be achieved.

BIOLOGICAL CONTROL

Because of the anxiety that has developed over the wide-scale use of insecticides, numerous attempts at biological control are being tried both in the laboratory and in the field. Biological control may be defined as the set of control measures designed to restrict the development of insect pests by:

- modifying their environment and food supply (ecological control);
- exposing them to their predators and parasites;
- disrupting their reproductive processes (genetic control).

ECOLOGICAL CONTROL

Alterations in the shelter and food supply of the vector may be effected through:

- *physical changes*, e.g. drainage of ponds, drying up of lakes, alteration in the speed and course of a river;
- *the fauna*, e.g. by driving away the big game from an area, there is a reduction in the food supply of *Glossina morsitans*, the vector of *Trypanosoma rhodesiense*;
- *the flora*, e.g. the clearance of low-level foliage to control *Glossina tachinoides* or of the water lily, *Pistia*, in the control of *Mansonia* larvae and pupae.

PREDATORS AND PARASITES

Biological agents have been extensively investigated for the control of arthropod pests. One successful application is the use of *Bacillus thuringiensis israeliensis* as a biological larvicide against the simulium fly.

GENETIC CONTROL

Sterilization of males by genetic manipulation has had limited success in field conditions, but a great deal of progress is being made at the laboratory level in the field of genetic control of malaria transmitting mosquitoes.

ARBOVIRUS INFECTIONS

The arthropod-borne viruses (arboviruses) may cause various syndromes in humans:

- fever, with rash, polyarthritis and myalgia;
- aseptic meningitis;
- encephalitis;
- haemorrhagic fever.

Alternatively, they may present as atypical or subclinical infections only recognizable by antibody studies. The majority produce non-fatal infections.

Virology

Three main groups of arboviruses have been serologically defined: groups A (alphaviruses), B (flaviviruses) and C (bunyaviruses). Phlebovirus infections include sandfly fever and Rift Valley fever; while coltivirus infections are typified by Colorado tick fever. The important arboviruses are given in Table 7.2.

Epidemiology

The majority are zoonoses, and about 70 of the many different arboviruses identified are known to cause disease in man.

Mosquitoes are the most common vectors of arboviruses, ticks the next most common, and *Phlebotomus* and *Culicoides* the least frequently involved. Because infection usually produces prolonged immunity, attack rates occurring throughout all age groups indicate the introduction of a new arbovirus, while disease confined to children implies re-introduction of a virus or overflow from a continuous animal cycle to susceptible humans.

Table 7.2: Classification of some clinically important arboviruses in the tropics

Alphaviruses (Group A)	Flaviviruses (Group B)	Bunyaviruses (Group C)	Phleboviruses	Coltiviruses
Chikungunya*	Yellow fever*	Apeu	Sandfly fever*	Colorado tick fever*
O Nyong-Nyong*	Dengue*	Caraparu	Rift Valley fever*	
Venezuelan equine encephalitis	Japanese B encephalitis*	Itaqui		
Western equine encephalitis	West Nile*	Marituba		
Eastern equine encephalitis	Kyasanur Forest disease*	Oriboca		
Ross River fever*	Murray Valley encephalitis	Ossa		
		Hantaviruses*		
		Nairoviruses* (Crimean–Congo haemorrhagic fever)		

*Infections described in this chapter.

Laboratory diagnosis

The definitive diagnosis depends upon isolation of the virus from patients early in the infection, with demonstration of a rise in antibody titre in the sera between the acute and convalescent stages of the disease. Other techniques include antigen capture ELISA, hybridization assays and polymerase chain reaction (PCR) assays.

Control

Control of the vector population, where practicable, will reduce the risk of infection. Steps can also be taken to avoid being bitten by vectors, for example impregnated nets – mosquito control methods.

ALPHAVIRUSES (GROUP A)

In the tropics infections usually occur in the rainy season which is the period of highest vector activity.

Chikungunya

The virus was isolated in 1952 during an outbreak in Tanzania, characterized by fever, rigors, arthralgias and myalgias. In the local language it means 'that which bends up'. The virus is transmitted by haematophagous mosquitoes of the *Aedes* group with secondary transmission by *Mansonia*. Non-human primates are the main reservoir of infection in Africa, while in Asia *Aedes aegypti* is responsible for maintaining a human to human cycle. The incubation period is short – 2–3 days. Antibody surveys have shown that subclinical infections are common – 20–90% of a given population may be immune.

O Nyong-Nyong (ONN)

The virus was isolated in 1959 during an epidemic in Uganda which then spread to Kenya, Tanzania, Malawi, Mozambique and elsewhere in Africa. In the local Ugandan dialect it means 'weakening of the joints'. The mosquito vectors are *A. gambiae* and *A. funestus*. ONN virus has been isolated only from humans. The clinical syndrome is similar to Chikungunya. The incubation period is 8 days.

Ross River fever

The first epidemic of epidemic polyarthritis was reported in 1928 from New South Wales, Australia. Epidemics occur periodically in Australia and the Pacific Islands where large proportions of the population (33–90%) have been infected. The principal vectors are species of *Aedes* and *Culex*. Natural reservoirs are large mammals, for example kangaroos, wallabies, as well as many other smaller animals. Human to human infection is important during epidemics.

FLAVIVIRUSES (GROUP B)

The diseases most important to man result from infections with arboviruses of this group, most of which have mosquitoes as their vectors, with the exception of a subgroup which are tick-borne. Antigenic cross-reactivity is marked in the group B viruses, so that in areas where there is a high endemicity, for example tropical Africa, serological diagnosis may be difficult, and the most rapid and definitive diagnostic method of active infection is by virus isolation.

Many infections are symptomless. The most important diseases are:

- yellow fever;
- dengue fever;
- Japanese B encephalitis;
- Kyasanur Forest disease;
- West Nile.

Yellow fever

Occurrence:	South America, tropical Africa
Organism:	Yellow fever virus
Reservoir:	Humans, monkeys
Transmission:	Aedes spp. bites
Control:	Isolation
	Vector control
	Immunization

Yellow fever is an acute infectious disease of sudden onset and variable severity caused by a virus transmitted by mosquitoes. It is characterized by fever, jaundice, haemorrhagic manifestations and albuminuria. The incubation period in humans is 3–6 days.

EPIDEMIOLOGY (PLATE 58)

Yellow fever is endemic in large areas of South America and tropical Africa. The endemic zone in Africa approximately covers that part of the continent which lies between latitudes 15°N and 100°S. In South America the endemic zone stretches from south of Honduras to the southern border of Bolivia and includes the western two-thirds of Brazil, Venezuela, Colombia, and those parts of Peru and Ecuador that lie east of the Andes. Certain towns are considered as not forming part of these zones provided they continuously maintain an *Aedes index* not exceeding 1%. This index represents the proportions of houses in a limited, well-defined area in which breeding places of *Aedes aegypti* are found (Plate 59).

Epidemics occur from time to time and have been described from various countries in Africa in recent years, resulting in considerable mortality.

Yellow fever does not occur in Asia or the Pacific region, though the urban vector is widespread (see dengue haemorrhagic fever). It is not clear whether this is because the disease has not been introduced or because of a peculiar racial immunity; in any case the risk of introduction must be avoided at all costs (yellow fever 'receptive areas').

Reservoir and transmission

There are two main epidemiological forms of yellow fever:

- urban type;
- sylvatic type.

Urban type

The virus cycle is man-mosquito-man; this method of spread requires large numbers of susceptible hosts, and hence tends to occur in large towns. Villages, with frequent passage of people from one village to another, will also be suitable for this type of spread.

The mosquito vector is *Aedes aegypti*, which is primarily a domestic mosquito which breeds in or near houses, with the female preferring to lay her eggs in water collecting in artificial containers, such as old tins, flower vases, etc.

Urban-type yellow fever can effectively be controlled by anti-mosquito measures. This has been achieved largely in South America. However, re-infestation is possible as has occurred in Santa Cruz, Bolivia. In this situation – towns near forest areas – uncontrolled migration and improved transport links provide the opportunity for unvaccinated rural residents to introduce the virus into urban centres re-infested with *A. aegypti*. In these circumstances, yellow fever should be included in any expanded programme of immunization (EPI), to minimize the risk of urban yellow fever.

Sylvatic type

This may occur in endemic or epizootic forms. In the endemic form, the disease, which is primarily one of monkeys, is almost constantly present, and sporadic cases of human infection occur from time to time. The primary spread of the virus is from monkey to monkey, via *Haemagogus* spp. in South America (Fig. 7.1) and *A. africanus* in Africa (Fig. 7.2): both these mosquitoes live in the tops of trees.

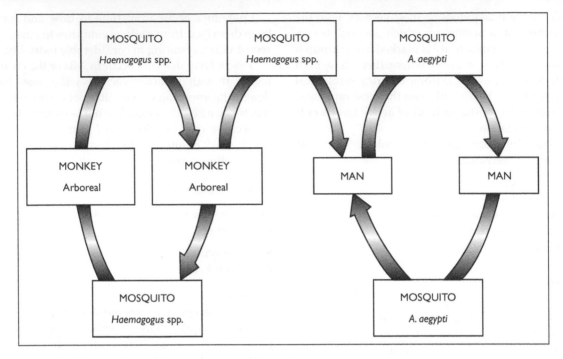

Figure 7.1: South American pattern of transmission of yellow fever.

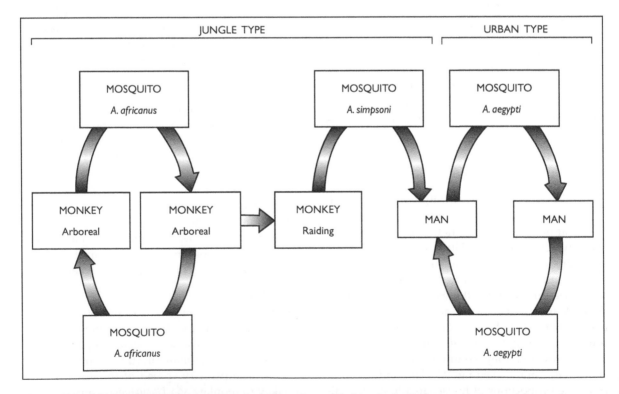

Figure 7.2: African pattern of transmission of yellow fever (Haddow's classical transmission cycle).

In South America, jungle yellow fever is transmitted to man when the *Haemagogus* species occasionally bites man, for example when a tree is felled.

In Africa, however, there is a different way in which jungle yellow fever virus can be transmitted from the monkey to man. Certain monkeys have the habit of raiding crops, particularly bananas. Another mosquito, *A. simpsoni,* occurs on the edges of forests, and becomes infected by biting infected raiding monkeys, and then later bites the humans when they collect their crops. *A. simpsoni* thus acts as a so-called 'link-host'.

In West Africa there are two main types of transmission of yellow fever:

- *horizontal* transmission by passage of virus between vertebrate hosts through a vector;
- *vertical* transmission by passage of virus from a vector to its progeny – also referred to as the 'vector reservoir'.

Two main epidemiological zones are described – the endemic area and the potential epidemic area. The endemic area is found in the rainforest and in the humid and semi-humid savannah microclimate, while the potential epidemic area occurs in the dry and sahelian savannahs where most of the major epidemics occur.

Humans may be infected with yellow fever in three ways:

- *Jungle yellow fever* involving monkeys and wild vectors. In this situation human cases are usually sporadic, resulting from infection occurring where humans enter the forest for a variety of occupational reasons.
- *Urban yellow fever* involves human to human infection generally by *A. aegypti* and severe epidemics may occur with a high fatality rate.
- *Intermediate yellow fever* was created to describe epidemics the pattern of which does not fit in with the above two ways of transmission. Here the main vectors are often wild mosquitoes with semi-domestic habits. Epidemics erupt simultaneously over a wide area. The most recent epidemics in West Africa were of this type.

Host factors

It is important to remember that, in endemic areas, many cases of yellow fever are mild illnesses resulting in subclinical infections leading to immunity among the indigenous population. There is evidence to suggest that the presence of extensive immunity to other group B viruses modifies the severity and spread of yellow fever.

Applied biology

Unmodified yellow fever virus attacks the cells of all three embryonic layers (pantropic). All strains show some degree of neurotropism, but the severity of the illness is largely due to the degree of viscerotropism shown; that is, the degree of affinity shown for the abdominal viscera, particularly the liver. The degree of virulence shown by the virus can be modified by serial passage through mouse brain, or by culture in chick embryos or in tissue culture and has led to the production of a live attenuated vaccine.

Mosquitoes, the only insects able to transmit infection, act as biological transmitters. The virus actually multiplies in the mosquito host: after biting an infected person or monkey, the mosquito itself becomes infective after an interval of about 12 days (extrinsic incubation period) and remains infective for the rest of its life.

LABORATORY DIAGNOSIS

Isolation

Virus isolation from the blood up to the 4th day of the disease is the diagnostic procedure of choice. Isolation of virus is by intracerebral inoculation of mice, or intrathoracic inoculation of mosquitoes.

Serology

After the 3rd day of the disease the mouse protection test can be used. This test involves demonstrating whether or not mice are protected from a challenge dose of the virus by antibodies in the patient's serum. A second protection test should be made some 5 days later. A significant rise of titre in the second sample would confirm the diagnosis, while an unaltered titre would only indicate an immunity due to a past infection or vaccination. It must be borne in mind that there may be a cross-reaction with other viruses of the group B arbovirus group.

Neutralization, complement fixation, or haemagglutination inhibition tests are also employed, depending on the particular circumstances and the likelihood of previous exposure to other group B viruses. ELISA techniques for the titration of specific IgM have been developed. Immuno-chemical methods and gene amplification are also now used.

Histology

Histology of the liver in fatal cases establishes the diagnosis. Occasionally, virus can be isolated from this organ.

CONTROL

The individual

Since the virus circulates in the blood during the first few days of the disease, a suspected case must be isolated for the first 6 days in a screened room or under a mosquito net. Steps should be taken at once to obtain laboratory confirmation of the diag-nosis, but institution of control measures should not await results from the laboratory. Domestic contacts should also be isolated under screened conditions for 6 days, and the patient's house and all premises within a radius of 55 m should be sprayed with a residual insecticide.

The first cases of yellow fever in an epidemic are likely to be mistaken for other illnesses, especially viral hepatitis. It is therefore very important always to remember the possibility of yellow fever in endemic areas and when in doubt to take blood for serological examination or specimens of the liver (if necessary with a viscerotome) from corpses. A life-long immunity follows recovery from the disease.

The vector

Breeding sites
In densely populated areas elimination of vector breeding must be undertaken at once. *A. aegypti is* a peridomestic mosquito and will breed in practic-ally anything that will hold water. This includes water containers such as jars and cisterns, as well as innumerable objects which may hold rainwater: defective gutters, old tins, jars and coconut shells (often hidden in the grass), old car tyres and the bottoms of small boats and canoes. These breeding foci should be reduced as far as possible by suitable measures: water containers covered or screened, tins and other rubbish buried, and so forth. This is unlikely to prevent all breeding, but it will simplify treatment of the remainder by regular oiling or by addition of insecticidal briquettes (e.g. Abate).

Insecticides
Residual spraying of the interiors of all houses and out-buildings or of all surfaces close to breeding places (perifocal spraying) will reduce the *Aedes* population rapidly. Epidemic transmission will cease when the *Aedes* index is reduced to below 1%. To prevent introduction of an infected mosquito into countries where the disease is absent but condi-tions exist for transmission, aircraft coming from the endemic zone must be disinsecticized (by insecti-cidal aerosol) as specified by the World Health Organization. This is particularly important in Asia, where vigorous antimosquito measures around airports should be carried out, international certifi-cates of all persons coming from endemic zones scrupulously checked and adequate quarantine of animal reservoirs such as monkeys instituted. International notification provides health author-ities with up-to-date information regarding the sta-tus of yellow fever throughout the world.

Immunization

Protection of scattered populations by vector con-trol is impracticable, and recourse must be made to vaccination of the whole community. This will afford protection for at least 10 years. The 17D strain maintained by passage in chick embryo or in tissue culture is now generally used; it is thermo-stable. The stabilization of the vaccine applies only to the lyophilized form, once reconstituted in diluent, it must be used within 1 hour. Mass vac-cination campaigns should be supplemented by incorporating yellow fever vaccine in the coun-try's expanded programme of immunization (EPI).

Contraindications

Infants under 1 year of age should preferably not be vaccinated, since encephalitis follows vaccin-ation in this age group more frequently than in adults. Some countries do not require vaccination certificates in the case of infants. Vaccination is contraindicated in patients whose immune responses are suppressed by steroids or immuno-suppressive drugs.

Certification

The spread of the disease is controlled by requiring all persons entering or leaving an endemic area to be in possession of a valid certificate of vaccination.

Those not in possession of such a certificate, on arrival in a non-endemic area, may be subjected to quarantine for a period of 6 days from the date of last exposure to infection or until the certificate becomes valid. (A vaccination certificate becomes valid 10 days after vaccination and remains so for 10 years. The certificate becomes valid on the day of revaccination if the person is revaccinated within 10 years of previous vaccination.)

Dengue viruses

Occurrence:	Wide distribution in the tropics Haemorrhagic epidemics, predominantly in South East Asia
Organisms:	Dengue viruses (serotypes 1–4)
Reservoir:	Humans
Transmission:	Aedes spp.
Control:	Vector control

Dengue viruses produce, in general, a non-fatal, short, febrile illness, characterized by severe myalgia and joint pains. The occurrence of haemorrhagic phenomena with a significant mortality, especially in childhood, has been a feature of epidemics predominantly in South East Asia, but have also occurred in the Caribbean and elsewhere. Dengue fever and dengue haemorrhagic fever (DHF) occur in over 100 countries and affect more than 2.5 billion people in urban, peri-urban and rural areas of the tropics and subtropics.

VIROLOGY

There are four main serotypes of dengue viruses, numbered 1–4.

EPIDEMIOLOGY

Dengue fever is widely distributed throughout urban areas of the tropics and subtropics. A pandemic of 'classical' dengue fever began in the Caribbean in 1977 and involved major outbreaks on many of the islands, including Puerto Rico. Epidemics of dengue with haemorrhagic phenomena have been reported from widely spaced regions Calcutta, the Philippines, Thailand, Malaysia, Indonesia, Burma and Cuba (Plate 60) – and all types of dengue viruses have been isolated from *A. aegypti* during these epidemics. The epidemics have an urban distribution with cases clustered in the crowded, poorer, central districts of cities. Open large water jars and discarded tyres provide ideal sites for egg-laying (Plates 61 and 62).

Although uncontrolled urbanization has been responsible for some of the epidemics that have occurred in South East Asia in recent years, the disease has now spread to rural areas as well. In 1988, a total of 1.2 million cases of dengue and DHF were reported to WHO, including 3442 deaths.

Some outbreaks of haemorrhagic fever have been caused by the arbovirus Chikungunya (group A). On the whole the syndrome associated with chikungunya infection is milder than haemorrhagic dengue. Important aspects of the epidemiology of dengue are: (i) the explosive growth of urban population in the tropics; (ii) deterioration of urban environments; (iii) improved transportation, and (iv) the intensity of transmission of dengue viruses. Asymptomatic or oligosymptomatic infections are common in endemic areas.

Reservoir and transmission

Man is the reservoir and *A. aegypti* the established mosquito vector of the dengue viruses responsible for dengue fever. The extrinsic incubation period of the virus in *A. aegypti* is about 2 weeks. Biting rates are highest during the day.

Host factors

Infection confers immunity to the homologous strain for about a year. The haemorrhagic form is usually seen in races of oriental origin, and haemorrhagic fatal manifestations are usually confined to those under 15 years of age, with a peak incidence in the 3–6 years age group. However, DHF can occur at any age.

LABORATORY DIAGNOSIS

Virus isolation in the early stages is achieved by inoculation of cell cultures. The serotype can be identified by complement-fixation, neutralization tests and immunofluorescence with type-specific monoclonal antibodies. Procedures for detection of dengue virus RNA or dengue virus antigens are now available.

CONTROL

The global strategy for prevention and control of dengue and DHF comprises of the following elements: (i) vector control; (ii) active disease surveillance; (iii) emergency preparedness; (iv) behaviour changes in the community; and (v) capacity building and training.

Control of both types of dengue fever is based on eradicating the urban vector mosquito *A. aegypti* in its aquatic or adult stages as described for yellow fever. This has been successfully achieved in Singapore where only sporadic cases now occur, in contrast to the epidemics reported some years ago. During an epidemic ultra-low volume application of insecticides can interrupt transmission; repeated weekly applications are required.

The prevention of mosquito bites by screening, impregnated nets, or repellents provides further protection. Vaccines are being developed but are not yet available for general use. In some countries (e.g. Indonesia, Vietnam and the Philippines) clinical management guidelines have been incorporated into integrated management of childhood infections (IMCI).

Japanese B encephalitis

The majority of infections are inapparent or mild.

EPIDEMIOLOGY

The disease occurs in Cambodia, Indonesia, Lao PDR, Thailand, Vietnam, China, Malaysia, Sri Lanka, Nepal and India. Vaccination has resulted in the near disappearance of Japanese B encephalitis (JE) in Japan and Taiwan and a reduction in other locations with high vaccine coverage, for example Thailand. The most efficient vector is *Culex tritaeniorhynchus,* and the preferred vertebrate hosts are birds and domestic animals (e.g. pigs), man being only an incidental host. The virus is spread from rural to urban areas by viraemic birds. The peak age specific prevalence in most areas is between 4 and 8 years of age. Patterns of transmission vary because of the seasonal occurrence of monsoons and vector composition, vector host preference, available vertebrate hosts and human behavioural factors. A bimodal pattern of age-related risk with increased susceptibility in the elderly is sometimes seen.

IgM capture ELISA of cerebrospinal fluid (CSF) and serum is the diagnostic procedure of choice. A dot-blot IgM assay suitable for field use has been developed while an RT-PCR assay of viral genomic material in CSF is being evaluated.

CONTROL

Control of the vector mosquitoes is not practicable on a large scale. Isolation of pig sties from human habitats reduces the mosquito/man contact. Vaccination for 'high-risk' persons is available. Immunization of pigs is also feasible.

A Hendra-like virus (Nipah virus) of the paramyxo family has recently been isolated in Malaysia. The virus seemed to be transmitted from pigs to humans through direct contact with body fluids of pigs. The epidemic affected around 300 persons, predominantly males and was at first diagnosed as Japanese B encephalitis; 1.5 million pigs had to be slaughtered to contain the epidemic.

Kyasanur Forest disease

The virus of Kyasanur Forest disease has to date been found only in Karnataka State, India. The disease occurs more frequently in the dry season and in persons working in the forest. It is characterized by fever and vesicular eruption in the palate.

The principal vector is the tick *Haemaphysalis spinigera*. Human infection is often preceded by illness and death in forest-dwelling monkeys, which act as amplifiers of the virus which is maintained in small mammals. Annual outbreaks of human and simian disease start in November, reach their peak in January and stop before the rainy season. Specific diagnosis is by virus isolation up to 10 days after onset. Serologic diagnosis with HI or CF is available, as is ELISA that detects IgM antibodies. Personal protection against the vector tick is the only practicable method of control.

West Nile

This virus was first isolated in the West Nile district of Uganda. However, it is widely distributed with a high prevalence in the southern portion of the Nile Delta in Egypt, the Sudan, South Africa, Central Africa, Nigeria and Pakistan. A few cases were recently reported in New York.

The transmission cycle involves *Culex* mosquitoes, migrating birds and humans.

Many infections are oligo or asymptomatic. The incubation period is between 2 and 6 days. Fever, rigors, myalgia, sore throat and diarrhoea occur. In the non-immune elderly the disease is more serious and may result in encephalitis.

Diagnosis is by isolation of the virus, serological tests or ELISA IgM antibody capture test.

Prevention is related to *Culex* control and aerial spraying during epidemics.

Bunyaviruses (group C)

These viruses produce a mild, self-limiting febrile illness and are mostly found in South America. They are mostly maintained in invertebrate–vertebrate–invertebrate cycles. Mammal-feeding mosquitoes transmit virus to small mammal hosts. Vector control is the only possibility of prevention.

Hantan virus infections

At least six distinct viruses of the family Bunyaviradae are known to cause human disease characterized by fever, renal dysfunction and haemorrhagic manifestations, also known as haemorrhagic fever with renal syndrome (HFRS). They have a worldwide distribution.

Human contact with rodents is responsible for transmission, predominantly by respiratory infection from aerosols of infectious virus in rodent urine, faeces and saliva.

Hantan virus infections are most often seen among rural populations and among military personnel in the field. It is a seasonal disease often associated with local agricultural practices and is thus a disease predominantly of adults.

Nairovirus infections

Nairoviruses also belong to the family of Bunyaviridae. The human disease produced is known as Crimean–Congo haemorrhagic fever, characterized by fever, severe headache and backache, myalgia and haemorrhage from any orifice. The disease is widely distributed in eastern Europe, Asia and Africa. Humans are infected by tick bites or from contact with blood or other tissues of infected livestock. The majority of patients are adult males working in the livestock industry, for example farmers, slaughtermen and veterinarians. Nosocomical infections also occur.

Phleboviruses

Phlebotomous fever group

The diseases caused by viruses in this group are usually non-fatal. The vectors are various species of *Phlebotomus* and the distribution of the disease is limited between the latitudes 25° and 45°N. There are two types of viruses, the Sicilian and the Neapolitan.

SANDFLY FEVER VIRUS

Sandfly fever appears epidemically over much of the tropics and subtropics, where it is transmitted by *Phlebotomus pupatasii*. Recovery from the disease is followed by a long-lasting immunity to the homologous strain of virus. Sandfly breeding can be controlled to some extent by clearing piles of rubbish and mending cracked and dilapidated walls. The insects are particularly susceptible to DDT, and have been drastically reduced in many places by residual house spraying employed for the control of mosquitoes.

RIFT VALLEY FEVER VIRUS

The first Rift Valley fever outbreak outside Africa occurred in the year 2000 in the Gizan province of Saudi Arabia and the adjoining Yemen. This virus usually causes a non-fatal disease in humans, characterized by fever, myalgia, severe headache, epistaxis and occasionally ocular complications. It is a cause of severe disease in sheep and cattle. Man is infected through handling sick animals or carcasses. Rift Valley fever virus has caused disastrous epizootics in the Sudan, Senegal River valley and Egypt. In the Egyptian outbreak in 1977 there were around 200 000 human infections and at least 600 deaths. The natural reservoir is unknown, but a high prevalence of antibodies in goats, sheep, bovines, camels and humans have been found; the vectors are mosquitoes of the *Aedes* and *Culex* groups. Epizootics are often associated with the rainy season and high mosquito density.

COLTIVIRUSES

Colorado tick fever group

Colorado tick fever virus is found in the USA, where small rodents are believed to be the normal hosts. Man, in whom it causes acute illness, becomes infected as the result of being bitten by the vector tick *Dermacentor andersoni*.

RICKETTSIAL INFECTIONS

Rickettsiae are intracellular organisms living and multiplying in arthropod tissues such as those of the lice, fleas, ticks and mites. The rickettsial diseases of man can be divided into five main antigenic groups as shown in Table 7.3. They have a worldwide distribution, and are not confined to the tropics. The most important diseases are:

- epidemic louse-borne typhus;
- murine typhus (flea-borne);
- scrub typhus (mite borne);

and to a lesser extent:

- African tick typhus;
- Q fever.

EPIDEMIC LOUSE-BORNE TYPHUS

Occurrence:	Worldwide
Organism:	*Rickettsia prowazekii*
Reservoir:	Humans
Transmission:	Contamination by infected louse faeces
Control:	Mass delousing Personal hygiene

This acute disease is caused by *R. prowazekii* and is transmitted by the louse *Pediculus humanus*. The incubation period is about 10 days.

Epidemiology

Epidemic typhus has a worldwide distribution but the disease is commoner in cold climates than in

Table 7.3: The main rickettsial diseases of man

Antigenic group	Disease	Agent	Vector	Reservoir	Distribution
Typhus fever	Louse-borne (epidemic) typhus	*R. prowazekii*	Louse	Man	Worldwide
	Murine (flea-borne) typhus	*R. typhi*	Flea	Rodents	Worldwide
Spotted fever	Rocky mountain spotted fever	*T. rickettsi*	Tick	Rodents, dogs	N and S America
	African tick typhus[a] Mediterranean tick typhus	*R. africae* *R. conori*	Tick	Rodents, dogs	Africa, India
	Rickettsial pox	*R. akari*	Rodent mite	Mouse	Asia, Africa, N America
Scrub typhus	Scrub (mite) typhus	*R. orientia tsutsugamushi*	Larval trombiculid mite		SE Asia, India Pacific Islands, Australia
Q fever[b]	Q fever	*Coxiella burnetti*	Ticks	Mammals	Worldwide
Trench fever[b]	Trench fever	*Rochailimaea quintana*	Body louse (*P. humanus*)	Man	Africa, Mexico, S America, Eastern Europe

[a]Also known as Boutonneuse or Marseilles fever.
[b]Q fever and trench fever are conventionally considered with the rickettsiae.

the tropics. Endemic foci exist in Central Europe, Russia, China, and North Africa. In the tropics it is common at high altitudes and in deserts: recently epidemics have occurred in Burundi and Rwanda, resulting in 100 000 cases and 10 000 deaths.

RESERVOIR

Man is the main reservoir of infection although in Tunisia serological evidence has been obtained that the rat may also be a reservoir of epidemic typhus.

TRANSMISSION

Biological transmission is by the louse *Pediculus humanus*. The louse becomes infected by feeding on a person with the disease during the period from 2 days before symptoms appear until the end of the fever. The rickettsiae multiply in the cells of the louse midgut, and when these rupture the organisms are discharged in the faeces. Human infection follows contamination of breaches of the skin surface by infected louse faeces. The rickettsiae can remain viable for months on dried louse faeces, and may possibly cause infection through the conjunctiva or by inhalation, as well as percutaneously.

HOST FACTORS

Recovery is followed by immunity, which persists for several years. In some patients the infection appears to remain latent after symptoms have subsided and to relapse some years later (Brill's disease).

Laboratory diagnosis

Serological assays are the most widely used and of these the indirect fluorescent antibody test (IFA) is the most popular. Early diagnosis can be established by ELISA or PCR. Serum specimens collected during the acute and convalescent phases showing a four-fold increase or greater are the mainstay of diagnosis.

Control

Delousing of the whole population with residual insecticidal powders is the principal control measure.

THE INDIVIDUAL

Sporadic cases are isolated and deloused, but isolation of infected persons is not practicable in epidemics. On admission to hospital, the patient should be bathed with soap and water or a 1% solution of lysol. The tetracyclines are highly specific and are given in a total dosage of 25 mg/kg, daily. They must be continued for 3 days after the temperature is normal. A single oral dose of 200 mg doxycycline is also very effective in controlling the disease. Chloramphenicol may be used for pregnant women and children under 8 years. Contacts should be deloused and kept under observation for 2 weeks. The patient's clothes and bedding should be sterilized and his or her house sprayed with residual insecticides.

THE COMMUNITY

Mass delousing of the entire population controls epidemic typhus. This is carried out by blowing insecticide (commonly 10% insecticidal powder) with a dusting-gun under the clothes next to the skin over the whole body, the operation occupying only a few minutes. In some areas lice have become resistant to DDT, and other residual insecticides, such as BHC, must be used.

MURINE TYPHUS

Occurrence:	Worldwide
Organism:	*Rickettsia typhi (mooseri)*
Reservoir:	Rodents
Transmission:	Contamination by infected rat faeces
Control:	Flea control, rat control

The disease is caused by *Rickettsia typhi* and transmitted by rat fleas. The incubation period is 10–12 days.

Epidemiology

Murine typhus has a worldwide distribution. Also known as flea-borne typhus, it occurs wherever the rat lives in close association with man, for example grain stores, irrespective of climate. In a serological survey carried out in the Ivory Coast, varieties of murine typhus had an overall frequency of 4.5% but were more prevalent among adults (6%) and also more frequent in the coastal regions (7%). Converted old rat-infested farmhouses are sometimes foci of infection.

RESERVOIR

Murine typhus is essentially a rodent infection which appears sporadically in man.

TRANSMISSION

The organism *Rickettsia typhi* is conveyed to man by the faeces of infected rat fleas of the genus *Xenopsylla* or rat-mite.

Laboratory diagnosis (see p. 189)

IgG and IgM are measured using haemagglutination inhibition or immunofluorescence antigen detection or PCR can be performed on biopsies of petechiae or skin rash.

Control

Control of murine typhus is rarely required, but if needed the anti-rat and anti-flea measures employed in plague will be effective. Individual patients should be treated with antibiotics as in epidemic typhus (see above).

MITE-BORNE TYPHUS (SCRUB TYPHUS)

Occurrence:	South East Asia, Far East
Organism:	*Rickettsia orientalis* (*tsutsugamushi*)
Reservoir:	Rodents
Transmission:	Bites of mites
Control:	Ecological
	Anti-mite measures
	Chemoprophylaxis

Scrub typhus (tsutsugamushi disease; Japanese river or flood fever; tropical typhus; rural typhus) is an acute febrile disease characterized by fever, a rash which appears on the 5th day, and an eschar at the site of attachment of the trombiculid mites which transmit the disease. The causative organism is *Rickettsia tsutsugamushi*. The incubation period is about 12 days.

Epidemiology

Mite-borne typhus occurs in Japan, Thailand, other countries in East and South East Asia, some Pacific Islands and Queensland in Australia (Fig. 7.3). The distribution of scrub typhus is closely related to certain physical and ecological factors which produce 'scrub typhus country', resulting in a recurring cycle of passage of rickettsia between rodents and mites with a spillover into man.

RESERVOIR AND TRANSMISSION

Scrub typhus is enzootic in wild rodents and the two most important vectors are the larvae of *Trombicula akamushi* and *T. deliensis* (Plate 63). In Indonesia the rat flea is the vector. The reservoir of infection is in rodents, and man becomes infected when the larval mites feed on blood. Only the larval mites feed on the vertebrate host's blood, and since the larva only feeds once, the rickettsiae persist through the nymph, adult and egg stages into the larval stages of the next generation, which are thus infective (transovarial transmission). Man contracts the disease by exposure, for example walking or resting in infected foci, particularly after slight rain or heavy dew. These include grassy fields, river banks, abandoned rice fields, forests or jungles, and the neglected shrubby fringes between field and forest.

The different epidemiological patterns of the disease are related to the influence of climatic variations on the life cycle of the trombiculid mite vectors. The seasonal occurrence of tsutsugamushi disease in Japan corresponds exactly with the time of appearance of each species of vector, *T. akamushi* in summer; *T. scutellaris* in autumn and winter; and *T. pallida* in winter and early spring. While the terrain of *T. akamushi* is limited to places along the rivers, other vectors seem to extend far beyond river banks. In Malaysia, scrub typhus occurs throughout the year. Man is only an accidental host, while field-mice, rats, possibly other small mammals, and ground-frequenting birds are the natural hosts responsible for the continuing transmission of *R. tsutsugamushi* from infected to uninfected mites. The mites function both as vector and reservoir since transovarial transmission of rickettsial infection occurs.

The presence of scrub typhus infection in rodents or trombiculid mites in unusual habitats in West Pakistan (e.g. alpine terrain at 3200 m, semidesert and desert 'oasis greenhouse') has been reported.

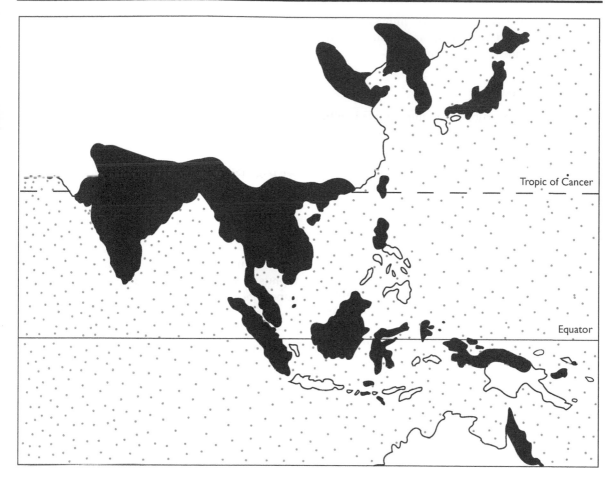

Figure 7.3: Distribution of scrub typhus.

Laboratory diagnosis

A diagnosis of scrub typhus can be made by recovering *R. tsutsugamushi* from the blood of a patient during the febrile period, by culture in living-tissue culture media or in the yolk-sac membrane of developing chick embryos. Intraperitoneal inoculation of blood or of tissue into white mice results in fatal illness, and on autopsy there is a white peritoneal exudate with numerous organisms in the peritoneal cells. The organism can also be recovered from human tissue taken at postmortem.

Control

Control measures are based upon:

- control of the ecology;
- anti-mite measures;

- chemoprophylaxis and treatment of individual cases.

CONTROL OF THE ECOLOGY

The ecology of scrub typhus must be clarified in each area where it occurs before control measures can be successful. The ecology will vary in different geographical areas, from the abandoned rubber plantations of Malaysia to the scrub typhus oases of Pakistan.

Known endemic regions which are often localized to small geographical areas should be avoided for the construction of camps and living quarters. These areas are frequently second-degree growths in deforested regions. Prospective camp sites may be prepared by cutting all vegetation level with the ground and burning it. After thorough clearing, the ground dries sufficiently in 2 or 3 weeks to kill the mites. If the site is required immediately, it should be sprayed with dieldrin or gamma benzene hexachlorine ($1\,kg/4000\,m^2$).

ANTI-MITE MEASURES

Clothing must be rubbed or impregnated with dimethyl or dibutyl phthalate, benzyl benzoate or benzene hexachloride. These kill the mites on contact. Particular care should be given to those parts of the clothing that give access to the interior of the garment.

CHEMOPROPHYLAXIS AND TREATMENT

Prophylactic tetracyclines 3 g orally once weekly, will permit individuals to remain ambulatory even though rickettsaemia will occur from time to time. The drug must be continued for 4 weeks after leaving the endemic area, otherwise clinical disease will occur within a week of withdrawal of the drug. Clinical cases respond to tetracyclines 3 g (loading dose) followed by 0.5 g 6-hourly until the temperature is normal.

Doxycycline is also effective in the treatment of individuals suffering from scrub typhus at a single dose of 200 mg orally, and is more convenient for obvious reasons.

AFRICAN TICK TYPHUS

Occurrence:	Africa
Organism:	*Rickettsia conorii*
Reservoir:	Wild rodents
Transmission:	Ticks
Control:	Reduce tick/man contact

African tick typhus (also known as Boutonneuse or Marseilles fever) is a mild disease in man and deaths are almost unknown. A primary eschar is found at the site of the tick bite. Inapparent infections do not occur, although mild abortive attacks without a rash are not uncommon.

Epidemiology

This is found in Africa south of the Sahara: West Africa, East Africa (Kenya), South Africa, the Sudan, Somalia and Ethiopia.

RESERVOIR AND TRANSMISSION

The disease is contracted by man from ticks in the bush, where the reservoirs are wild rodents. Occasionally, the infection may be brought into suburban areas by dog ticks on domestic dogs. Transovarial transmission occurs in the tick.

Diagnosis

See page 189.

Control

TREATMENT

Tetracyclines are specific in treatment as for scrub typhus. If antibiotic therapy is given at the time of appearance of the primary eschar, the attack will be aborted.

ANTI-TICK MEASURES

Breaking the tick/man contact is the most effective control measure. Known endemic areas should be avoided during the tick season when they are most active. When camping in these areas, individuals should sleep off the ground on camp beds. Where dogs act as tick carriers, then the animals, if they are household pets, should be regularly examined for ticks, which must be removed. Proper clothing should be worn, and the shirt tucked inside the trousers. Socks and high boots should be worn outside the trousers. Since ticks rarely transmit the infection until they have fed for several hours, an important precaution is to remove the clothes and search both body and clothing twice daily, removing the ticks gently with a gloved hand or with forceps.

Q FEVER

Occurrence:	Worldwide
Organism:	*Coxiella burnetii*
Reservoir:	Wild mammals, birds, domestic animals
Transmission:	Milk, droplet, transconjunctival
Control:	Immunization of man and animals Pasteurization of milk at high temperature

The disease normally presents as an acute febrile illness, with chest symptoms but minimal clinical signs; involvement of the lungs occurs in the form of atypical pneumonia. Spontaneous recovery is common. The incubation period is 14–21 days.

Epidemiology

This infection due to *Coxiella burnetii* has a worldwide distribution. The epidemiology varies in different parts of the world, according to the local geographical and environmental factors present.

RESERVOIR

The rickettsiae are distributed widely in nature in ticks, human body lice, small wild mammals, cattle, sheep, goats, birds and man.

TRANSMISSION

The infection is maintained in man through contact with domestic animals, man acquiring the infection as an occupational hazard by direct contact with milk, or transconjunctival entry (e.g. in abattoirs). Secondary cases are caused by the inhalation of infected dust or from human carriers, when the infection is transmitted from man to man via the respiratory tract. Many mild and inapparent infections undoubtedly occur.

Microbiology

Coxiella burnetii survives adverse physical conditions, for example drying; pasteurization at 60° for 30 min.

Laboratory diagnosis

The organism can be recovered on culture in eggs or animal inoculation of blood taken soon after the onset of the illness.

Control

ANIMALS

Control of the disease on a community basis rests upon control of the disease in domestic animals either by immunization or by antibiotics. This requires a large economic effort.

Milk from goats, sheep and cows should be pasteurized at high temperature (62.9°C for 30 min or 71.7°C for 15 min). Calving and lambing processes in endemic areas should be confined to an enclosed area which can be decontaminated after the products of parturition have been disposed of. Immunization is the most effective control measure.

MAN

Treatment with chloramphenicol or tetracycline is effective. Vaccination will prevent infection with Q fever amongst high-risk laboratory workers and in heavily exposed industrial groups, for example farm workers in endemic areas and workers handling farm products such as meat and milk. A standard vaccine Q-34, prepared by Cox's method from formalized *C. burnetii* and containing 10 complement fixing units/ml is given in 1-ml doses as 3-weekly subcutaneous injections. Preliminary skin testing with 0.1 ml of a 1/50 dilution of the vaccine should be performed to avoid reactions. Successful vaccination is shown by the development of a positive skin reaction after 40 days.

BACTERIAL INFECTIONS

PLAGUE

Occurrence:	South East Asia, South America, Middle East, Africa
Organisms:	*Yersinia pestis*
Reservoir:	Rats (bubonic), man (pneumonic)
Transmission:	Fleabite (bubonic), droplet (pneumonic)
Control:	Isolation
	Notification
	DDT for elimination of fleas
	Rat destruction
	Raising standards of environmental hygiene
	Immunization, chemoprophylaxis

Plague is a rapidly fatal disease due to *Yersinia pestis* which can manifest itself in a variety of

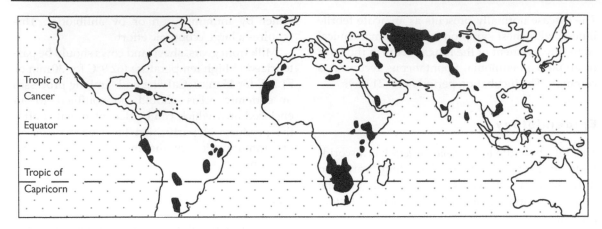

Figure 7.4: Known and probable foci of plague.

ways – bubonic, pneumonic and septicaemic forms. The incubation period is 2–4 days. It is a notifiable disease.

Bacteriology

The organisms are small, Gram-negative, ovoid bacilli showing bipolar staining. *Y. pestis* is easily destroyed by disinfectants, heat and sunlight but in cold or freezing conditions it can survive for weeks or months.

Epidemiology

Although the number of cases of plague have gradually declined, foci of the disease still exist in the Indian subcontinent, China, South East Asia, Africa, South America and the Middle East (Fig. 7.4). A noteworthy feature has been the continuing importance of the disease in Vietnam. The principal endemic foci are India, China, Manchuria, Mongolia, Burma, Vietnam, East Africa, Malagasy Republic, Brazil, Bolivia, Peru and Ecuador.

BUBONIC PLAGUE

The reservoirs of infection are rats and non-domestic rodents. The bubonic disease, which is the commonest, is transmitted by the bite of an infected rat flea *Xenopsylla cheopis* while pneumonic plague spreads from a human reservoir, person to person by droplet infection (see below).

The occurrence of bubonic plague in a human population is always preceded by an enzootic in the rat population and hence any unusual mortality among rats should be looked into promptly. Plague spreads rapidly within the human population when conditions are insanitary and congested and where rats are numerous and have access to food.

When a flea ingests infected blood the plague bacilli multiply in its gut and may gradually block the flea's proventriculus. As a result, the flea cannot feed, becomes hungry and tries repeatedly to bite, regurgitating plague bacilli into the puncture at each attempt. These so-called 'blocked fleas' are a very important factor in the dissemination of human disease. In temperate climates plague is common in the warmer months (i.e. summer), while in the tropics it appears in the colder months (i.e. winter). The efficiency of flea transmission declines with increasing temperatures. All ages and either sex may be infected. Serological evidence indicates that there are a substantial number of asymptomatic plague infections.

Plague also occurs in non-domestic rodents – wild rodent plague – and epizootics affect many different species throughout the world. The infection is transferred to rats living in urban areas from wild rodents and thence to man. In rural areas man, for example hunters and trappers, can be infected in the field, bring the disease home, infect their own domestic rats and fleas and thereby their families.

PNEUMONIC PLAGUE

Pneumonic plague is transmitted from person to person by 'droplet infection' from patients suffering from primary pneumonic plague or from individuals with bubonic plague who develop terminal plague pneumonia. Neither rats nor fleas play a part in the spread of the disease. Overcrowding favours dissemination of pneumonic plague. Some years ago in Vietnam, a mixed pneumonic/bubonic plague outbreak occurred and *Y. pestis* was recovered from the throats of asymptomatic healthy carriers.

Laboratory diagnosis

Y. pestis may be detected in smears of material aspirated from buboes and from sputum, by immunofluorescence assays and even from the blood stained by Gram's method. Culture and animal inoculation should be performed. Smears from the spleen are positive at necropsy. Specimens of material aspirated from buboes, throat swabs and sputa can now be placed in a special holding medium which maintains the organisms in a viable condition during transport to distant laboratories, where DNA probes or polymerase chain reaction (PCR) may be available. The serological test most commonly used is the passive haemagglutination assay.

Control

Plague, one of only three diseases – together with cholera and yellow fever, is a notifiable and quarantinable disease and the quarantine period laid down by the International Health Regulations is 6 days.

THE INDIVIDUAL

Bubonic plague

Cases should be removed to hospital and isolated. Care should be taken in the nursing of patients in case they develop pneumonia and hence masks and gowns should be worn by attendants. Contacts should be under surveillance for 6 days and dusted with DDT powder. Most authorities have also recommended chemoprophylaxis for all contacts: tetracyclines 2 g daily for 1 week or sulphadimidine 3 g daily for 1 week.

Streptomycin is the drug of choice but chloramphenicol and tetracycline have often been used. Regardless of the choice of the antibiotic, treatment should continue for at least 3 days after the patient is afebrile. The overall fatality rate of untreated bubonic plague is between 20 and 75%, while untreated pneumonic plague is almost invariably fatal. Prompt and adequate therapy reduces the overall mortality to less than 5%.

All personnel engaged in flea or rat control during an epizootic must wear protective clothing impregnated with DDT, while dead rats should be sprinkled with DDT, and handled and disposed of carefully.

Pneumonic plague

This is a highly infectious disease and immediate and strict isolation is vitally important. The patients' clothing, their house and everything they have been in contact with must be disinfected. Medical and nursing staff attending such patients must wear protective clothing, including goggles. Strict surveillance of all contacts must be carried out daily and prompt isolation and treatment of infected cases carried out. Chemoprophylaxis for all contacts, as described for bubonic plague, has been recommended. While in hospital the strict current disinfection must be done throughout the course of the disease.

THE COMMUNITY

Elimination of fleas

The immediate and widespread use of dusts of DDT (10%) and benzene hexachloride (BHC) (3%) in rat-infested areas to eliminate the fleas is the most important single control measure that interrupts transmission. In areas where resistance to one or both of these occurs, dusts of carbanyl (2%), diazinon (2%) or malathion (5%) should prove effective. An evaluation of the efficiency of the dusting programme is mandatory.

Rat control

The elimination of fleas must precede the systematic destruction of rats; which should commence on lines extending radially from the centre of infection in order to delimit the enzootic area. All rats caught should be examined for evidence of plague and any new foci of infection treated with DDT. The systematic rat trapping and destruction is followed by measures such as rat-proofing of houses and buildings, protection of food and sanitary disposal of refuse. Since the spread of plague from region to region is chiefly through rats in ships, rat-proofing of ships and general maintenance of ship hygiene should be encouraged. Port health authorities are particularly responsible for supervising this and constant vigilance is required, especially in busy ports such as Singapore.

Immunization

Protection for groups at risk is provided by the use of a dead vaccine or attenuated live vaccine of *Y. pestis*. The latter is given in a single dose while two doses of the dead vaccine are required at weekly intervals. Protection commences a week after inoculation and lasts for about 10 months. Most authorities also recommend chemoprophylaxis for all contacts of both forms of plague.

THE RELAPSING FEVERS

Relapsing fever is due to infection of the blood by morphologically indistinguishable strains of spirochaetes, which are transmitted by ticks and lice, resulting in endemic disease. The louse-borne spirochaete is known as *Borrelia recurrentis* while the tick-borne spirochaete is commonly *B. duttoni*.

Tick-borne relapsing fever

Occurrence:	Endemic in Africa, Middle East; sporadic in South America
Organism:	Borrelia duttoni
Reservoir:	Rodents, humans
Transmission:	Tick
Control:	Personal protection
	Vector control
	Rehousing

Non-epidemic relapsing fever is due to infection with *Borrelia duttoni* and is transmitted by a number of ticks, of which the African *Ornithodorus moubata* is one of the most important. Three or more elapses may occur, with a rapid drop in temperature, drenching sweats, intense thirst, bradycardia and hypotension.

The incubation period is 3–10 days, and recovery is followed by immunity lasting about a year.

EPIDEMIOLOGY

The disease occurs in Central, East and South Africa as well as in North Africa, North, Central

and South America, the Middle East and northern India.

Reservoir

In most areas *B. duttoni* normally affects rodents and occurs only accidentally in man, while in Central Africa it primarily affects man, in whom it is endemic.

Transmission

The vector in South America is *Ornithodorus rudis*. The other vector species are not domestic in habit, and they feed primarily on rodents and other small mammals. The disease, therefore, is highly endemic where the vector is domestic in habit and very sporadic in areas where human contact with the tick is in open country or caves. The tick lives in the soil of the floor, or the mud-plaster walls of African huts; they are also found in caves and in the soil of bush or scrub country.

The female lays batches of eggs, each of which hatches to produce a larval tick with three pairs of legs. The larval forms pass through about five moults at intervals of 2 weeks. Larval forms and adults feed by sucking blood. A proportion of the offspring of infected female ticks is infected transovarially, thus the infection may persist through several generations. During feeding a saline fluid, called coxal fluid, is excreted from glands near the attachment of the legs. It is generally believed that the infected fluid exuded by the coxal glands, saliva and bowel contaminates the wound made by the bite of the tick and spirochaetes enter the bloodstream.

Although *B. duttoni* will infect lice, no large-scale change in vector has been proved to occur under natural conditions.

Host factors

Humans entering caves, working in bush country, living in infected African huts, or sleeping in rest houses in the vicinity of infected villages are liable to acquire the infection. It seems that babies and little children are very susceptible to the disease and it appears that immunity is acquired with increasing age by those living in endemic areas. There are several reports in the literature of newborn infants developing relapsing fever within the first few days after birth, but no case of congenital infection has been recorded. It has been suggested that infection is transmitted after birth during the process of suckling, possibly from cracks in nipples, to abrasions in the child's mouth.

LABORATORY DIAGNOSIS

Blood films show the circulating spirochaete *B. duttoni*.

CONTROL

The individual

In areas where transmission is by non-domestic vectors, control consists of wearing protective clothing, such a high-legged boots, or in using repellents.

The vector

Domestic vectors can be controlled by treating the interiors of houses with BHC or dieldrin. Spray treatments (usually suspensions) have been used in dosages of 0.2–6 g BHC/m^2; the higher dosage will give protection up to a year or more.

The community

The most satisfactory control results from rehousing the people in buildings which provide no harbourage for ticks.

Louse-borne relapsing fever

Occurrence:	Epidemic in parts of Africa, India, South America; endemic in Ethiopia
Organism:	*Borrelia recurrentis*
Reservoir:	Humans
Transmission:	Body louse
Control:	Mass delousing

Borrelia recurrentis produces fever, headache, skeletal and abdominal pain, and the usual symptoms of acute infection are common. Tachypnoea, upper abdominal tenderness with a palpable liver and spleen, jaundice and purpura occur. Hyperpyrexia, hypotension and cardiac failure can be fatal.

In an attack of louse-borne relapsing fever there are one or two relapses, and death, in contrast to tick-borne relapsing fever, is often in the first attack.

The incubation period is usually from 2 to 10 days.

EPIDEMIOLOGY

Louse-borne relapsing fever has a similar geographical distribution to epidemic typhus and is more common in temperate than in tropical climates. However, outbreaks of epidemic louse-borne relapsing fever have occurred in parts of Africa, India and South America. The disease is endemic in Ethiopia.

Reservoir

Man is the only reservoir of louse-borne relapsing fever, and an endemic focus, as is present in Ethiopia, is capable of starting a widespread epidemic. African epidemics in the past seem to have occurred every 20 years, the last being in 1943. Little is known of where relapsing fever lurks between epidemics and how it suddenly springs up after silent intervals of several years.

Transmission

Disease is conveyed from one man to another by the human body louse, *Pediculus humanus*. The blood of a patient suffering from relapsing fever contains spirochaetes only during febrile periods and lice become infected at this time. In contrast to ticks, no transovarial transmission occurs in lice. Infection is transmitted from louse to man not by the bite, as in tick-borne disease, but by contamination of the wound (made by scratching) with the body fluids of the louse, following crushing on the skin.

Host factors

Like epidemic typhus fever, which it may accompany, it is associated with poor sanitation and personal hygiene, particularly overcrowding, undernutrition and lice-infested clothing.

LABORATORY DIAGNOSIS

Blood should be taken during the pyrexial period and examined either by dark-ground illumination or after staining with a Romanovsky stain. *B. recurrentis* is about 15 µm long and made up of spiral turns occupying 2–3 µm. The numbers present in blood films vary from case to case; at the height of the first pyrexial attack they are often numerous. Blood infection is less heavy in tick-borne than in the louse-borne disease. The organisms may be recovered by culture or by intraperitoneal inoculation of blood into laboratory animals (e.g. mouse or rat). Relapsing fever antibodies may cross-react with syphilis antigens to produce a positive reaction in non-treponemal antigen tests. The commonly used serological test is the immunofluorescent antibody assay (IFA). PCR and other molecular biology techniques are also available.

CONTROL

This essentially consists of mass delousing by residual insecticidal powers, as in epidemic typhus.

The individual

The safest, most effective and economical method of treating louse-borne relapsing fever is one injection of 300 000 units of procaine penicillin followed the next day by an oral dose of 250 mg tetracycline. Severe reactions of the Jarisch–Herxheimer type can occur.

The community

The only effective measure is to control lice infestation with DDT as has been described for epidemic typhus.

BARTONELLOSIS

Occurrence:	Bolivia, Peru, Colombia, Ecuador
Organism:	Bartonella bacilliformis
Reservoir:	Humans
Transmission:	Sandflies (Phelbotomus spp.)
Control:	Insecticides
	Repellents and nets
	Salmonella prophylaxis

Bartonellosis appears in two distinct forms:

- Oroya fever – an acute, febrile illness associated with a rapidly developing anaemia and a high mortality.
- Verruca peruana – a non-fatal disease exemplified by generalized cutaneous lesions. It usually occurs following recovery from the Oroya fever stage although it occasionally arises apparently spontaneously.

Epidemiology

The infection is limited to Bolivia, Peru, Colombia and Ecuador. The causative organism is Bartonella bacilliformis. Although known since 1905 it was first cultured in 1928 by Noguchi from an acute case of Oroya fever and the culture produced the nodules of verruca in monkeys. Oroya fever is also known as Carrion's disease, since Carrion, a medical student, inoculated himself with material from a verruca lesion and died from Oroya fever 39 days later.

RESERVOIR AND TRANSMISSION

The disease is transmitted from man to man by the bites of various species of Phlebotomus sandflies, which live at altitudes of 600–2400 m feet and bite only at night. The disease is most prevalent at the end of the rainy season when these insects are most numerous. When a susceptible person is bitten infection follows, usually in 3–4 weeks.

HOST FACTORS

The principal cause of mortality is a particular susceptibility of patients with Oroya fever to septicaemic infections with salmonella organisms, commonly S. typhimurium. Recovery confers some resistance to reinfection, so that in endemic areas the disease is most prevalent in children.

Laboratory diagnosis

The organisms are pleomorphic Gram-negative coccobacilli and are found in blood smears, either free in the plasma or within red cells, in Oroya fever. They are sparse in the nodules in verruca and culture of material on serum agar is the most reliable method of isolation.

Control

The disease has been successfully controlled by applying residual insecticides to the interior of houses and outbuildings. Personal prophylaxis consists in the use of repellents and impregnated nets. As soon as Oroya fever is diagnosed the patient should be given chloramphenicol in standard doses as for salmonella infections.

PROTOZOAL INFECTIONS

MALARIA For late addenda on Malaria
see p. 233.

For late addenda on Malaria
see p. 233.

Occurrence:	Worldwide (60°N–40°S)
Organisms:	Plasmodium falciparum, P. vivax, P. malariae, P. ovale
Reservoir:	Humans
Transmission:	Bite of Anopheles mosquitoes
Control:	Early diagnosis and treatment
	Chemoprophylaxis
	Impregnated nets and curtains
	Vector control
	Personal protection

Human malaria is a disease of wide distribution caused by sporozoa of the genus *Plasmodium*. There are four species of parasites that infect man: *P. falciparum*; *P. vivax*; *P. malariae*; *P. ovale*.

The burden of disease malaria causes is considerable, amounting to 300–500 million clinical cases per year – 80% of which occur in Africa. It is responsible for 1 million deaths per year – virtually all due to *P. falciparum* and 90% of which are in Africa. In Kenya 1 in 15 children suffers from one episode of severe malaria before the age of 5 years; in the Gambia 1% of children under 5 years die of malaria while in Malawi malaria is responsible for one-third of paediatric admissions and one-third of hospital deaths.

The differentiation of the species depends on the morphology and staining of the parasites and associated changes in the containing cells. The most common and important infections are those caused by *P. falciparum* and *P. vivax*. Mixed infections occur.

The arthropod hosts are females of certain species of *Anopheles* mosquitoes. Of the 60 species of *Anopheles* mosquitoes that are vectors for malaria, only 30 are of major epidemiological importance (Plate 64).

Clinically, malaria is characterized by fever, hepatomegaly, splenomegaly, varying degrees of anaemia, and various syndromes resulting from the involvement of individual organs. Multiorgan failure is common. Death is usually due either to anaemia, usually in children 6 months–2 years; cerebral malaria in children 2–5 years; metabolic acidosis in both groups; or a combination of these severe manifestations.

The complete life cycle of the human malaria parasite embraces a period of development within the mosquito – extrinsic incubation period – and a period of development in humans (Fig. 7.5). In *P. vivax* and *P. ovale* infections hypnozoites (dormant forms) are found in the liver following sporozoite invasion. These are responsible for both the long incubation period seen with some *P. vivax* strains (e.g. North Korean) and the relapses that occur with these two infections. The relapses due to *P. malariae* are now thought to be the result of persistent low-grade blood parasitaemia. It follows therefore that adequate treatment of the asexual phase (blood stages) should prevent recrudescences of the infection – as is the case for *P. falciparum*.

Epidemiology

Malaria is found in regions lying roughly between latitudes 60°N and 40°S. It is still commonly found throughout most of Africa, the Middle East, South East Asia, the western Pacific and South America (Fig. 7.6). Autochthonous malaria is reoccurring in the southern states of the former USSR and eastern Turkey.

The four factors that determine the epidemiology of malaria are: environmental, vectorial, parasite and host factors. Their interplay determines the two polar epidemiological extremes – stable and unstable malaria (Table 7.4). It must be appreciated, however, that the transmission pattern of malaria does vary within the same country, sometimes within short distances.

ENVIRONMENTAL FACTORS

Temperature, humidity, rainfall and altitude all affect the transmission of malaria. Thus, *P. falciparum* requires a minimum temperature of 20°C to develop in the female mosquito, while the other species of human malaria parasites can develop in temperatures as low as 16°C.

A relatively high humidity is required for survival of adult vectors while rainfall is essential to provide breeding sites. The threat of global warming presents a risk of serious epidemics through an extension of malaria into the highlands and plateau areas of Africa previously considered free from the disease.

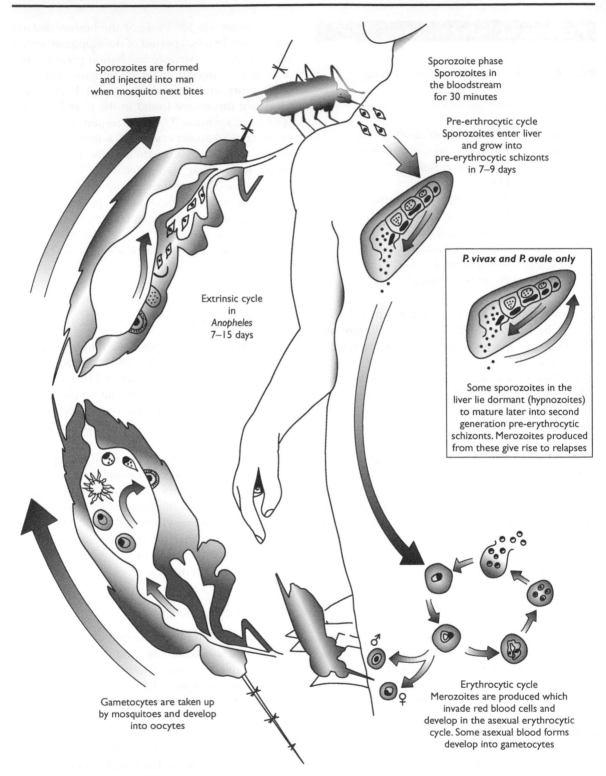

Figure 7.5: Life cycles of *Plasmodium* spp.

Sporozoites are formed
and injected into man
when mosquito next bites

Sporozoite phase
Sporozoites in
the bloodstream
for 30 minutes

Pre-erthrocytic cycle
Sporozoites enter liver
and grow into
pre-erythrocytic schizonts
in 7–9 days

P. vivax and P. ovale only

Some sporozoites in the
liver lie dormant (hypnozoites)
to mature later into second
generation pre-erythrocytic
schizonts. Merozoites produced
from these give rise to relapses

Extrinsic cycle
in
Anopheles
7–15 days

Gametocytes are taken up
by mosquitoes and develop
into oocytes

Erythrocytic cycle
Merozoites are produced which
invade red blood cells and
develop in the asexual erythrocytic
cycle. Some asexual blood forms
develop into gametocytes

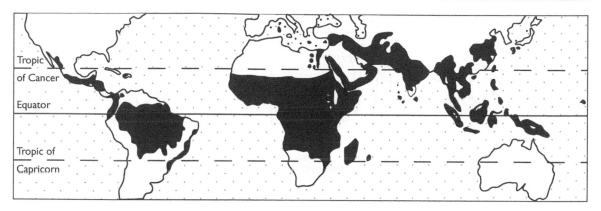

Figure 7.6: Distribution of malaria.

Table 7.4: The epidemiological features of stable and unstable malaria

	Stable malaria (Plate 65)	Unstable malaria
Transmission pattern	Transmission occurs throughout the year. Fairly uniform intensity of transmission. Pattern repeats annually, with astonishing regularity	Seasonal transmission. Variable intensity of transmission. Liable to flare up in dramatic epidemics
Immunity	Potent resistance in the community due to prevailing intense transmission	General lack of immunity in the community due to low level of transmission, which only occasionally becomes intense
Age	Mainly young children	All age groups
Control	Difficult to eradicate	Eradicated with greater ease than stable malaria
Occurrence	West Africa, Lowlands of New Guinea	Ethiopia, Highlands of New Guinea, Plateau of Madagascar

VECTORIAL FACTORS

These are behavioural factors and susceptibility to infection. Some species are anthropophilic, others zoophilic (prefer animal blood); some prefer to bite indoors, others outdoors (endophagy, exophagy); some prefer to rest during the day indoors, others outdoors (endophily, exophily). Malaria vectors bite between dusk and dawn and generally choose well-oxygenated water rather than stagnant polluted pools to lay their eggs.

PARASITE FACTORS

The prepatency period – time from infection to appearance of parasitaemia – is shortest in *P. falciparum*, 6–25 days, and longest in *P. malariae*, 18–59 days.

The time of appearance of gametocytes in the peripheral blood after the initial asexual parasitaemia, occurs simultaneously in *P. vivax* but not until 8–15 days in *P. falciparum*.

The duration of infection is usually 1 year for *P. falciparum*, 5 years for *P. vivax/P. ovale* and 50 years for *P. malariae*, after acquiring the original infection.

P. vivax and *P. ovale* relapse because of the presence of intrahepatic parasites with retarded development. *P. falciparum* and *P. malariae* only recrudesce if parasitological cure has not been achieved.

Sporozoite loads may not vary significantly as a function of transmission intensity; not all naturally infected mosquitoes transmit sporozoites and the numbers of sporozoites transmitted per blood-feeding are quite low. The species with the largest multiplication of the parasite is *P. falciparum* with

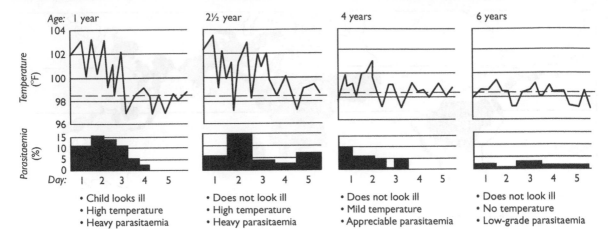

Figure 7.7: The natural history of falciparum malaria in a highly endemic area showing how clinical immunity develops in a child. With each subsequent phase there is both a decline in the febrile response to infection and in parasitaemia as immunity develops.

infection rates up to 30% of the erythrocytes while for *P. vivax* infection rates rarely rise above 5%, due to the fact that *P. falciparum* tends to infect parasites of any age, while the other species are more selective, for example *P. vivax* prefers reticulocytes and young cells.

Finally, mature forms of *P. falciparum* are able to sequestrate in the deep vascular beds.

HOST FACTORS

The following four factors influence the epidemiology of malaria – genetic, immune, nutritional and behavioural.

Genetic factors (see p. 248)

There is now considerable evidence that several genetic factors protect against severe disease and mortality from *P. falciparum* malaria. These include HbS heterozygotes; alpha-thalassaemia homozygotes and heterozygotes; B-thalassaemia heterozygotes; HbC homozygotes and heterozygotes; G6PD deficiency; HLA-BW53; HLA-DRB[1] 1302 and ovalocytosis. Conversely, some TNF alleles and haptoglobin types increase the susceptibility to severe malaria.

Immune factors

The mechanisms involved are complex and beyond the scope of this book. In areas of stable malaria, infants born to immune mothers are partially protected from clinical malaria for

4–6 months, due to a combination of passive immunity via maternal antibodies and high levels of haemoglobin F, which does not sustain parasite growth as well as haemoglobin A.

From about 6 months to 5 years or longer, the child is susceptible to severe attacks of malaria resulting in death. After this, and into adult life, attacks of malaria become less frequent and less severe and mortality is extremely rare. The substantial immunity persists throughout life providing antigenic stimulation continues by repeated inoculation of parasites by vectors, as occurs in stable areas of malaria (see Fig. 7.7). However, this immunity can be lost if a previously immune person lives in a non-endemic area for more than 2 years; if he or she is immunosuppressed, is on steroid therapy, or has had a splenectomy. There is some evidence that HIV-infected adults have an increased susceptibility to malarial fever but, paradoxically, severe malaria does not seem to occur.

In areas of unstable malaria, antigenic stimulation is not strong nor constant enough for the development of a substantial immunity.

Nutritional factors

The influence of nutrition on malaria susceptibility is complex. There is good evidence from animal and autopsy studies that severe malnutrition – Kwashiorkor – may be antagonistic to malaria. In contrast, mild–moderate malnutrition is a risk factor for severe malaria. This paradox could be explained by postulating that in severe malnutrition a specific nutrient crucial to parasite growth is absent.

Behavioural factors

Many elements of human behaviour profoundly affect the epidemiology of malaria – uncontrolled urbanization; subsistence agriculture; population movements; wood-gathering in the forest; open-cast mining; gem – silver and other mining, legal or clandestine; agricultural production of cotton, sugar cane, rubber and rice (Plate 66).

Behavioural patterns emerge in different communities and are influenced by cultural, ethnic and religious backgrounds.

The introduction of electricity into rural areas has resulted in promoting late-night outdoor human activities and thus increased biting opportunities for mosquitoes.

Health impact of *P. falciparum* malaria

Attempts are now being made to define and measure the epidemiology of disease and provide more accurate measurements of malaria morbidity and mortality.

The methodology known as population attributable fractions (PAF) increases the sensitivity and specificity of defining morbid events. Since geometric parasite densities differ in various age groups, stratification for age is required.

PAF together with active and passive case detection are providing more reliable data. Weekly active case detection, which is feasible, obtains 75% of the information acquired from daily visits, which are impractical in most countries. Malaria-specific mortality is obtained by using detailed demographic surveillance systems (DSS) of large populations (120 000 or more).

The critical components of DSS are: (i) community sensitization; (ii) mapping including Global Positioning Systems (GPS), which provide spatial maps of households in relation to physical, environmental and health service features; (iii) census; and (iv) multiround household visits and verbal autopsy. The sensitivity of verbal autopsy has varied between 45 and 72% and its specificity between 77 and 89%.

Using the above methods in the Kilifi area of Kenya, it has been estimated that children under 5 years will suffer 1.2 attacks of malaria per year; children between 5 and 9 years one attack every 18 months and persons over 10 years one attack every 3–4 years. Mortality would be 8.3, 1.2 and 0.1 per thousand respectively per year.

A conceptual diagram of the morbidity and mortality of malaria is shown in Plate 67. In stable areas a huge proportion of the population will have an asymptomatic parasitaemia; a number of individuals will suffer from uncomplicated malaria; a proportion will develop severe disease and some of these will die.

The ecological approach

A pragmatic approach to the epidemiological stratification of malaria has been described, encompassing eight different paradigms which are self-explanatory namely: (i) African savannah malaria; (ii) plains and valleys outside Africa (malaria associated with traditional agriculture); (iii) forest; (iv) forest fringe malaria; (v) desert fringe and highland fringe malaria; (vi) urban slums malaria; (vii) malaria associated with agricultural developments; and (viii) malaria resulting from socio-political disturbances.

The above paradigms were designed to make the epidemiology of malaria (and its control) more understandable and possibly more reproduceable.

Mathematical models to characterize the events of malaria transmission have been developed.

Transmission of malaria

Apart from the most common method of transmission – the bite of many species of *Anopheles* mosquitoes – other forms of transmission have occurred, namely: (i) by blood transfusion; (ii) congenital from mother to foetus; (iii) sharing needles and syringes among drug addicts; (iv) accidental among health workers through needle and instrument puncture; and (v) plasmapheris and organ transplantation.

Vectors surviving journeys from endemic to non-endemic areas have been responsible for transmitting malaria to airport workers or individuals living around airports ('airport malaria'), or in baggage originating from endemic areas ('baggage malaria'), or in taxis emanating from endemic areas ('taxi-rank malaria').

HIV and malaria

The prevalence and intensity of malaria in pregnancy are higher in women who are HIV positive. In areas of moderate or high transmission, HIV renders multigravidae as susceptible to malaria as primigravidae. Both HIV infection and malaria are independent risk factors. In lower birth weight and maternal anaemia, a common occurrence especially in subsaharan Africa, the risks for both mother and baby are high.

In non-pregnant women and all other persons exposed to malaria, HIV paradoxically does not seem to increase the severity of the disease nor significantly enhance the intensity of parasitaemia.

Epidemic malaria

Severe epidemics have occurred in Africa and elsewhere, as recently as 1996. They are often the result of exceptional meteorological conditions or massive destruction as a consequence of war or natural disasters followed by population movements. The following risk factors have been identified: (i) abnormally prolonged rains; (ii) extensive floods; (iii) global warming; (iv) colonization of tropical jungle areas by agricultural settlers; (v) explosive growth of urban areas; (vi) open-cast mining; (vii) arrival of a non-immune population into a malarious area (e.g. refugees); (viii) the introduction of a number of infected individuals into a malaria-free area where both the *Anopheles* vector and conditions for transmission exist; (ix) admixtures of large numbers of immunes and non-immunes living under primitive conditions (e.g. labour camps); (x) sudden increase in *Anopheles* densities; (xi) agricultural development schemes; (xii) failure to maintain previous control; (xiii) breakdown of health services (e.g. Afghanistan); and (xiv) progressive spread of drug resistance to antimalarials (see p. 205).

Epidemiology of *Plasmodium vivax*

It is opined that among the malaria parasites of humans, *P. malariae* is the most ancestral, followed by *P. vivax/P. ovale*, with *P. falciparum* the most recent from an evolutionary point of view.

Shute explained the mechanism of latency by proposing that there must be two different populations of sporozoites that are genetically programmed to produce either a short or a long incubation period. Lysenko in 1977 propounded the theory of *P. vivax* sporozoites polymorphism. When a Yemeni strain of *P. vivax* was inoculated into 11 volunteers infected by *A. atroparvus*, 7 developed malaria; 5 of the cases had short incubations while two of them developed malaria after 164 and 175 days respectively.

Recent research from Thailand, Sri Lanka and Vanuatu has provided new information into the health impact of *P. vivax* under unstable and stable transmission conditions and where *P. vivax* and *P. falciparum* coexist.

UNSTABLE *P. VIVAX* MALARIA

Missiroli in the 1930s had demonstrated that in southern Italy vivax malaria had a seasonal incidence and was characteristically a disease of infancy and early childhood; the incidence declined in adolescence and was lowest in adults. However, this early exposure to *P. vivax* did not protect adults from acquiring severe clinical attacks when *P. falciparum* infections developed later in life.

In the well-documented epidemic in Ceylon in 1934–35, *P. vivax* played a predominant part during the early stages of the epidemic, but gave place to *P. falciparum* towards its close. The toll of life was approximately 100 000 while probably one-third to one-half of the total population of the island was clinically infected. During the acute stage of the epidemic infants and young children were mainly involved, whilst towards the decline of the epidemic the mortality was almost exclusively confined to persons over 40 years of age. Virtually all deaths were due to *P. falciparum*.

Scientists in Sri Lanka described the characteristics of 'unstable' malaria transmission in a *P. vivax* endemic region, where this species accounted for more than 95% of malaria cases and where the incidence of *P. falciparum* was usually low, although severe epidemics occur at 7–10 year intervals. The focus at Kataragama was being subjected to a *P. falciparum* epidemic at the time of their study.

They noted that both adults and children developed acute symptoms of malaria; moreover there was a low clinical tolerance to *P. falciparum* malaria, to which the population had only recently been at risk, compared to *P. vivax* to which most had had a life-long exposure.

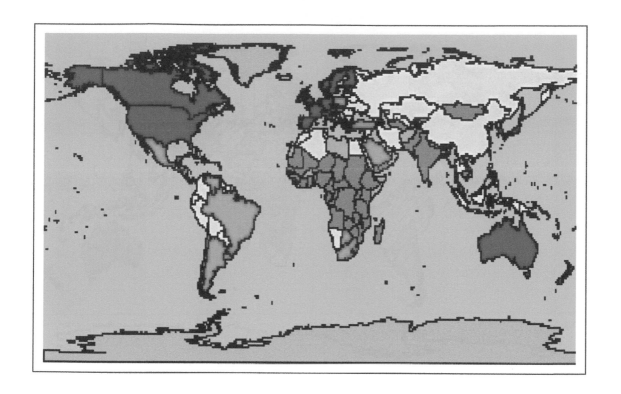

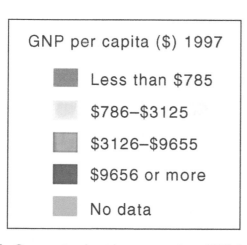

GNP per capita ($) 1997

Less than $785

$786–$3125

$3126–$9655

$9656 or more

No data

Plate 1: Gross national products per capita – 1997. Source: World Bank (2001).

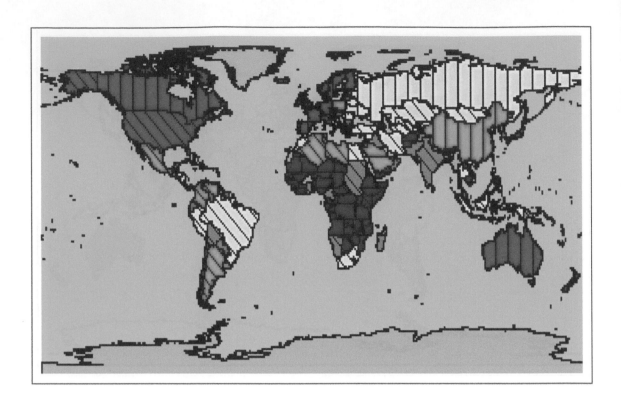

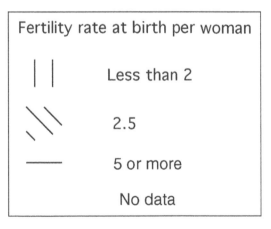

Fertility rate at birth per woman

Less than 2

2.5

5 or more

No data

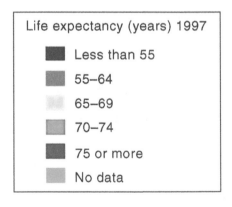

Life expectancy (years) 1997

Less than 55

55–64

65–69

70–74

75 or more

No data

Plate 2: Life expectancy and Fertility – 1997.

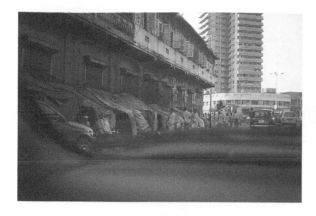

Plate 3: Uncontrolled urbanization in a street in Mumbai not too distant from a high rise flat complex.

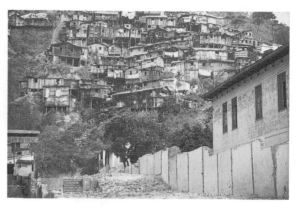

Plate 4: Hill slums in Rio de Janeiro are a source of socio-economic depravity, crime and drug trafficking.

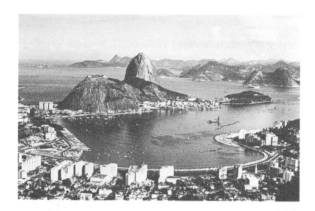

Plate 5: The conditions shown in Plate 4 are in marked contrast to the luxury flats within view of the beautiful entrance to Rio de Janeiro harbour.

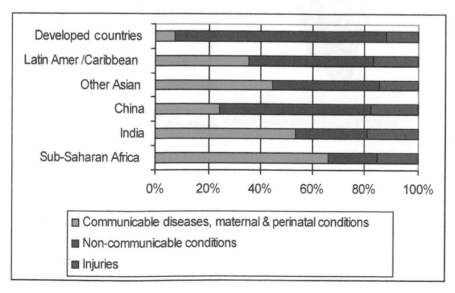

Plate 6: Burden of disease by region. Source: WHO.

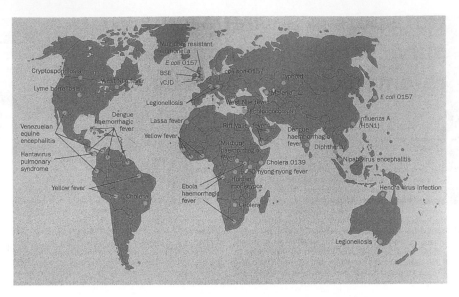

Plate 7: Emerging and re-emerging infectious diseases 1996–2001. Source: WHO (2001).

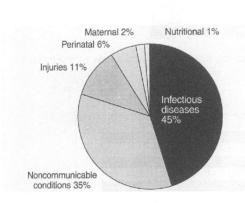

Plate 8: Main causes of death in low income countries in South East Asia and Africa, 1998. Source: WHO (1999).

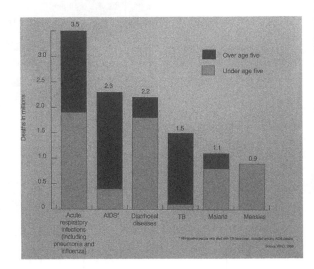

Plate 9: Leading infectious killers. Millions of deaths, worldwide, all ages, 1998. Source: WHO (1999).

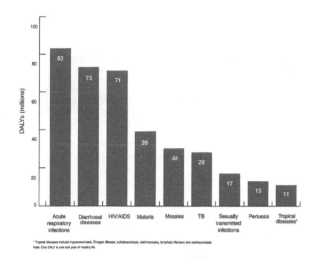

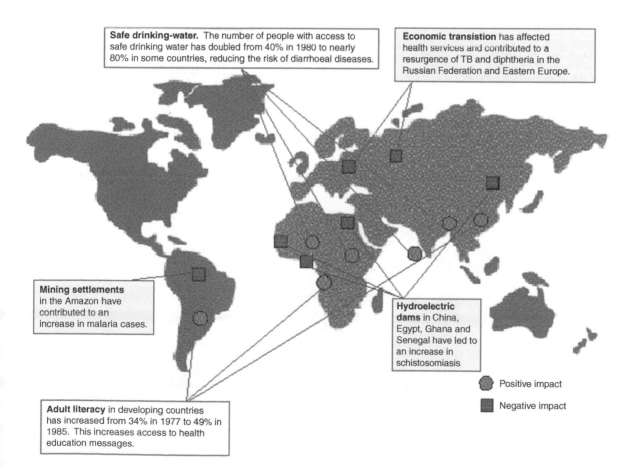

Plate 10: Burden of disease – disability-adjusted life years (DALYs) lost in 1998 due to infectious diseases, millions, all ages. Source: WHO (1999).

Plate 11: Health policy void. Source: WHO.

Safe drinking-water. The number of people with access to safe drinking water has doubled from 40% in 1980 to nearly 80% in some countries, reducing the risk of diarrhoeal diseases.

Economic transistion has affected health services and contributed to a resurgence of TB and diphtheria in the Russian Federation and Eastern Europe.

Mining settlements in the Amazon have contributed to an increase in malaria cases.

Hydroelectric dams in China, Egypt, Ghana and Senegal have led to an increase in schistosomiasis

Adult literacy in developing countries has increased from 34% in 1977 to 49% in 1985. This increases access to health education messages.

Positive impact

Negative impact

Plate 12: Impact of development on infectious disease control. Source: WHO, 1999.

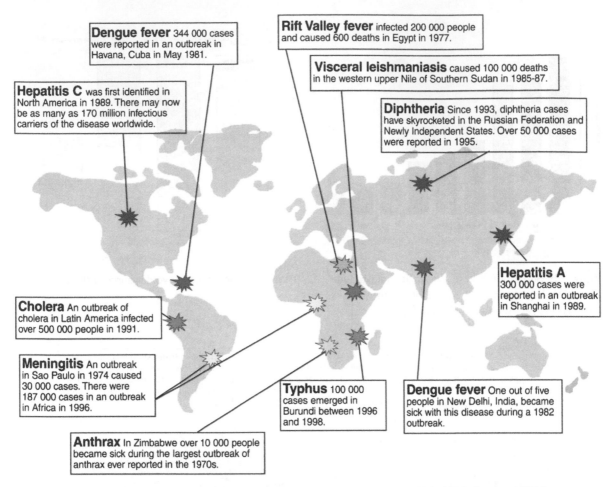

Plate 13: Large outbreaks – selected outbreaks of more than 10,000 cases, 1970–1990. Source: WHO.

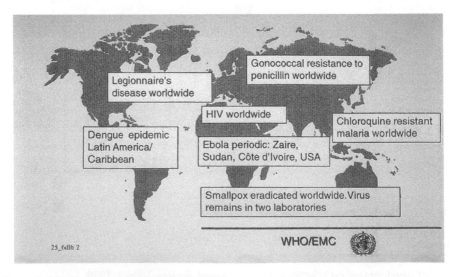

Plate 14: Infectious diseases in transition, 1996 (WHO).

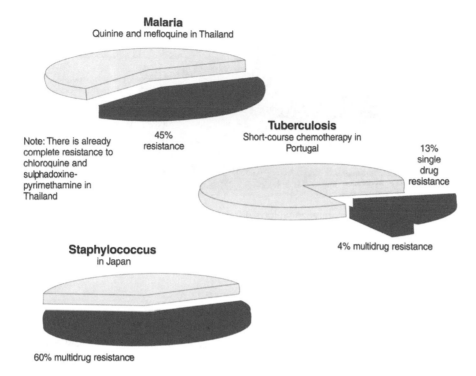

Malaria
Quinine and mefloquine in Thailand

Note: There is already
complete resistance to
chloroquine and
sulphadoxine-
pyrimethamine in
Thailand

45%
resistance

Tuberculosis
Short-course chemotherapy in
Portugal

13%
single
drug
resistance

4% multidrug resistance

Staphylococcus
in Japan

60% multidrug resistance

Plate 15: Antimicrobial resistance. Source: WHO (1997b).

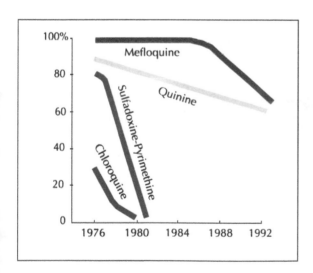

Plate 16: Declining response to antimalarial drugs.
Source: *Southeast Journal of Tropical Medicine and Public
Health*, Mekong Malaria, Vol. 30, Supplement 4, p. 68,
1999.

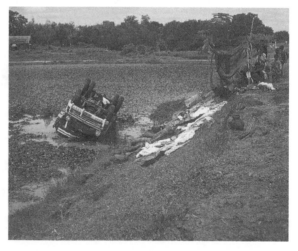

Plate 17: Road accidents are an important cause of
adult deaths in the tropics.

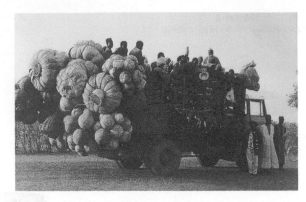

Plate 18: Gross overloading, poor maintenance, long distance and tiring drivers are some of the factors responsible.

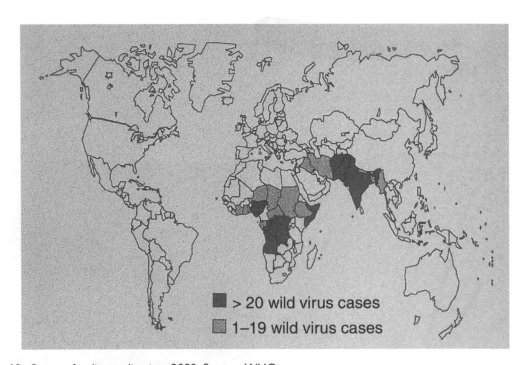

Plate 19: Status of polio eradication, 2000. Source: WHO.

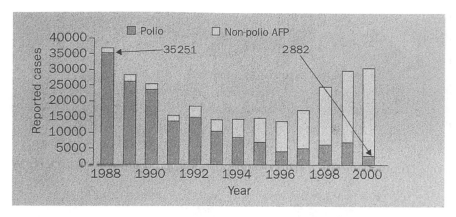

Plate 20: Global annual reported acute flaccid paralysis (AFP) and polio cases, 1988–2000. Source: WHO.

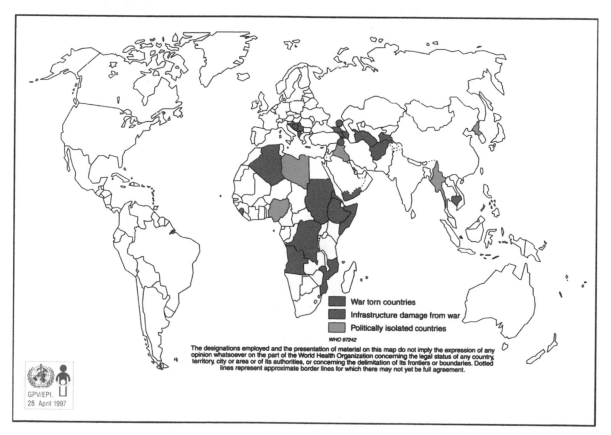

Plate 21: Polio-endemic areas affected by war. Source: WHO.

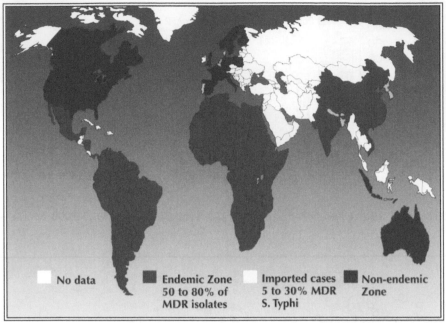

Source: World Health Organization/VRD

Plate 22: Multiresistant *Salmonella typhi*. Source: WHO/VRD.

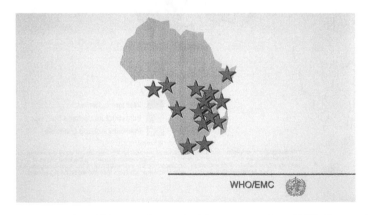

Plate 23: Shigella dysentary type 1 in Africa: epidemics in 15 countries since 1979. Source: WHO.

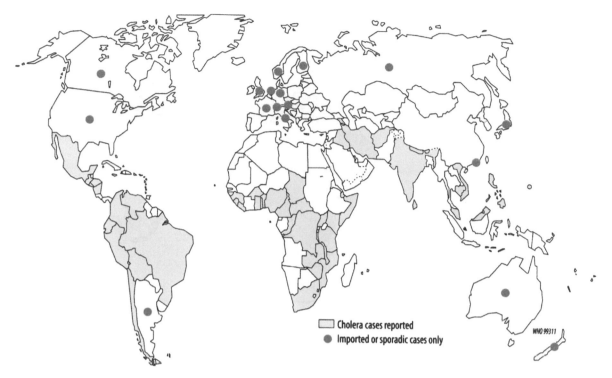

Legend: Cholera cases reported / Imported or sporadic cases only

WHO 99311

Plate 24: Countries/areas reporting cholera, 1998. Source: WHO.

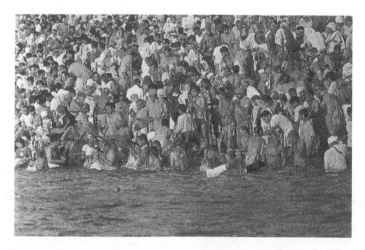

Plate 25: Mass assemblies of pilgrims for religious activities as that seen here on the River Ganges are an important source of cholera.

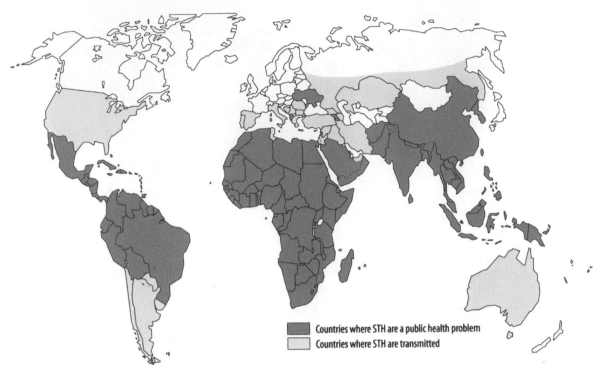

Plate 26: Soil-transmitted helminths (STH), 1999. Source: WHO.

Countries where STH are a public health problem
Countries where STH are transmitted

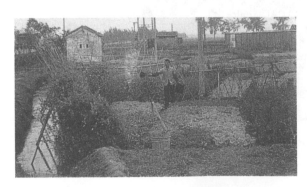

Plate 27: Use of fresh nightsoil to fertilize green-leaf vegetables are a common cause of *Ascaris* and *Trichuris* infection.

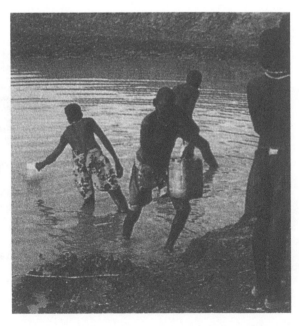

Plate 28: Small collections of fresh water in which cyclops are breeding are major sources of infection with *Dracunculus medinensis*. In the southern Sudan and subsahelian countries these are sometimes the only source of drinking water.

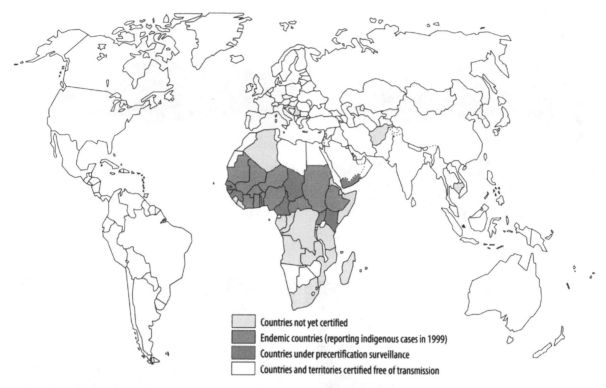

Countries not yet certified
Endemic countries (reporting indigenous cases in 1999)
Countries under precertification surveillance
Countries and territories certified free of transmission

Plate 29: Certification of dracunculiasis eradication status, 2000. Source: WHO.

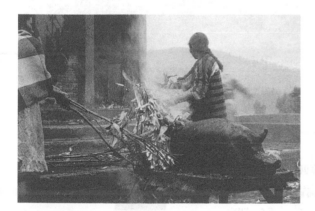

Plate 30: Roasting of pigs in the open often results in the undercooking of meat and the development of *Taenia solium* infection when meat is eaten.

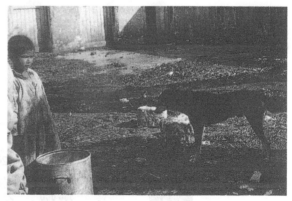

Plate 31: Dogs eating infected offal from the uncontrolled slaughter of animals are a common source of hydatid disease.

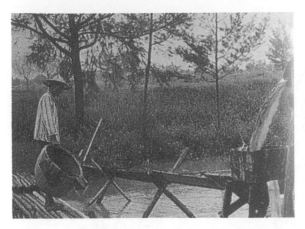

Plate 32: Pouring nightsoil into fish ponds is an ideal way of infecting cultivated fish with *Clonorchis sinensis*.

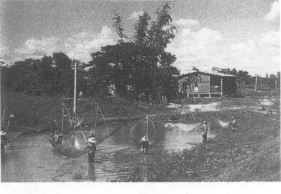

Plate 33: A pond in North East Thailand where cyprinoid fishes are grown. Many of these are infected with metacerceriae of *Opisthorchis viverrini*.

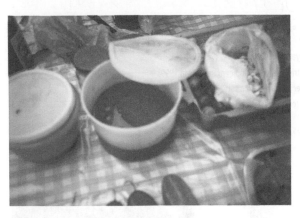

Plate 34: 'Koi-pla' is a favourite fish dish in North East Thailand. The raw fishes of which it is made are contaminated with *Opisthorchis viverrini*.

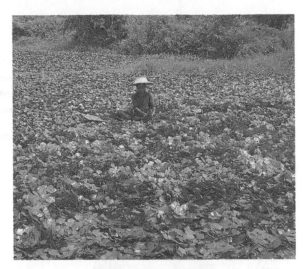

Plate 35: A water calthrop farm in Thailand, an ideal reservoir for fasciolopsis infection.

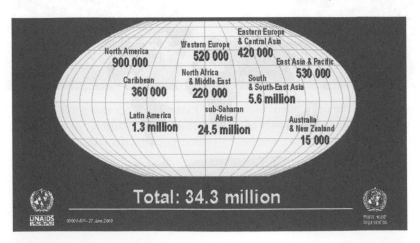

Plate 36: Global distribution of HIV infection. Source: WHO.

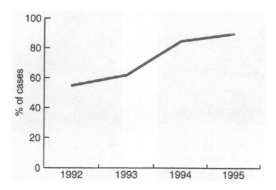

Plate 37: Penicillin-resistant gonorrhoea in Vietnam. Source: WHO.

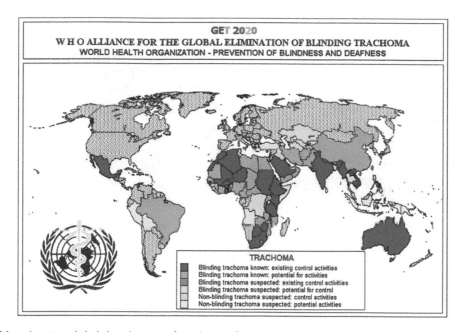

Plate 38: Map showing global distribution of trachoma. Source: WHO.

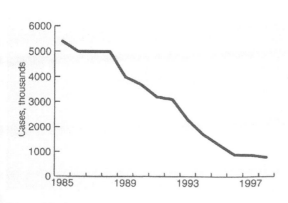

Plate 39: Leprosy nearly eliminated. Source: WHO.

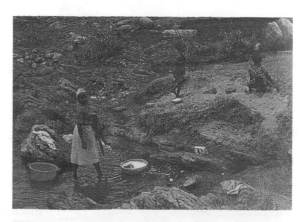

Plate 40: This woman and her children became infected by cercariae of *Schistosoma mansoni* while washing clothes in contaminated fresh water.

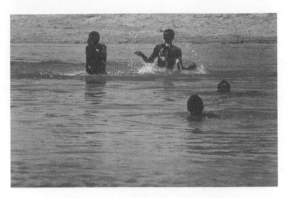

Plate 41: Children and young adults often use freshwater pools to swim in the hot summer months. They are also favourite breeding grounds for *Bulinus* snails that transmit *Schistosoma haematobium*.

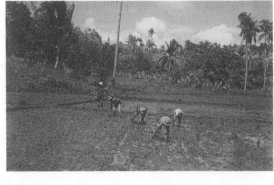

Plate 42: Human infection of *Schistosoma japonicum* occurs in farm workers, for example when planting rice in contaminated paddy fields.

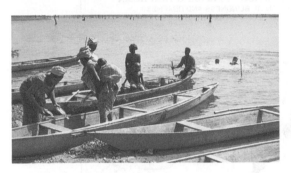

Plate 43: Fishermen on Lake Volta are at risk of contracting schistosomiasis when going out or bringing back their catch.

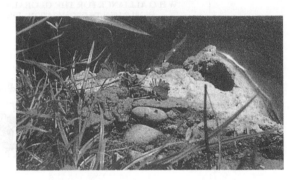

Plate 44: Human faeces deposited at the edge of a pond or irrigation canal are washed by rainfall and infect snail hosts of *Schistosoma mansoni* breeding in them.

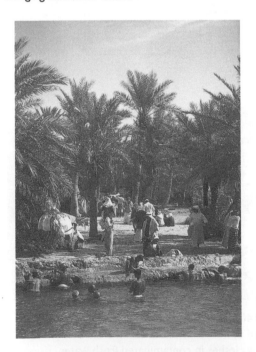

Plate 45: In the villages of the Nile Delta irrigation canals are the main source of plentiful water. Human/snail contact is maximal in the summer months.

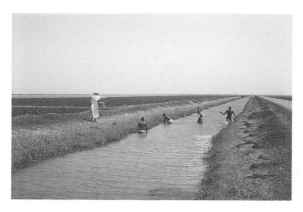

Plate 46: In the Gezira, Sudan, persons engaged to remove vegetation from the irrigation canals are at maximal risk to develop schistosomiasis.

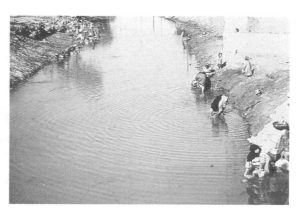

Plate 47: Egyptian women washing their utensils in an irrigation canal in the Nile Delta infested with *Schistosomasis mansoni* and *S. haematobium*.

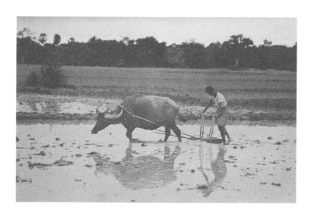

Plate 48: The water-buffalo often used to plough the land in the Philippines are a potent reservoir of *Schistosoma japonicum* infection.

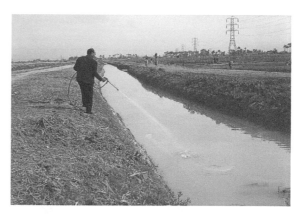

Plate 49: Focal mollusciciding with Baylucide is now preferred to wide scale mollusciciding.

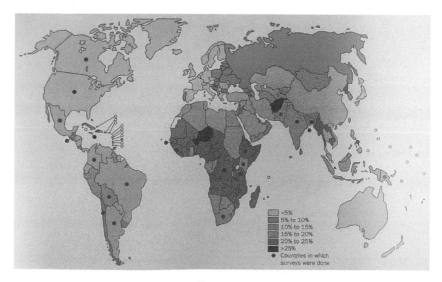

Plate 50: Estimate of the percentage of children that die from lower acute respiratory infections (ARI).
Source: WHO.

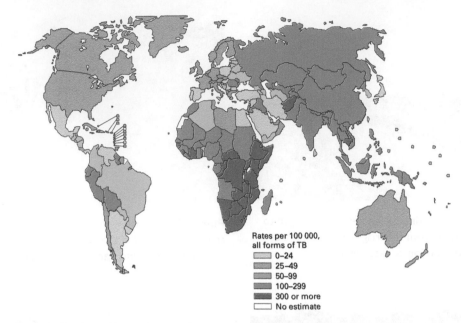

Plate 51: Estimated TB incidence rates, 2003. Source: WHO.

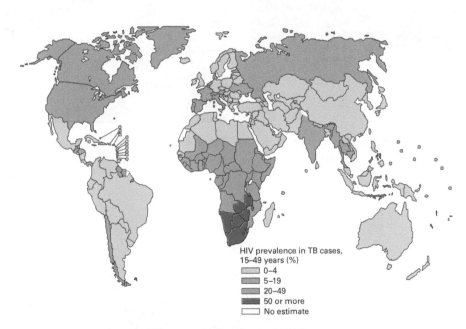

Plate 52: Estimated HIV prevalence in TB cases, 2003. Source: WHO.

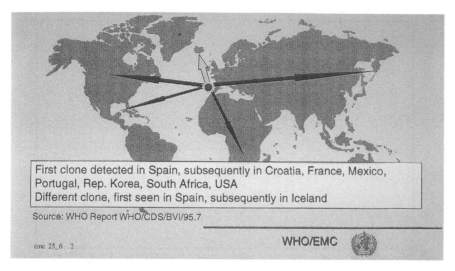

Plate 53: *Streptococcus pneumoniae.* Probable spread of two multiresistant clones. Source: WHO.

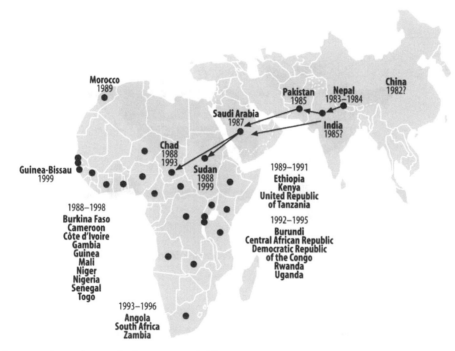

Plate 54: Intercontinental spread of serogroup A *Neisseria meningitidis* (clonal group III-1). Source: WHO.

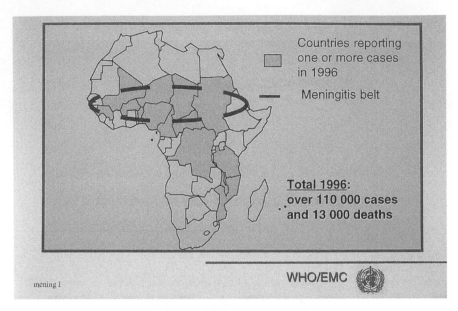

Plate 55: Epidemic meningococcal disease, Africa 1996–1999. Source: WHO.

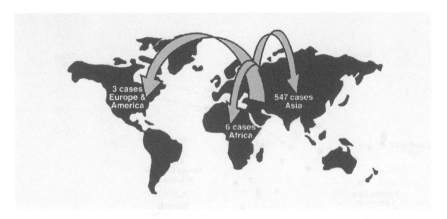

Plate 56: Spread of meningococcal meningitis by pilgrims returning from the Haj, 1987. Source: WHO.

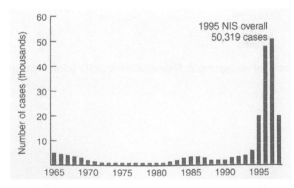

Plate 57: Diphtheria in the Russian Federation and Newly Independent States. Source: WHO.

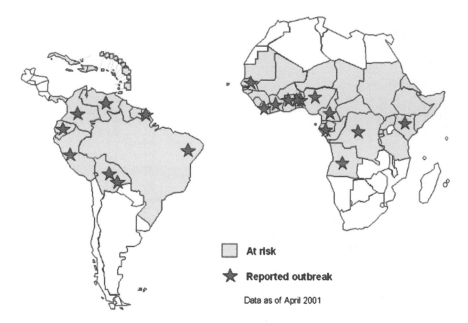

Plate 58: Countries at risk for yellow fever and having reported at least one outbreak, 1985–1997. Source: WHO.

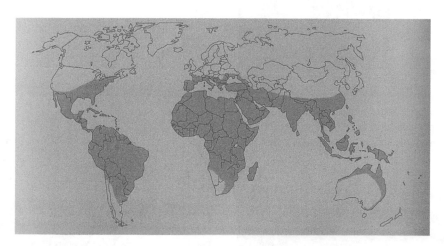

Plate 59: Actual and potential distribution of *Aedes aegypti*, 1998. Source: WHO.

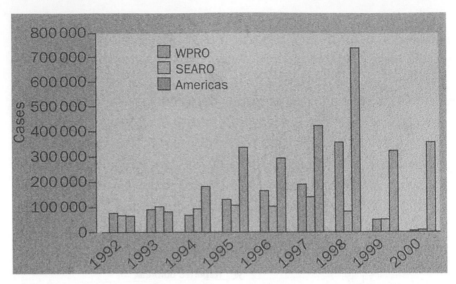

Plate 60: World DF/ DHF reported cases 1992–2000 by WHO region. Source: WHO.

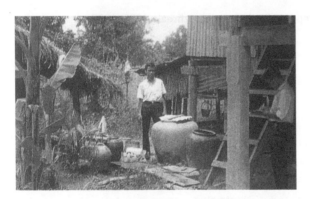

Plate 61: Open large water jars and jars with ill-fitting covers provide ideal breeding habitats for *Ae. egypti* as seen in this village in Thailand.

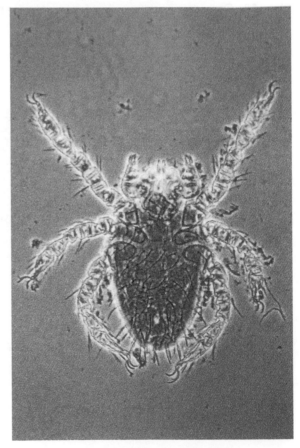

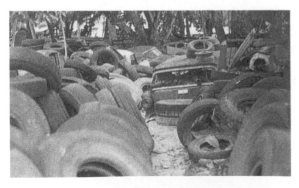

Plate 62: Discarded motor tyres left in dumps exposed to the rain provide ideal site for egg-laying.

Plate 63: Larval mites transmit scrub typhus and also act as reservoirs of infection since transovarial transmission of *R. tsutsugamushi* occurs.

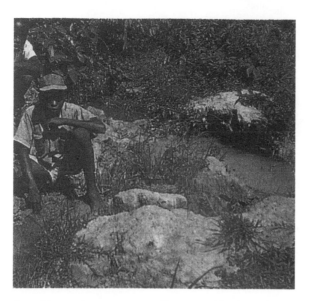

Plate 64: *Anopheles gambiae* breed in small temporary collections of fresh surface water exposed to sunlight on residual pools in drying river beds.

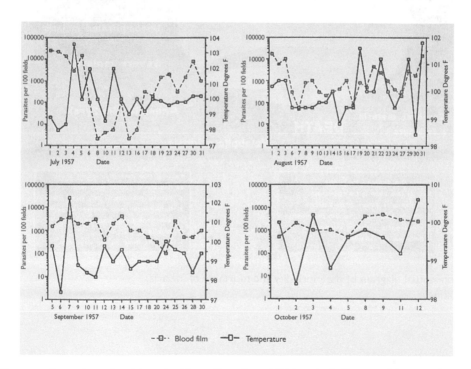

Plate 65: Pattern of parasitaemia with and without fever in a child 1 and a half years old in a stable area of malaria. This long-standing oligosymptomatic parasitaemia is an important cause of anaemia in infants and young children.

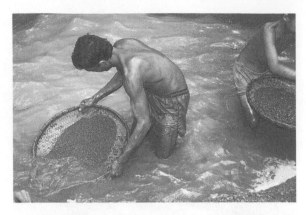

Plate 66: Legal or clandestine gem mining provides breeding sites for mosquitos.

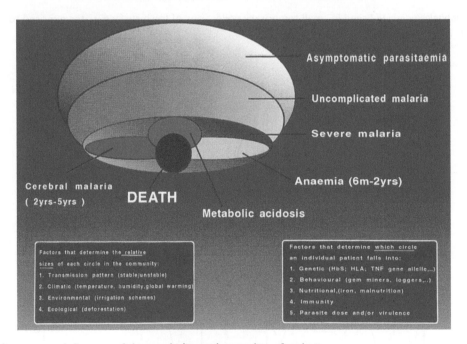

Plate 67: A conceptual diagram of the morbidity and mortality of malaria.

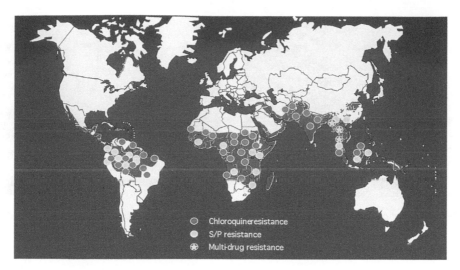

Plate 68: Widespread parasite resistance to anti-malarials. Source: WHO.

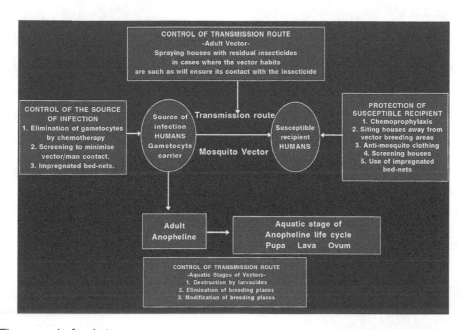

Plate 69: The control of malaria.

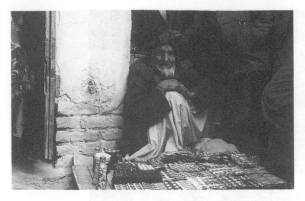

Plate 70: Private vendor of drugs in a street in Afghanistan.

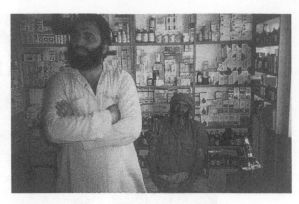

Plate 71: Well-stocked pharmacy with drugs of uncertain quality and long passed expiry dates (Afghanistan).

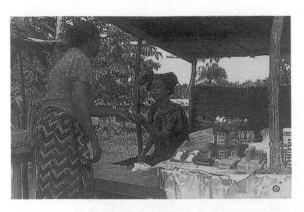

Plate 72: Market vendor of drugs in a Nigerian market. Source: WHO.

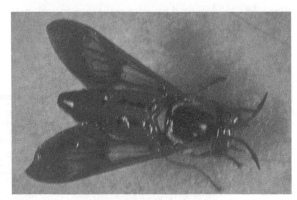

Plate 73: Various species of *Glossina* transmit African trypanosomiasis.

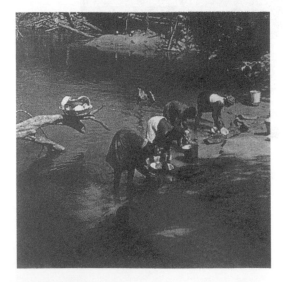

Plate 74: Riverine species of *Glossina* transmit *Gambiense trypanosomiasis*. Man-fly contact is intimate when villagers congregate around pools for collecting water or washing.

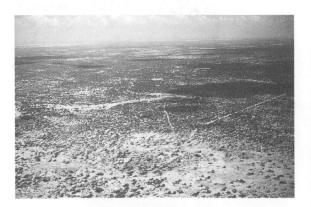

Plate 75: Woodland savannah provides an ideal habitat for *Glossina* species that transmit *Trypanosoma rhodesiense*.

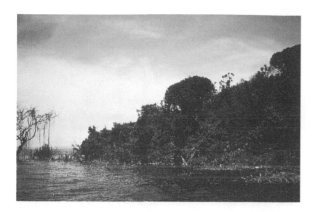

Plate 76: Riverine species of tsetse that transmit *Trypanosoma gambiense* thrive in a moist shady environment.

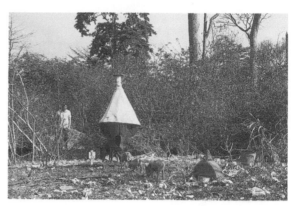

Plate 78: Conical traps such as this one have been used effectively to control tsetse flies.

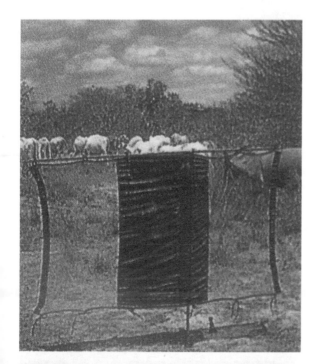

Plate 77: Two of the most successful methods of *Glossina* control is the use of various types of target traps with an odour attraction in a bottle, for example screens treated with long-lasting synthetic pyrethroids. Cattle can be used as a bait for tsetse control, after the animal has been dipped in a synthetic pyrethroid preparation.

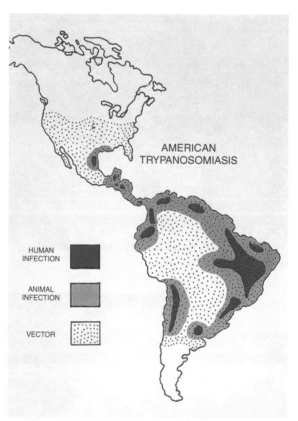

Plate 79: Map of distribution of Chagas' disease and its vectors.

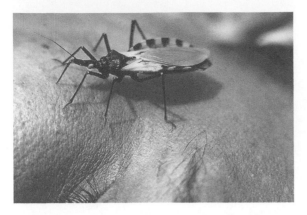

Plate 80: Various species of reduviid bugs transmit Chagas' disease.

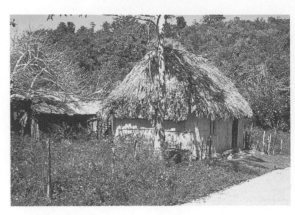

Plate 81: Typical poor housing in a rural area of Brazil provides ideal habitat for reduviid bugs.

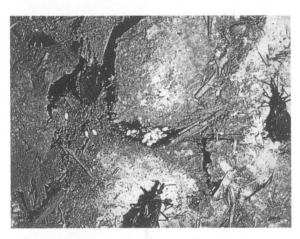

Plate 82: Cracks in the walls of the mud huts in poor rural areas are the favourite habitats of reduviid bugs.

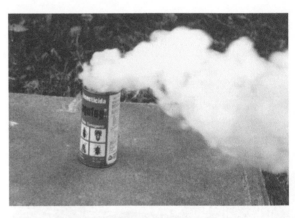

Plate 83: Fumigant cans have proved to be effective in the control of Chagas' disease.

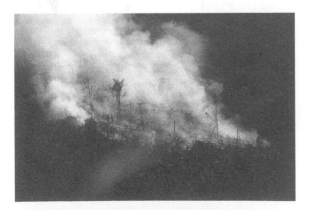

Plate 84: Risk factors for leishmaniasis. (a) Slash and burn in the Amazonian forest, Brazil (courtesy of P. Dejeux).

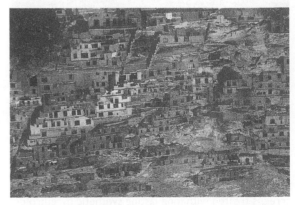

Plate 85: Risk factors for leishmaniasis. (b) Suburbs with poor sanitary conditions, Kabul, Afghanistan (courtesy of P. Dejeux).

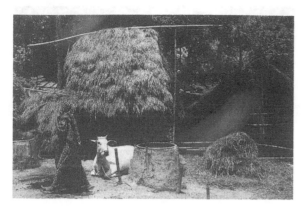

Plate 86: Risk factors for leishmaniasis. (c) Sandfly breeding sites in India, in cowsheds near houses (courtesy of P. Dejeux).

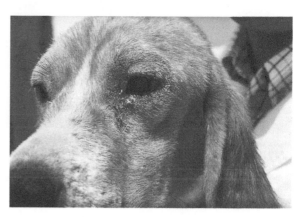

Plate 87: Dogs are the most important reservoir for *Leishmania infantum*. Source: WHO.

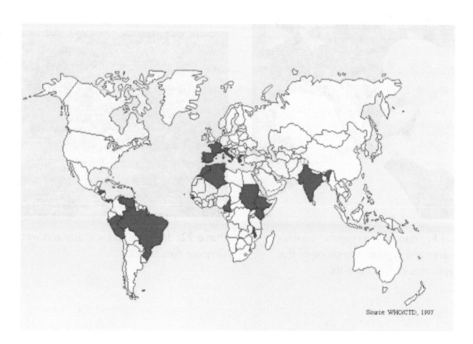

Source WHO/CTD, 1997

Plate 88: Countries reporting leishmaniasis/HIV co-infection. Source: WHO.

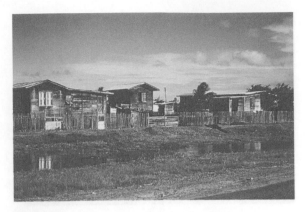

Plate 89: A typical breeding site for *Culex quinquefasciatus* is polluted water.

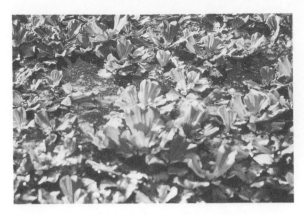

Plate 90: *Pistia* plants provide excellent breeding sites for *Mansonia* species that transmit *Brugia malayi*.

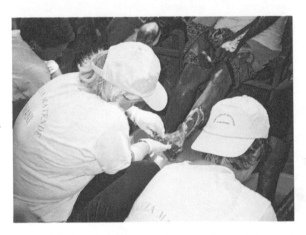

Plate 91: Simple hygiene such as regular washing with soap and water and regular exercising of the limbs prevents episodes of lymphangitis.

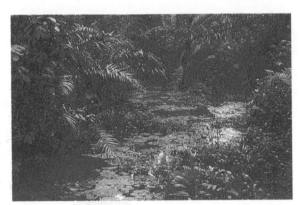

Plate 92: Ideal habitat – shady and wet – where *Chrysops* flies breed.

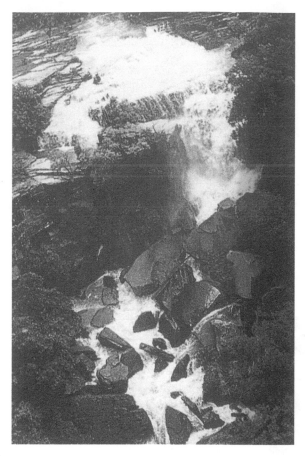

Plate 93: Fast-moving, highly oxygenated water in streams, rivers etc. provide ideal breeding places for *Simulium* species.

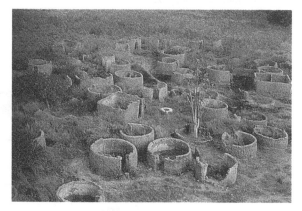

Plate 94: High blindness rates in some areas resulted in the past in the depopulation of entire villages. The success of the OCP programme has resulted in these villages being repopulated. Source: OCP.

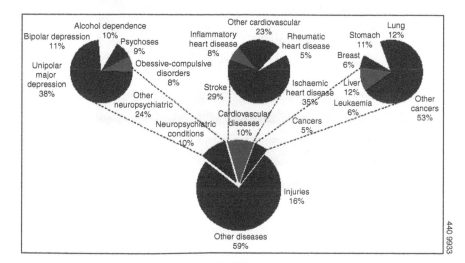

Plate 95: The emerging challenges: DALYs attributable to non-communicable diseases in low- and middle-income countries, estimates for 1998.

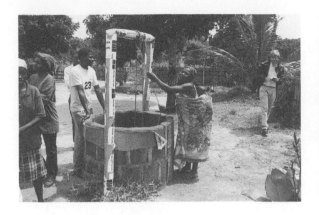

Plate 96: Shallow well – Open – Maputo Province, Mozambique, February 2000.

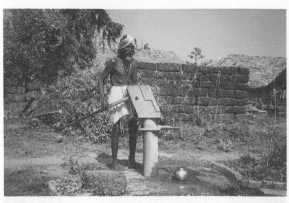

Plate 97: Shallow well – Handpump, Orissa State, India, November 1999.

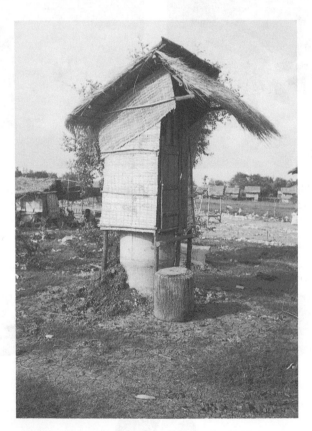

Plate 98: Raised pit latrine – Banteag Mearchey Province, Cambodia, 1993.

In contrast, other scientists also reporting from Sri Lanka noted that while infection with *P. vivax* did not protect patients from developing subsequent infections with *P. falciparum*, the subjective symptomatic scores of such patients were lower than of patients who had not suffered *P. vivax* infection.

'STABLE' *P. VIVAX* MALARIA

On Espiritu Santo, Vanuatu there has been a long established stable coexistence of *P. vivax* and *P. falciparum* in the population. Scientists from Oxford conducted weekly active case detection in 10 villages where malaria was hyperendemic, on all children <10 years from consenting families resident in these villages, for a period of 2 years. *P. falciparum* predominated in the wet season while *P. vivax* predominated in the dry season.

In 1992–93, *P. vivax* morbidity reached a peak in the age group 0–1 years and caused little morbidity beyond the age of 6 years. In 1993–94 the peak of *P. vivax* shifted slightly to 1–2 years, but again fell in the older age group. The densities of *P. falciparum* associated with clinical malaria were very low. There was a strong negative correlation between haemoglobin level and parasite density for *P. vivax*, which they attributed to the selective invasion of reticulocytes by this species. There was a reciprocal relationship between *P. falciparum* and *P. vivax*, suggesting that infection with the former species may inhibit erythrocyte infection or relapse of *P. vivax*; while cerebral malaria and malaria specific morbidity was low.

Although the homozygous state for α-thalassaemia is protective against the serious manifestations of *P. falciparum* malaria, they paradoxically found that on the island of Espiritu Santo, both the incidence of uncomplicated malaria and the prevalence of splenomegaly were significantly higher in young children with an α-thalassaemia and that the effect was most marked in the youngest children and for *P. vivax*. They postulated that early exposure to *P. vivax* modulates the outcome of subsequent infections with *P. falciparum* and protects against severe disease and mortality. In support of the hypothesis is evidence of cross-species immunity in animal models.

Several workers have in the past reported that immunity to *P. vivax* in endemic areas is rapidly developed and is of a permanent and effective character. Moreover, the greater the degree of immunity, the fewer will be the gametocytes produced.

Recent studies have confirmed that symptom-free cases of *P. vivax* are not uncommon in the western border of Thailand, among native Amazonians and in Sri Lanka.

P. vivax malaria has re-emerged in some of the states of the former USSR (Armenia, Tajikistan, Azerbajan) and near the demilitarized zone of the Republic of Korea.

Diagnosis

The diagnosis of malaria is clinical, parasitological, immunological and molecular. Clinically, a high index of suspicion is the most important feature while parasitological diagnosis remains the most certain means of diagnosing all four species of human malaria parasites.

Detection of antibodies by various serological techniques is useful for epidemiological purposes. Antigen detection tests in dipstick format are now available, while molecular methods have a place as a research tool or in central laboratories to perform quality control checks on microscopic diagnosis.

Antimalarial drug resistance

Widespread resistance to chloroquine and other antimalarials has now occurred in many endemic countries (Plate 68). WHO have now developed a test for antimalarial resistance that is a major advance on its predecessors and clinical rather than solely parasitological response to treatment, is the prime test outcome.

Overall classification of therapeutic response

There are three categories of therapeutic response, namely early treatment failure (ETF), late treatment failure (LTF) and adequate clinical response (ACR). These are defined as follows:

1 The therapeutic response will be classified as early treatment failure (ETF) if the patient develops one of the following conditions during the first 3 days of follow-up:

- development of danger signs or severe malaria on day 1, day 2 or day 3, in the presence of parasitaemia;
- axillary temperature $\geq 37.5°C$ on day 2 with parasitaemia > day 0 count;

- axillary temperature ≥37.5°C on day 3 in the presence of parasitaemia;
- parasitaemia on day 3 ≥ 25% of count on day 0.

2 The therapeutic response will be classified as late treatment failure (LTF) if the patient develops one of the following conditions during the follow-up period from day 4 to day 14:
   - development of danger signs or severe malaria in the presence of parasitaemia on any day from day 4 to day 14, without previously meeting any of the criteria of early treatment failure;
   - axillary temperature ≥37.5°C in the presence of parasitaemia on any day from day 4 to day 14, without previously meeting any of the criteria of early treatment failure.

3 The response to treatment will be classified as adequate clinical response (ACR) if the patient shows one of the following conditions during the follow-up period (up to day 14):
   - absence of parasitaemia on day 14 irrespective of axillary temperature, without previously meeting any of the criteria of early or late treatment failure;
   - axillary temperature <37.5°C irrespective of the presence of parasitaemia, without previously meeting any of the criteria of early or late treatment failure.

Over a period of 12 years a study was conducted on three rural populations in the sahel, savannah and forest areas of Senegal, West Africa. As a result of chloroquine resistance, the risk of dying from malaria in children aged 0–9 years increased by 1.2-, 2.5- and 5.5-fold respectively. Chloroquine was still being used as the first-line drug in these villages. Resistance to *P. vivax* has been reported but is still very uncommon.

Control

Control measures are aimed at the individual, against the vector or to provide communal protection (Plate 69).

THE INDIVIDUAL

Individual protective measures include: (i) regular chemoprophylaxis; (ii) impregnated mosquito nets and clothing; and (iii) repellents.

Chemoprophylaxis

The following points must be emphasized:

- No antimalarial drug is 100% protective.
- Persons on prophylaxis are less likely to develop malaria than those without.
- The risk of malaria must be balanced against the risk of adverse effects of the drug used.
- If a person has been exposed to malaria and feels unwell, malaria should not be excluded even if he or she has been taking regular chemoprophylaxis.
- Malaria can be acquired at relatively short stops, e.g. refuelling the aeroplane.
- Although many of the big cities in South East Asia are malaria free, this is not the case for the majority of cities in Africa.

The antimalarials available for prophylaxis are: (i) chloroquine/proguanil; (ii) (in very limited areas of the tropics), mefloquine; (iii) doxycycline; and (iv) atovaquone/proguanil (malarone). Which of these to use depends on the endemic area to be visited. Since national recommendations change, advice from specialized institutions should be sought.

Chemoprophylaxis in pregnancy

In non-immunes, malaria is more severe in pregnant women than non-pregnant women and the mortality is higher. It is a major cause of abortion, stillbirth, premature delivery and low-birth weight. They are particularly vulnerable to hyper-insulinaemic hypoglycaemia, even when the malaria is otherwise uncomplicated.

In semi-immunes and particularly in primigravidae, there is increased parasitaemia, maternal anaemia, placental accumulation of parasites, low birth weight of infants due to both prematurity and intrauterine growth retardation. However, the other manifestations of severe malaria are uncommon. There is good evidence of impaired parasite control in HIV-infected pregnant women, irrespective of their parity.

The most effective intervention – instead of weekly chloroquine as given in the past – is to administer a curative dose of sulphadoxine – pyrimethamine (Fansidar) (3 tablets) in the second trimester, repeated in the third trimester. In areas where Fansidar resistance is widespread, for example South East Asia – weekly mefloquine (250 mg) can be used in the second and third trimesters. *It must not be given in the first trimester.* Meticulous personal protection is mandatory during this period when chemoprophylaxis is not available. In areas where chloroquine is still effective, or partially effective, chloroquine weekly can safely be used in the first trimester and throughout the rest of the pregnancy.

THE VECTOR

Control of the vector can be carried out by destroying the adult (imagicidal control) or the larvae (larval control).

Imagicidal control

Residual indoor spraying constituted the backbone of the global malaria eradication campaign. The effect of spraying results in a selective killing of vectors that rest indoors. Its effectiveness was greatly reduced because of insufficient coverage, exophily, development of resistance and poor compliance by the community.

Indoor spraying of residual insecticides no longer has the predominant role given it in the past. It is still indicated, in situations where its use could be clearly targeted, limited in time and in the control of epidemics.

DDT is still effective in many endemic countries and its use is justifiable for malaria control.

Larval control

The indications for larval control are limited to densely populated areas with relatively few breeding places, such as urban or irrigated arid areas. The classical larvicides include Parisgreen, larvicidal oils and polystyrene beads. Larvicidal fish, for example *Gambusia*, have had limited success in some areas.

Peridomestic sanitation for appropriate vectors, for example care of water tanks, is a complementary measure.

Environmental sanitation

This constitutes the most effective and sustainable measure for mosquito control but in most tropical countries it remains a desirable though long-term objective.

THE COMMUNITY

The WHO global malaria strategy has now moved from eradication and control to reduction of morbidity and mortality. The cornerstone of this strategy formulated in Amsterdam in 1992 is early diagnosis and treatment of affected persons. The prepackaging of antimalarials improves compliance, and reduces waiting time at dispensaries and drug wastage.

Roll back malaria (RBM)

In June 1997, Heads of States of Africa met in Harare and issued a declaration on malaria prevention and control in the context of African economic recovery and development. This political commitment was endorsed by the leaders of the industrialized G8 nations.

Upon taking office in July 1998, Dr Gro Harlem Brundtland, WHO's new Director-General, decided that malaria was to be one of WHO's top priorities and announced the introduction of a new initiative 'roll back malaria' (RBM).

The goals of RBM include: (i) support to endemic countries in developing their national health systems as a major strategy for controlling malaria; (ii) developing the broader health sector, i.e. all providers of health care to the community including the private sector (drug vendors and traditional healers, pharmacists and others); and (iii) encouraging the required human and financial investments for health system development, nationally and internationally.

A functioning partnership with a range of organizations at global, regional and country levels is being established to ensure a sustained capacity to address malaria and other priority health problems. WHO's partners in RBM include malaria endemic countries, other UN organizations, development banks including the World Bank, bilateral development agencies, non-governmental organizations and the private sector.

WHO's role in this global partnership is:

- to provide strategic direction and catalyse actions;
- to provide an RBM secretariat at its Geneva headquarters;
- to work to build and sustain country and global partnerships;
- to arrange the provision of technical endorsement for both a collective strategy and for individual partners' action;
- to ensure that all aspects of progress of RBM are monitored;

- to provide global accountability for RBM;
- to broker technical assistance and finance;
- to undertake responsible advocacy for the RBM approach to reducing malaria-related suffering and poverty.

The RBM campaign focuses first on Africa, where the impact of malaria morbidity and mortality is greatest. The general objective of RBM is to significantly reduce the global burden of malaria through interventions adapted to local needs and by reinforcement of the health sector. Performance indicators are used to assess the RBM project.

It will build upon existing initiatives, such as the African Initiative on Malaria (AIM), the WHO Special Fund for Africa, Medicines for Malaria Venture (MMV) and the Multilateral Incentive on Malaria (MIM). Although the need for new drugs, insecticides and vaccines still remains, major gains can still be made through better application of current knowledge and best practice.

The elements of the RBM strategy are: (i) early detection; (ii) rapid treatment; (iii) multiple prevention; (iv) well-co-ordinated action; (v) dynamic global movement; and (vi) focused research.

Impregnated treated nets (ITN)

Considerable evidence has now accumulated that insecticide-treated materials, for example bed nets, curtains nets (for persons who do not sleep on beds) and (screens) can substantially reduce childhood malaria mortality and are effective both in high- and low-endemicity areas. Moreover, protection is good even in areas where the vector has developed strong pyrethroid resistance. To be fully effective nets have to be treated once or twice a year. A kit designed to allow families to safely and effectively dip their own bed-nets at home, irrespective of their degree of literacy, has now been produced.

The problem of sustainability and cost recovery seems to have been successfully tackled using a pragmatic approach involving the public and private sectors in Ifakara, Tanzania. Nets distributed through a social marketing programme involving: (i) the identification of a suitable brand and logo as well as the most effective message for the promotional campaign; (ii) adjustment of the price and insecticide according to the ability of people to pay; and (iii) distribution of nets by shopkeepers, community leaders and health workers, resulted in

a dramatic impact on childhood mortality; anaemia in children under 2 years as well as parasitaemia. The challenge to this approach is whether it can be sustained in the absence of a research team to stimulate the social marketing, and whether the Ifakara methods work elsewhere in Africa.

Since vaccines are provided free of charge, a strong case could be made to provide free or heavily subsidised ITNs. Cost-effective calculations have shown that ITNs and childhood vaccination are of similar value. Long-lasting insecticide-treated mosquito nets (LLNs) are being developed. They are treated only once at factory level and can resist multiple washes. The insecticide is released over time to the surface of the netting fibres.

Screening of houses is an established method of reducing human/vector contact.

Zooprophylaxis

This is an old method of protection of variable efficacy, depending on the habits of the vectors involved, which should be predominantly zoophilic. Similarly, cattle sponging with insecticide every 6 weeks may be used in areas where transmission is seasonal and the vector zoophilic.

Vaccines

Vaccines and transgenic mosquitoes offer exciting possibilities for the future. The topic of malaria vaccines is vast and complex and beyond the scope of this book. A number of vaccine candidates are undergoing clinical trials but none is likely to be available at an operational level for many years.

Current trends are geared towards 'cocktail' vaccines including a combination of multiple epitopes from different malarial antigens and from different stages of the parasite life cycle.

The private sector

It is well known that in many of the endemic malaria countries the private sector provides more antimalarials than the public sector (Fig. 7.8). Counterfeit drugs, drugs which have long passed their expiry date, and improper dosaging are common occurrences (Plates 70–72).

WHO is embarking on an extensive programme to train drug sellers and teach them to optimize the use of antimalarial drugs.

No. of CQ tablets

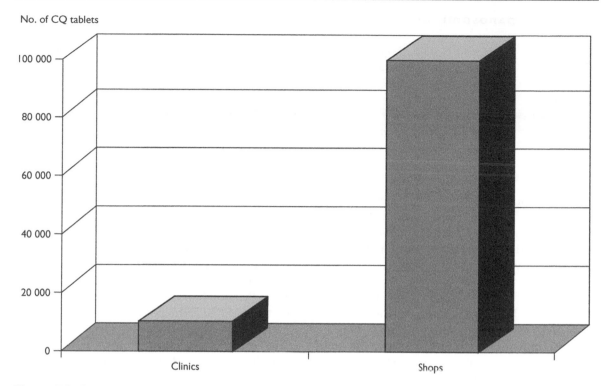

Figure 7.8: Sale of antimalarials in the public and private sector (of a district in Nigeria). Source: WHO.

Economic impact

It is estimated that 40 million disability adjusted life years (DALYs) are lost annually. Cross-country regressions covering a 25-year period confirm the relationship between malaria and economic growth. Taking various factors into account countries with endemic malaria grew 1.3% lower per year, and a 10% reduction in malaria was associated with 0.3% higher growth per year.

CONTROL OF EPIDEMICS

Ideally, malaria epidemics should be forecast and prevented, not detected and controlled. Such forecasting may be possible if based on a dynamic information system capable of identifying well-established risk factors.

The containment of an epidemic will require the implementation of the following measures:

- mass drug administration to all the population considered at risk, especially young children and pregnant mothers;
- presumptive treatment of all fever cases;

- space spraying of insecticides using thermal foggers, mist-blowers, ultra low volume (ULV) sprayers;
- indoor residual spraying – DDT, deltamethrin, lambda-cyhalothrin;
- reimpregnation of bed-nets – in areas where bed-nets are already widely used.

THE TRYPANOSOMIASES

The *Trypanosoma* species are flagellate protozoa transmitted by blood-sucking insects. Those pathogenic to man can be classified into two groups causing the clinically and geographically distinct diseases:

- African trypanosomiasis (sleeping sickness) caused by *Trypanosoma brucei gambiense* or *T.b. rhodesiense* and transmitted through the bite of a blood-sucking tsetse fly.
- South American trypanosomiasis (Chagas' disease) caused by *T. cruzi* and transmitted by faecal contaminaion by blood-sucking reduviid bugs.

African trypanosomiasis

Occurrence:	Africa 10°N–25°S of equator
Organisms:	Trypanosoma brucei gambiense, T.b. rhodesiense
Reservoir:	Humans
Transmission:	Bite of tsetse fly
Control:	Active and passive surveillance Tsetse control by trapping or spraying

African trypanosomiasis (sleeping sickness) has two clinically distinct forms, caused by either *Trypanosoma brucei gambiense* or *T.b. rhodesiense*. The incubation period is usually between 2 and 3 weeks but can be very much longer (6 years).

In humans, *T.b. gambiense* and *T.b. rhodesiense* are morphologically identical and have similar life cycles. When blood containing trypanosomes is ingested by a suitable species of *Glossina,* the trypanosomes reach the intestine of the fly and undergo cyclical development, eventually producing infective metacyclic forms in the salivary glands. These are transmitted to man when saliva is injected into the puncture wound while feeding. Multiplication of the trypanosomes occurs in the blood. The entire cycle of development in the fly, after feeding on blood containing trypanosomes, is about 3 weeks (extrinsic incubation period).

The main vectors of gambian sleeping sickness are the riverine species of *Glossina: G. palpalis* and *G. tachinoides;* while the chief vectors of Rhodesian sleeping sickness are *G. morsitans, G. swynnertoni* and *G. pallipides.*

EPIDEMIOLOGY (PLATES 73–76)

African trypanosomiasis is confined to that part of Africa lying between latitudes 10°N and 25°S (Fig. 7.9). *T.b. rhodesiense* infection is limited to southern Sudan, Ethiopia, Kenya, Tanzania, Uganda, Malawi, Zambia, Rhodesia, Mozambique, northern Botswana and South East Angola, while *T.b. gambiense* is more widespread, extending from West Africa through Central Africa to Uganda, Tanzania and Malawi. Comparatively recent epidemics of *T.b. rhodesiense* have been reported from Botswana, the southern Sudan, Ethiopia, Zaire and Uganda. It is estimated that 55 million people in 36 countries and about 25 million cattle are exposed to the risk of infection. Some 300000 new cases occur each year, although only a few of these are reported.

The maintenance of human trypanosomiasis in Africa depends on the interrelations of three elements – the vertebrate host, the parasite and the vector responsible for transmission. Sleeping sickness is essentially a disease of rural populations and its prevalence is largely dependent on the degree of contact between man and tsetse; this is

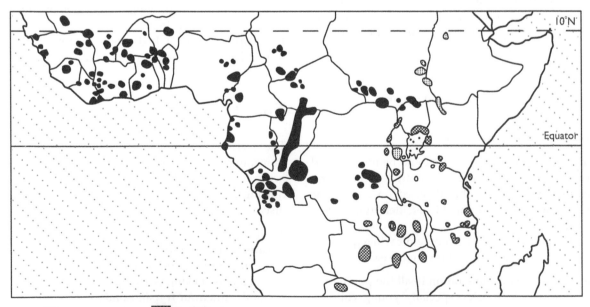

Key: ■ *T.b. gambiense*   ▨ *T.b. rhodesiense*

Figure 7.9: Distribution of African trypanosomiasis.

particularly so with gambiense sleeping sickness in which man is the principal reservoir of infection. Thus, at the height of the dry season, riverine species of fly are often restricted to isolated pools of water which are essential to the local human population for so many of their activities, for example collecting water and firewood, washing, fishing and cultivation. The sacred groves of some religions may also provide foci of intimate man–fly contact. Over recent years there has been an increasing incidence and dispersion of *T.b. rhodesiense* sleeping sickness on the north-east shores of Lake Victoria, associated with increased fishing activity and increasing and irregular settlement of the tsetse-fly belt of south-east Uganda. It has been recognized that *T.b. rhodesiense* may also be transmitted by riverine species of tsetse fly. Population movements have long been known to play a role in the spread of trypanosomiasis, for example as a result of civil wars.

Reservoir

T.b. rhodesiense was isolated from a bushbuck in 1958, and so a reservoir in wild animals, long suspected, was proved. This wild animal reservoir plays an important role in the epidemiology of the human disease, man being the incidental host. *T.b. rhodesiense* has been found in lion, hyena, hartebeest, giraffe, hippopotamus, reedbuck, waterbuck, warthog and domestic cattle, sheep, goats and dogs.

Man is the major reservoir of *T.b. gambiense* infection. However, there is now increasing evidence confirming the suspicion that there is also an animal reservoir for *T.b. gambiense*. Organisms indistinguishable from *T.b. gambiense* have been found in domestic and wild animals using the technique of biochemical characterization of strains. It remains to be shown what part these infections in animals play in the epidemiology of the human disease. The classical man–fly–man cycle is likely to be the predominant cycle for *T.b. gambiense* in West and Central Africa.

Vector

Each species of tsetse has particular requirements, with regard to climate and vegetation, which determine its distribution. All of them tend to concentrate seasonally in habitats offering permanent shade and humidity. The distribution of the fly thus varies with the season, and in addition it advances and retreats spatially at intervals of years.

Adverse environmental climatic conditions can affect the mean period between emergence of the young fly (pupa) and the taking of the first blood meal as well as the period of development of trypanosomes in the vector; these factors can influence the chance of transmission of the disease.

Host factors

Population density affects the incidence of the disease, which is sporadic at densities below 50 per km^2, and is liable to become epidemic at densities up to around 500 per km^2, above which it disappears because tsetse habitats are eliminated.

In general, in endemic conditions, the incidence of sleeping sickness is greater in males. In contrast to this usual picture, it has been reported that in the Gambia the women and older girls were most affected because they were exposed while working in the rice fields. In epidemic conditions no sex difference in incidence occurs and the proportion of children affected rises sharply.

LABORATORY DIAGNOSIS

Microscopical examination of blood, lymph fluid, serous fluids, bone marrow or CSF with or without concentration techniques may reveal the organism in fresh or suitably stained preparations. Indirect methods, such as the detection of antibodies or circulating antigens, are useful in establishing a suspicion of trypanosomiasis and in mass surveys for the preselection of individuals most likely to be infected. This strategy has been shown to reduce the workload and the cost of surveillance. Several serological tests are available, namely fluorescent antibody test (FAT); indirect haemagglutination; ELISA; and counter-current immunoelectrophoresis. The card agglutination trypanosomiasis test (CATT) has been successfully used for mass surveys of *T.b. gambiense*. Antigen detection has been developed with the card-indirect-agglutination test (CIAT). IgM is increased. DNA probes are available in research laboratories. Serological screening is followed by parasitological confirmation.

CONTROL

The leading principles for sleeping sickness control are suppression by surveillance combined with vector control. The choice of methods depends on the local epidemiological situation, the available personnel, the structure of the health services concerned, and financial considerations. Each country has to find the most appropriate compromise. Basically control and surveillance include case detection and treatment, and vector control using impregnated traps and screens.

The individual

Protective measures

The wearing of long trousers and of long-sleeved shirts gives some protection against the bites of tsetse flies. Vehicles which have to pass through heavily tsetse-infected country should be fly-proofed with mosquito gauze. Individuals who are sensitive to insect bites may find repellents (dimethylphthalate or diethyl toluamide) useful quite apart from the protection that they may give against infection, for a severe local reaction to the tsetse bite is not uncommon. Chemoprophylaxis is no longer recommended since it may mask a second stage infection and may enhance the development of drug resistance. Strategies for case detection are based either on passive surveillance, or active screening by mobile teams or health workers. Usually, a combination of both is used.

Chemotherapy

The commonly used drugs for African trypanosomiasis are pentamidine, suramin and melarsoprol. Pentamidine is not active against *T.b. rhodesiense*. Melarsoprol is the only drug used for the routine treatment of patients with CNS involvement. Alpha-difluoromethylornithine (DFMO; eflornithine) can be used in melarsoprol refractory *T.b. gambiense* patients.

The fly

Chemical control

Selective ground spraying of resting sites with synthetic pyrethroids (e.g. deltamethrine) has replaced DDT and the older insecticides. Aerial spraying techniques have been developed applying aerosols or ultra low volume (ULV) formulations.

Land-use management

The need to integrate tsetse control programmes into rural development has long been recognized. Thus, organized land settlement has been used to control sleeping sickness in both East and West Africa. Large-scale tsetse reclamation projects are motivated by the current impact of urbanization and the need to accommodate a rapidly expanding human population aspiring to a higher standard of living – the development of tsetse is modified by this type of ecological control.

Biological methods

These include the use of predators and parasites as well as genetic control. The genetic methods explored include hybridization, the production of heterozygotes for chromosomal translocations, and the release of males sterilized by irradiation or chemical means.

Insecticide-impregnated traps and screens (Plates 77 and 78)

Insecticide-impregnated traps and screens are playing an increasing role in the control of vectors of trypanosomiasis (Fig. 7.10). They are effective, simple, non-polluting and ideally suited to the primary health care concept. The numbers of traps required depends on the density of the vegetation and the abundance of the fly. Traps can be concentrated at points of known man–fly contact. Odour attractants have been additionally used to lure G. *morsitans* group flies (Fig. 7.10b). The trap chosen must be appropriate for the tsetse species present in the area – for the palpalis group the biconical, vavova or pyramidal trap are used, while for the morsitans group the Beta or F-2 traps are used.

The community

Passive surveillance involves individuals who present at health centres. This is an effective method for *T.b. rhodesiense* provided the centres are adequately staffed and equipped. Active screening of the population once yearly using serological tests – CATT or immunofluorescence (IF) – on blood samples collected on blotting paper and using specialized community health workers is another option. Often, the two strategies are combined. The integration of sleeping sickness control within the primary health programmes is yet another option. All the choices have advantages and disadvantages and the choice of strategy will depend on many local factors, for example finance, human resources, and epidemiological conditions.

The *biconical target and trap* has an upper cone of mosquito netting and an electric-blue cloth lower cone, with black internal screens. As a target, it must be impregnated with residual insecticide. A trapping device can be attached to the apex of the upper cone.

WHO 851682

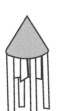

The *monoconical target and trap* has a plastic cone with four electric-blue cloth bands attached to it and black cloth internal screens. As a target, it must be impregnated with residual insecticide. A collection device can be attached to the apex of the cone.

WHO 851680

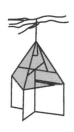

The *pyramidal target and trap* has two electric-blue and two broad black screens made of cloth at the base. The pyramid is made of mosquito netting. If impregnated with residual insecticide, it can be used as a target but it is normally used with a permanent trapping device at the apex of the pyramid, consisting of a plastic bottle containing kerosene.

WHO 851681

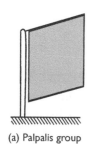

The *screen* consists of royal blue cloth, approximately one metre square, hanging from a gallows. It must be used with residual insecticide.

WHO 851676

(a) Palpalis group

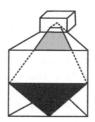

The *Beta trap* is a prism made of black-and-white cloth stretched on a frame. There is internal mosquito netting placed in such a way as to direct flies to a trapping device.

WHO 851674

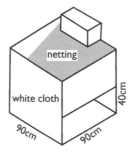

The *F-2 trap* is a cube made of black-and-white cloth stretched over a frame. Internal mosquito netting directs the flies to a trapping device.

WHO 851675

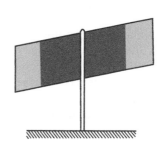

The *target* is made of two pieces of electric-blue cloth stretched at the ends of a rectangular frame hinged on a verticle support. It must be used with residual insect-icide. The inclusion of acetone, CO_2, or 1-octen-3-ol considerably enhances catches of *G. morsitans* by these traps.

WHO 851673

(b) Morsitans group

Figure 7.10: Traps, targets and screens used for the control of *Glossina palpalis* and *G. morsitans* (after WHO, 1986).

South American trypanosomiasis (Chagas' disease)

Occurrence:	South America
Organism:	*Trypanosoma cruzi*
Reservoir:	Humans and animals
Transmission:	Rubbing infected reduviid bugs' faeces into skin
Control:	Synthetic pyrethroids
	Community vigilance
	House improvement
	Screening of blood donors

Chagas' disease may present as congenital, acute or chronic forms. It is endemic in the New World, infecting around 16 million people and with about 90 million at risk. The main impact of the infection especially in children is on the heart. Entero-megaly is common in chronic Chagas' disease. The incubation period is about 2 weeks.

APPLIED BIOLOGY

The adult trypanosomes in human blood are ingested by blood-sucking reduviid bugs. After a period of development in the invertebrate host's intestinal canal lasting 8–10 days, trypanosomes, known as metacyclic forms, reappear in the hindgut and are passed with the faeces of the insect. Infection of man takes place when faecal matter is rubbed into scratch wounds or the wound caused by the bite of the insect. Certain trypanosomes leave the bloodstream and invade various organs, especially the myocardium. Here they assume a leishmanoid appearance and rapid multiplication by binary fission takes place forming nests of Leishmanoid–Donovan bodies. At a later stage these forms elongate and are eventually transformed into trypanosomes, which make their way through the tissues and into the bloodstream.

EPIDEMIOLOGY

The infection is found in Central and South America, especially in Brazil, Venezuela, Colombia and northern Argentina (Plate 79).

Reservoir

The reservoir of infection is man. A large number of animal species have been described as naturally infected and this enzootic cycle is especially important in recently colonized areas. Chagas' disease can, however, be maintained in domestic cycles without participation of wild reservoir hosts.

Transmission

The most important vector bugs belong to the genera *Triatoma*, *Panstrongylus* and *Rhodnius*. These reduviid bugs are largely disseminated throughout the rural areas of Latin America where the mud huts of the agricultural workers are their favourite habitats. The usual mode of transmission is by rubbing infected faeces into cuts or abrasions or into the intact skin or mucous membrane. Transmission occurs predominantly at night since reduviid bugs attack only in darkness. Other methods of infection are by blood transfusion, transplacental, and laboratory transmission from infected syringes or blood (Plates 80–82).

Host factors

The disease is observed at any age, although children are mainly affected.

T. RANGELI

Infections with another trypanosome, *T. rangeli*, have been found in various animals, and human infections with this trypanosome have occasionally also been reported. In contrast to *T. cruzi* the transmission of this disease is by the actual bite of the reduviid bug rather than through its excreta.

LABORATORY DIAGNOSIS

Trypanosomes may be demonstrated in wet and stained thick blood films, in lymph gland juice, or in CSF and may be cultured on NNN medium. Immunofluorescence, IHAT and ELISA are used in the diagnosis of Chagas' disease. DNA probes and PCR have been developed and are available in research laboratories.

CONTROL

Chagas' disease flourishes only where social and economic levels are low, and long-term control measures involve economic rehabilitation, in particular, better housing. Control of Chagas' disease has been given a high priority in Latin America and the disease has been eliminated from Chile and Ecuador.

The individual

Personal prophylaxis consists of avoiding sleeping in houses liable to harbour the vectors. In endemic areas blood donors should be carefully screened and rejected if infected. If screening is not possible, the addition of gentian violet to stored blood (1:4000) for 24 hours will kill any flagellates.

The community

Mud hovels with thatched roofs need to be replaced by houses constructed from materials giving no harbour to bugs. Synthetic pyrethroids (e.g. deltamethrin, lambda-cyhalothrin) have been a major advance in controlling domestic Triatominae. Large-scale spraying of all premises in the target area should be carried out regardless of whether or not an individual house is known to be infected. Community-based vigilance is emphasized. Fumigant cans have been proved successful, convenient and economical (Plate 83); as well as insecticide paints.

THE LEISHMANIASES

It is convenient (though not strictly justifiable) to subdivide the leishmaniases into clinical types according to the site affected (see Table 7.5).

APPLIED BIOLOGY

There are two phases in the life cycle of leishmania each associated with a different form of the protozoa:

- An aflagellate: *amastigote* (leishmanial) – rounded form occurs in man and in animal reservoir hosts.
- A flagellate: *promastigote* (leptomonad) – form is found in the vector sandfly and in culture media.

The former is oval ($2\,\mu m \times 3\,\mu m$) and consists of cytoplasm, a round nucleus and a small, more deeply staining, rod-shaped kinetoplast or rhizoplast and a vacuole. It is known as the Leishman–Donovan (L–D) body. In man leishmania multiply by binary fission. They are most commonly found in the large mononuclear cells of the reticuloendothelial system, especially in the liver, spleen and bone marrow; leishmanial forms are also found in the leucocytes of the circulating blood.

Table 7.5: Classification of leishmania species into various 'complexes' and the diseases they cause. After Chance and Evans (1999)

Leishmania (Leishmania) donovani complex	
L. (L.) donovani	Visceral leishmaniasis
L. (L.) infantum	Visceral and cutaneous leishmaniasis
L. (L.) chagasi	Visceral and cutaneous leishmaniasis
Leishmania (Leishmania) tropica complex	
L. (L.) tropica	Cutaneous leishmaniasis
Leishmania (Leishmania) major complex	
L. (L.) major	Cutaneous leishmaniasis
Leishmania (Leishmania) aethiopica complex	
L. (L.) aethiopica	Diffuse cutaneous leishmaniasis
Leishmania (Leishmania) mexicana complex	
L. (L.) mexicana and other species	Cutaneous and diffuse cutaneous leishmaniasis
Leishmania (Viannia) braziliensis complex	
L. (V.) braziliensis and other species	Cutaneous and mucocutaneous leishmaniasis

LIFE CYCLE

Visceral

When the appropriate sandfly feeds on an infected person, it ingests the parasites with the blood meal. These develop in its gut into the flagellate (promastigote) forms: these migrate forwards, multiply and form a mass which may block the pharynx of the sandfly.

When the sandfly next feeds, some of these leptomonads become dislodged and are injected into the new host in the process of feeding; they again assume the leishmanial form. They are phagocytosed by macrophages, multiply by simple division and cause the cells to rupture. They are then carried in the circulation to sites already referred to where they give rise to the characteristic lesions. Following specific treatment in some cases they pass from their visceral habitat (liver, spleen, etc.) back to the skin, giving rise to the condition described as post-kala-azar dermal leishmaniasis.

Cutaneous and muco-cutaneous

In cutaneous and muco-cutaneous leishmaniasis, the multiplication of the amastigote forms takes place in the skin and the appropriate sandfly vectors become infected by feeding on a cutaneous lesion.

TAXONOMY

Biochemical taxonomy, using the excreted factor (EF) serotyping, enzyme analysis and DNA buoyant density determination is being used to identify leishmanial strains from different geographical areas and to subdivide the various complexes.

EPIDEMIOLOGY

The leishmaniases occur over wide areas of the globe from China across Asia, India, Persia and Afghanistan, the Caucasus, the Middle and Near East, the Mediterranean basin, East and West Africa, the Sudan and South America (see Figs 7.11–7.13). There is an increasing awareness of the importance of the leishmaniases as public health problems, and of the seriousness of recent outbreaks in South America, Asia and Africa. A conservative estimate of the number of new cases is 400 000/year. *L. infantum* is replaced in Africa and South Asia by

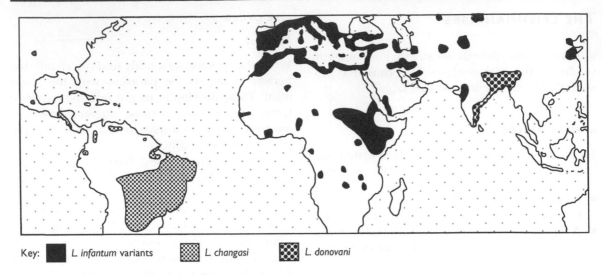

Key: ▮ *L. infantum* variants ▨ *L. changasi* ▩ *L. donovani*

Figure 7.11: Distribution of visceral leishmaniasis.

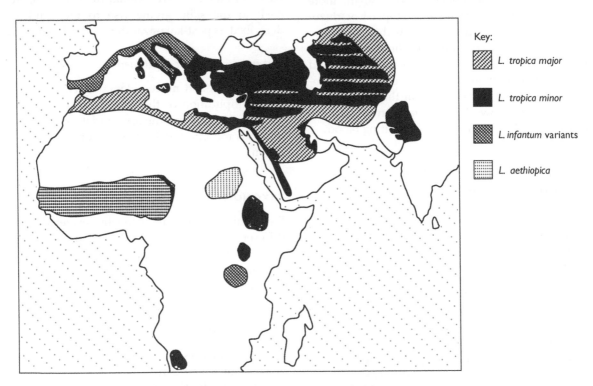

Key:

▨ *L. tropica major*

▮ *L. tropica minor*

▩ *L. infantum* variants

░ *L. aethiopica*

Figure 7.12: Distribution of cutaneous leishmaniasis in the Old World.

L. donovani, while the two forms occur sympatric-ally in the Sudan and south west Arabia.

The epidemiology of the leishmaniases, whether visceral, cutaneous or muco-cutaneous, is in every case determined by a reservoir of infection (animal,

man or both) from which local *Phlebotomine* sand-flies infect themselves by ingesting amastigote forms from blood or infected tissues. The climatic conditions of the various foci of leishmaniasis range from arid to tropical humid and the terrain and

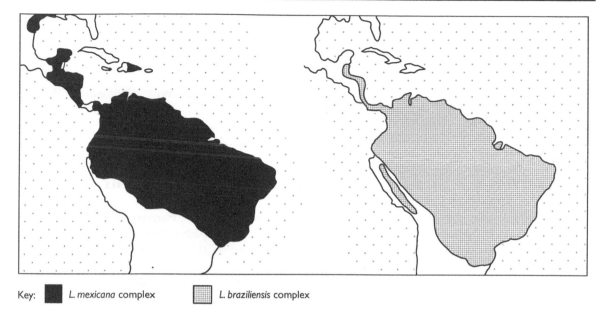

Key: ■ *L. mexicana* complex   ▦ *L. braziliensis* complex

Figure 7.13: Distribution of New World cutaneous and muco-cutaneous leishmaniasis.

altitude are equally variable. Modes of transmission other than by sandflies, for example sexual, blood transfusion, and intrauterine infection, are of little epidemiological significance. With the possible exception of Indian kala-azar it is recognized that in most endemic foci the leishmaniases are zoonoses. Extensive studies in France and North Africa have demonstrated close links between vector numbers and bioclimatic zones. In Brazil, it was found that young age and poor nutrition were the most important factors determining who developed serious disease.

The reservoir systems – the gerbil and the fat sand rat – produce stable and continuous sources of *L. major* infection. *L. tropica*, for which man is the only reservoir, requires an adequate number of sandflies and susceptible people for its maintenance. In areas where transmission is intense, the majority of people are immune and only young children and immigrants are susceptible.

New World cutaneous and muco-cutaneous leishmaniasis are forest fringe zoonoses that have shown a remarkable potential to adapt and can exist in different ecological situations ranging from tropical rainforest to peri-urban areas.

Reservoirs include ground-dwelling rodents, two-toed sloths, wild mammals and humans (Plates 84–86).

Visceral leishmaniasis

Occurrence:	India, Mediterranean, Middle East, Africa, South America
Organisms:	*Leishmania donovani, L. infantum, L. chagasi*
Reservoir:	Humans, dogs, rodents
Transmission:	Sandfly bite (*Phlebotomus* spp.)
Control:	Treatment of cases
	Control of vector and of animal reservoir

There are three distinct types of visceral leishmaniasis:

- Indian kala-azar, human reservoir;
- kala-azar associated with a canine reservoir (Plate 87);
- African kala-azar.

Kala-azar is essentially a rural disease, and the *L. donovani* complex is now accepted as the cause of most forms of kala-azar; *L. infantum* is responsible for cases of kala-azar in children. Post-kala-azar dermal leishmaniasis occurs as a sequel of visceral leishmaniasis. The incubation period of visceral leishmaniasis ranges from 2 weeks to more than 1 year or longer. A large epidemic occurred in the southern Sudan between 1984 and 1994, with an estimated 100 000 deaths.

INDIAN KALA-AZAR

Indian kala-azar is unique in so far as man is the only known natural host of the infection. The vector *P. argentipes* breeds in close proximity to human habitations and feeds readily on man. All age groups are susceptible with a peak incidence at 10–20 years. Devastating epidemics may occur. The lesions of post-kala-azar dermal leishmaniasis are of epidemiological importance since they contain numerous L–D bodies in the dermis and are readily accessible to sandflies. They are a feature of Indian kala-azar but are also seen elsewhere.

KALA-AZAR PREDOMINANTLY ASSOCIATED WITH A CANINE RESERVOIR

In the Mediterranean basin, Portugal, North Africa, the Caucasus, China, Brazil and other parts of South America, the domestic dog, fox and jackal are very important reservoirs of human infection.

Visceral leishmaniasis associated with a canine reservoir is predominantly a disease of children under 10 years. The most important vector sandflies are *Phlebotomus chinensis* in China, *P. longipalpis* in Brazil, and *P. perniciosus* in the Mediterranean.

AFRICAN KALA-AZAR

The epidemiology of the disease in the Sudan and Kenya presents unique features differing from those described above. There is a primary stage in the skin (leishmanoma) which lasts for some time before the symptoms of kala-azar develop, and this is of prime epidemiological importance. Rodents may form a reservoir of infection. A definite relationship was shown in Kenya some years ago, between the proximity of homes to termite hills and the incidence of kala-azar. The most important vectors are *P. martini* in Kenya and *P. orientalis* in the Sudan. Both these vectors are out-of-doors biters. The disease attacks all age groups but is commoner in adults than in children. The human distribution is affected by immunity as well as by relative exposure to infection. Development projects in many endemic areas of the Old and New World may introduce non-immune individuals into the region which can result in a large number of new infections.

VISCERAL LEISHMANIASIS AND HIV

Many cases of visceral leishmaniasis in HIV patients have been described presenting with atypical manifestations and poor response to conventional treatment (Plate 88).

Cutaneous leishmaniasis

Occurrence:	India, Mediterranean, Middle East, Africa, Central and South America
Organisms:	*Leishmania major, L. tropica, L. mexicana, L. peruviana*
Reservoir:	Humans, rodents, dogs
Transmission:	Bite of sandfly (*Phlebotomus* spp.)
Control:	Breaking man/vector contact
	Rodent control
	Immunization

Several varieties of cutaneous leishmaniasis have been described. From the Old World these include:

- oriental sore;
- Ethiopian cutaneous leishmaniasis;
- lupoid leishmaniasis.

From the New World:

- chiclero ulcer;
- uta;
- leishmaniasis tegumentaria diffusa.

OLD WORLD

Oriental sore

Alternative names include: tropical sore; bouton d'Orient; Aleppo, Baghdad or Delhi boil; Pendah sore. The infection is widely distributed in the Indian subcontinent, the Middle East, the Sudan, Ethiopia, southern Russia, the Mediterranean countries, the Sahelian Belt, parts of East Africa and China.

The most important vectors are *P. papatasii* and *P. sergenti*. The disease is most commonly seen in children, and in high endemic areas most of the adult population have been infected in childhood. The parasites responsible are *L. (L.) tropica* and *L. (L.) major*.

L. (L.) major is an infection of rodents occasionally transmitted to man which produces a disease with a short incubation period, rapid course of about 3 months, much inflammatory reaction and the 'moist' lesion it produces contains few parasites.

L. (L.) tropica is anthroponotic, characterized by a 'dry' lesion containing many parasites with a long incubation period, course of over 1 year and a mild inflammatory reaction.

Immunity to L. (L.) tropica and L. (L.) major follows spontaneous cure and experimental attempt at re-infection very often (but not invariably) gives negative results; moreover, 98% of cases of ori-ental sore show a delayed hypersensitivity test (Montenegro reaction) in response to the intradermal inoculation of dead and washed leptomonads.

Ethiopian cutaneous leishmaniasis

This is an antimony-resistant cutaneous leishmaniasis which is endemic in Ethiopia and clinically is very similar to leprosy. The Montenegro test is negative in the pseudo-lepromatous type of the disease and positive in the tuberculoid type. Two species of hydrax are reservoir hosts.

Lupoid leishmaniasis

This is a relapsing form of cutaneous leishmaniasis which is common in the Middle East, and resembles lupus vulgaris. Leishmania are scarce in biopsies and the leishmania test is positive.

NEW WORLD

The cutaneous leishmaniases of the New World – chiclero ulcer, uta, and leishmaniasis tegumentaria diffusa – are scattered in Central and South America over an area extending from 22°N to 30°S of the equator. They are characterized epidemiologically by the fact that they are zoonoses and predominantly non-urban diseases, usually confined to the forest regions or jungles.

Chiclero ulcer

L. mexicana is the cause of 'chiclero's ulcer' in Mexico and neighbouring countries. The infection is virtually restricted to people who habitually live and work in the forests, with the result that women and children are rarely infected. It is an 'occupational disease' of the chicleros who spend a considerable time in the forests bleeding the Sapodella trees for chewing-gum latex. The disease is almost always limited to a single dermal lesion, usually in the ear. Forest rodents are the important animal reservoirs and man is an accidental host. Transmission of L. mexicana is by P. pessoanus in British Honduras.

With L. mexicana, a solid and long-lasting immunity is developed from the infection and the development of this immunity occurs very early in the course of the disease.

Uta

L. peruviana causes cutaneous lesions on exposed sites such as the face, arm and leg. The disease is known as uta in Peru. The infection occurs primarily in dogs, which are the reservoir from which man acquires the disease. House-dwelling sandflies, for example P. peruensis, are the vectors of infection.

Leishmaniasis tegumentaria diffusa

L. pifanoi causes a disseminated form of cutaneous leishmaniasis in Bolivia and Venezuela. The leishmania intradermal test (Montenegro) is always negative.

Although the traditional activities associated with disease transmission of cutaneous leishmaniasis in the New World continue to be cutting timber and vegetation in small clearings and collecting chincona bark and chickle, in recent years road building, petroleum exploration, mining operations and military training have become important additions to the list.

Muco-cutaneous leishmaniasis (espundia)

Occurrence:	South and Central America
Organism:	Leishmania (Viannia) braziliensis
Reservoir:	Rodents
Transmission:	Bite of sandfly (Phlebotomus spp.)
Control:	Break man/vector contact

Espundia is widely distributed through South and Central America (see Fig. 7.13). It is caused by L. braziliensis and the sandflies P. whitmani, P. passoai and *P. mignei* are proven vectors of the disease. The most important animal reservoir of infection is the spiny rat. Espundia occurs mainly among men working in virgin forest. Human infections are acquired when new settlements are started in jungle areas and small clearings are made. At first, these settlements have an intimate contact with the forest, but after a time the wild rodents are driven away and the disease dies out. The infection is often confined to the skin but metastases to mucous membrane often occur through the bloodstream. The parasite has a predilection for the nasopharynx.

It appears that clinical immunity to heterologous strains of leishmania does occur, an observation in keeping with the finding that although *L. (L.) braziliensis*, *L. (L.) tropica* and *L. (L.) mexicana* can easily be distinguished from each other serologically, they share certain common antigens. It seems, moreover, that chiclero's ulcer, oriental sore and uta produce low levels of circulating antibody in the serum despite the fact that they result in lifelong immunity in most patients, while patients suffering from muco-cutaneous leishmaniasis possess high levels of circulating antibody.

Laboratory diagnosis of the leishmaniases

VISCERAL LEISHMANIASIS (VL)

Examination of lymph node, spleen, bone marrow aspirate and blood demonstrate the parasite. Blood examination in immunocompetent persons is often unproductive while parasites are commonly seen in HIV patients, thus offering a simple and easy method of diagnosis.

Non-specific tests such as the formal gel or Chopra's are still used in remote areas.

Several serological tests are also available, for example direct agglutination, indirect immunofluorescence, ELISA, immunoblot, counter-current immunoelectrophoresis, complement-fixation and indirect haemagglutination test. The leishmanin or Montenegro test is an important epidemiological tool which measures cell-mediated immunity. In active primary VL it is negative, as is the lymphocyte proliferation test. New techniques include monoclonal antibodies, nucleic acid hybridization and PCR.

CUTANEOUS LEISHMANIASIS (CL)

Parasites may be demonstrated by needle aspiration or in a biopsy from the edge of cutaneous lesions. Serological tests as above with variable sensitivity and specificity can be used.

The leishmanin test becomes positive 2–3 months after the lesion appears and remains positive for life. The new techniques referred to above are also available.

MUCO-CUTANEOUS LEISHMANIASIS (MCL)

Smears or biopsies and culture are used, as well as the new techniques, particularly PCR. Serological tests are of more value in MCL than in CL. The leishmanin test is usually strongly positive as well as the lymphoproliferative response.

Control of the leishmaniases

VISCERAL

Control of visceral leishmaniasis consists of identifying and treating infected persons, including cases of dermal leishmaniasis, and in attacking the sandfly as well as the animal reservoir of infection.

The individual

Pentavalent antimonials are the initial treatment of choice for visceral leishmaniasis. They are easy to administer and toxic effects are generally low. The dose is 20 mg of Sb^v/kg body weight intravenously or intramuscularly, for a minimum of 20 days for all forms of visceral leishmaniasis. Resistant cases occur and are on the increase, especially in India. Other drugs available are pentamidine, aminosidine and lipid-associated amphotericin B and miltefosine. Case detection and treatment will reduce transmission.

Sandfly bites can be partially avoided by sleeping on the upper floors of houses and using repellents. Impregnated bed-nets and curtains should also be effective.

The vector

The breeding places of sandflies in walls can be plastered over and the rubble of broken-down houses cleared away. The indoor biting *Phlebotomus* species are very susceptible to DDT and residual spraying of dwellings eradicates the sandfly. Insecticide-impregnated dog collars are being developed.

The animal reservoir

The detection and treatment of dogs with *L. infantum* has been disappointing, as asymptomatic seroneg-ative dogs are infective to sandflies. Elimination of symptomatic dogs was successfully used in China, but this method is not generally accepted.

The community

Villages should be sited away from ecological environments favourable to outdoor biting sand-fly vectors. Thus, in northern Kenya, houses should be sited more than 90 m from termite hills, which can be destroyed or treated with DDT.

Mass surveys and treatment of the human pop-ulation should be undertaken. Army and police personnel working in endemic areas should con-sist of leishmanin-positive persons. When a large number of leishmanin-negative persons is intro-duced into endemic areas, an epidemic of kala-azar can be expected. This is a particularly pertinent point to remember when populations are moving from one area to another as a result of the building of dams, or in the wake of civil wars.

CUTANEOUS: OLD WORLD

Control of cutaneous leishmaniasis of the Old World (tropical sore) is achieved by breaking the man/sandfly contact, rodent destruction and immunization.

Man/sandfly contact

Sandfly eradication by DDT spraying of houses and breeding places as above has markedly reduced the prevalence of cutaneous leish-maniasis. If this cannot be done, sleeping at night on the roof or the second floor of a house will reduce infection, since sandflies do not readily move above the ground floor. *Leishmania (L.) major* which is zoonotic, mainly results from sandfly bites out of doors, and house spraying is not as effective as in *L. (L.) tropica*, which is anthro-ponotic. The use of impregnated curtains and nets is indicated for peridomestic vectors.

Animal reservoir

Since the main reservoir of infection in Asia is a communal rodent, rat destruction for a radius of 5 km around villages should be carried out. Uzbekistan and Turkmenistan rodents were elimi-nated by ploughing their burrow networks with a deep plough. Alternatively, a combination of poi-soned grain and anticoagulants is also effective.

Immunization

Since rodents cannot be eradicated from remote areas, travellers and nomads should be protected by immunization. The deliberate inoculation of live amastigotes or promastigotes in the upper arm or buttock has been practised in endemic areas for years. The leishmanization with *L. (L.) major* para-sites of high virulence is recommended and also protects against *L. (L.) tropica*. The ulcerating lesion heals quickly and gives rise to life-long immunity. A vaccine is currently undergoing extensive trials. The Montenegro test becomes positive.

CUTANEOUS: NEW WORLD

Chiclero ulcer

Since both eradication of the rodent reservoir and spraying to destroy the sandflies in the forest canopy high above the ground are impracticable, immunization of gum collectors and forest work-ers is the only sensible remedy. Vaccination using a live culture of *L. mexicana* protects against the chronic disfiguring lesions found on the ears.

Uta

Residual spraying of dwellings with DDT eradi-cates the disease.

MUCO-CUTANEOUS

Muco-cutaneous leishmaniasis, being a sporadic jungle forest disease with an animal reservoir, is extremely difficult to control. Dwellings in new settlements in the forest should be concentrated away from the forest edge so that a barrier of clear land is maintained between the village and the for-est. Temporary spraying of the forest edges with insecticides can be carried out and travellers into forests should wear protective clothing and use repellents.

HELMINTHIC INFECTIONS

THE FILARIASES

Under this generic title are grouped a variety of diseases which bear little relation to each other pathologically, although they are produced by nematode worms all belonging to the superfamily Filariodea. Man is the definitive host of several filarial nematodes. Their embryos (microfilariae) are taken up by insect vectors when feeding on man. They pass through a developmental cycle lasting about 2 weeks, at the end of which infective larvae are present in the proboscis. When the insect next feeds, the larvae escape and pass through breaches of the skin surface into the tissues.

Filariasis (Bancroftian and Malayan)

Filariasis results from infection with the parasite nematodes *Wuchereria bancrofti* and *Brugia malayi*. It is estimated that at least 120 million people throughout the world are infected and 1 billion are 'at risk' of infection in about 90 countries. Indeed, the prevalence is increasing worldwide due to uncontrolled urbanization in many of the endemic countries. The life cycle is shown in Figure 7.14.

The features of the life cycles of these two filariae are practically identical (*Brugia malayi* alone may also infect animals as well as man). The adult worms live in the lymphatic system where the female worms, which are viviparous, produce sheathed microfilariae which are about 200–300 μm long. Many species of mosquitoes, belonging to the genera *Culex, Aedes, Anopheles* and *Mansonia*, can act as intermediate hosts of *W. bancrofti* and *B. malayi*.

The microfilariae of *B. malayi* can be distinguished from those of *W. bancrofti* on morphological grounds and by their staining reaction to Giemsa.

Microfilariae of both *W. bancrofti* and *B. malayi* appear in the peripheral blood at distinct times of the day – a characteristic referred to as periodicity. The controlling mechanism for this periodicity has never been satisfactorily explained. It does not appear to depend on the parasympathetic system, nor is the microfilarial count influenced by alterations in the corticosteroid level in the blood of man, or by a general anaesthetic.

B. timori is a nocturnal periodic species found in Indonesia and transmitted by *A. barbirostris*.

Epidemiology

The geographical distribution of the parasites is determined largely by climate and the distribution of their mosquito vectors (see Fig. 7.15).

Whereas *W. bancrofti* has so far been found only in man, *B. malayi* is a parasite of both man and animals.

The most consistent sign of infection is the appearance of microfilariae in the peripheral blood but many microfilaria carriers are apparently symptom-free and remain so for many years or for life. Severe disabling symptoms or deformity are usually due to a long period of exposure and re-infection.

Males are usually more frequently affected than females. This higher incidence of microfilaraemia in males is probably due to a greater chance of infection; it is possible, however, that a hormonal influence may be responsible. Most surveys for either form of *W. bancrofti* have shown low microfilaria rates in children below the age of 5 years, probably because *W. bancrofti* takes a long time to produce a patent microfilaraemia. In contrast, it has been shown that high microfilarial rates occur in children under 5 years with both forms of *B. malayi*; thus, a low infection rate among children under 5 years usually implies low transmission for *B. malayi* in the area surveyed.

Rapid mapping techniques have been developed as well as indirect methods, such as the use of key informants responding to self-administered questionnaires about the prevalence of hydrocele and lymphoedema; and the use of mobile health workers to examine an established number of persons for lymphoedema and hydrocele, have been successfully employed to assess the endemicity of filariasis in Ghana and elsewhere.

WUCHERERIA BANCROFTI

Occurrence:	Worldwide in the tropics
Organism:	*Wuchereria bancrofti*
Reservoir:	Humans
Transmission:	*Culex* and *Anopheles* spp.
Control:	Treatment with diethylcarbamazine and Albendazole
	Ivermectin and Albendazole (in areas where onchocerciasis coexists)
	Vector control

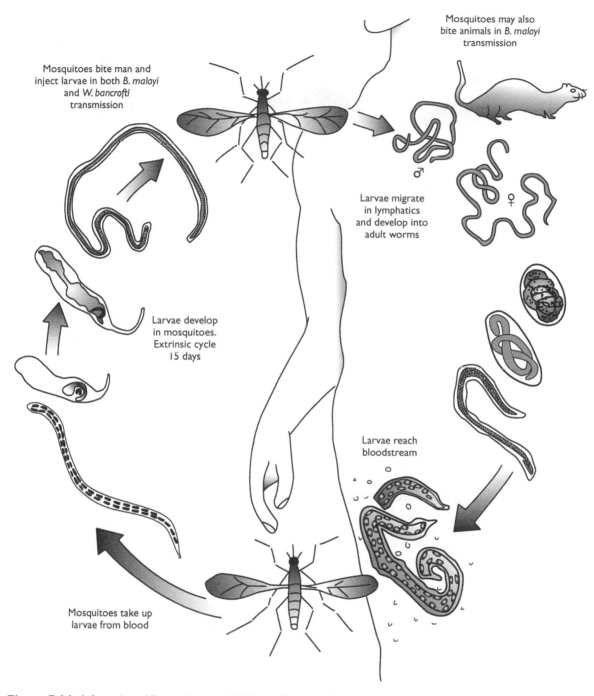

Mosquitoes may also
bite animals in *B. malayi*
transmission

Mosquitoes bite man and
inject larvae in both *B. malayi*
and *W. bancrofti*
transmission

Larvae migrate
in lymphatics
and develop into
adult worms

Larvae develop
in mosquitoes.
Extrinsic cycle
15 days

Larvae reach
bloodstream

Mosquitoes take up
larvae from blood

Figure 7.14: Life cycles of Bancroftian and Malayan filariases. *Brugia malayi* may also infect animals.

Two biologically different forms of *W. bancrofti* exist:

- nocturnal periodic;
- diurnal subperiodic.

Nocturnal periodic

The microfilariae appear in the peripheral blood between 10 pm and 2 am. This form is predominantly an infection of urban communities, transmitted by

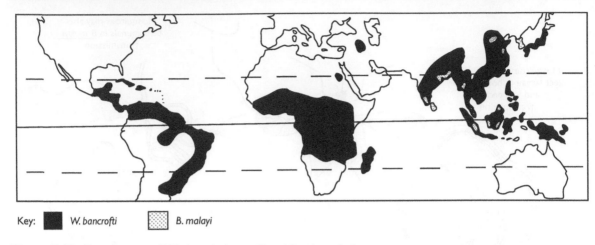

Key: ■ *W. bancrofti*   ▨ *B. malayi*

Figure 7.15: Distribution of *Wuchereria bancrofti* and *Brugia malayi*.

the domestic night-biting mosquito *Culex quinque-fasciatus*; as well as by *Anopheles* species in the African region and elsewhere (Plate 89). It has an almost worldwide distribution, occurring in Central and South America, West, Central and East Africa, Egypt and South East Asia (see Fig. 7.15).

Diurnal subperiodic

In this form, microfilariae are present in appreciable numbers throughout the 24 hours but show a consistent minor peak diurnally (usually sometime in the afternoon). It is restricted to Polynesia and is transmitted mainly by day-biting mosquitoes (*Aedes* spp.). The growth of the human population, uncontrolled increasing urbanization and migration have all contributed to an increase in the prevalence of *W. bancrofti*.

BRUGIA MALAYI

Occurrence:	South East and East Asia
Organism:	*Brugia malayi*
Reservoir:	Humans, animals
Transmission:	*Mansonia* and *Anopheles* spp.
Control:	Treatment with diethylcarbamazine and Albendazole
	Vector control

Human infection with *B. malayi* has only been recognized in Asia (see Fig. 7.15), where it is predominantly an infection of rural populations, in contrast to the usual urban distribution of *W. bancrofti*. There are two forms of *B. malayi*:

- nocturnal periodic;
- nocturnal subperiodic.

Nocturnal periodic

The microfilariae show markedly nocturnal periodicity in the blood (10 pm to 2 am). This form has a tendency to occur in small endemic foci in countries extending from the west coast of India to New Guinea, the Philippines and Japan. It is transmitted by the *Mansonia* mosquitoes of open swamps (Plate 90), lakes and reservoirs, which bite mainly at night and also *Anopheles* species. The periodic form is found mainly in man, and animal infections are rare.

Nocturnal subperiodic

In the subperiodic form the microfilariae tend to be present throughout the 24 hours with a minor nocturnal peak from 10 pm to 6 am. This nocturnally subperiodic form has been found, to date, only in Malaysia, Borneo and Palawan Island in the Philippines. It is transmitted by the *Mansonia* of swamp forest, mosquitoes which will bite in shade at any time and also by *Coquillethidia crassipes*. In contrast to the periodic form, the subperiodic form is found in many animals (primates, carnivores, rodents, etc.) as well as man.

LABORATORY DIAGNOSIS OF FILARIASIS

Isolation

The finding of microfilariae in the blood provides the certain diagnosis of filarial infection. It is important to realize that microfilariae may be absent in the very early or late stages of the infection – thus in only 4% of patients with elephantiasis and 30% with hydrocoeles are microfilariae found in the blood.

Thick blood films should be taken at the appropriate times (e.g. at night for microfilaria of *W. bancrofti*) and fresh cover-slip preparations examined. Simultaneously, dried, stained specimens should be made and the microfilariae identified. Many techniques are available for concentrating blood microfilariae.

Microfilariae may also be found in fluid obtained from hydrocoeles, varices, pleura, joints and in ascitic fluid. Eosinophilia is usually present. Occasionally the adult filarial worms may be found in biopsy of lymph glands, or by X-ray when calcified.

Antigen detection tests on children's blood have shown that 2% are infected by the age of 2 years and 16% by the age of 4 years in endemic areas. They also obviate the use of taking night blood films. A rapid dipstick method for the diagnosis of *B. malayi* is available.

Serology

Serodiagnostic methods for the diagnosis of filariasis have been widely used. There is a range of variation in the results obtained and these variations derive partly from differences in technique of antigen preparation. These immunodiagnostic methods are group specific (i.e. positive in any filarial infection) and on the whole still unsatisfactory, especially as they are unable to discriminate between past exposure, treated cases and current infection. Circulating filarial antigens can be detected in a drop of blood with the use of monoclonal antibodies using a dot ELISA technique which can be carried out without sophisticated equipment.

In central laboratories DNA-based technology can be used for diagnosis of filarial infection, both in humans and in the mosquito vectors by PCR-based assays, which provide excellent sensitivity and specificity.

CONTROL OF FILARIASIS

The filariases may be controlled by reducing the human reservoir with mass drug administration (MDA) and attacking the vector mosquitoes.

In 1997, the World Health assembly called for the elimination of lymphatic filariasis as a public health problem. The major thrust of the programme is MDA, which has been greatly facilitated by the free donation of Albendazole by Glaxo Smith Kline and Mectizan (Ivermectin) by Merck & Co., for as long as they are needed for the elimination of the disease.

MDA can be achieved either by the distribution of diethylcarbamazine (DEC)-fortified salt as has been successfully used in China and India, or by single annual or semi-annual treatment of DEC plus albendazole as is being envisaged in the global filariasis elimination programme. In areas where filariasis coexists with onchocerciasis and loaiasis, DEC 6 mg/kg plus Ivermectin 400 g/kg will be co-administered. The aim of the MDA programme is to reach the entire global at-risk population over the next 20 years.

Community involvement could be enhanced by simultaneously providing symptomatic treatment for lymphoedema based on regular washing of skin with soap and water, limb elevation, topical application of antibiotics and antifungal creams (Plate 91). The delivery of drugs could be either through existing health services or community directed. Mathematical models could provide powerful tools for analysis, prediction and control strategies.

The vector

Control measures may be taken against the aquatic stages of the mosquito by eliminating breeding places, using insecticides to kill aquatic forms; or in the case of *Mansonia* mosquitoes, destroying, by herbicides or hand collection, the water vegetation on which the insect is dependent. The insecticidal control of most adult culicine mosquitoes is important. Where the vectors are anophelines, malaria control methods are effective. Larval control of *C. quinquefasciatus* is now only possible by using pyrethroids such as permethrin, since resistance to the organophosphorus insecticides is now widespread.

Other measures such as insect growth regulators, biological competitors, the use of larvivorous fish, and environmental management have been used with variable success. Integrated control using a combination of the above methods is required.

Reduction of man–vector contact can be achieved by house-screening and the use of impregnated nets and curtains. Biocides and polystyrene beads for larval control have been also effective in certain areas.

ELIMINATION OF FILARIASIS

The task of eliminating lymphatic filariasis (LF) is being undertaken by the L F Global Alliance, a coalition of 37 bodies which includes three international organizations (WHO, World Bank, Unicef); two pharmaceutical multinationals – Glaxo Smith Kline who are donating Albendazole and Merck who are donating Ivermectin; eight NGOs; two academic institutions – The Liverpool School of Tropical Medicine and Emory University's Rollins School of Public Health, CDC and Ministries of Health of endemic countries.

The time scale to eliminate the disease is 20 years, 70–80% of the at-risk community (1.2 billion) have got to be treated if transmission is to be broken.

In Africa Albendazole and Ivermectin will be given. DEC will not be used because of the risk of eye complications. In the rest of the world, the combination of Albendazole and DEC will be used.

Loaiasis

Occurrence:	West Africa
Organism:	*Loa loa*
Reservoir:	Humans
Transmission:	*Chrysops* spp.
Control:	Prophylactic DEC

This is an infection due to the filarial worm *Loa loa* and is characterized by transient subcutaneous swellings.

APPLIED BIOLOGY

The adult worms live in the connective tissue of man. They are about 70 mm long and produce microfilariae which pass into the bloodstream. The microfilariae (sheathed and about 300 μm in length) appear in greatest numbers in the blood during the day. When the circulating microfilariae are taken up by suitable species of *Chrysops*, they

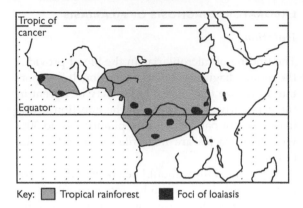

Key: ▨ Tropical rainforest   ■ Foci of loaiasis

Figure 7.16: Distribution of loaiasis.

pass from the stomach to the thoracic muscles and after a period of development, lasting about 12 days, present in the proboscis. When the fly next feeds on a human host the larvae penetrate the skin and migrate in the connective tissues, reaching maturity in about a year.

EPIDEMIOLOGY

Loaiasis is found in the equatorial rainforest belt of Africa stretching from the Gulf of Guinea in the west to the Great Lakes in the east (Fig. 7.16).

Transmission

Various species of *Chrysops* are the only known vectors of loaiasis and they breed in densely shaded, slow-moving streams and swamps (Plate 92). The adults live in the tree tops, the females coming down to attack man at ground level or to lay their eggs on the mud and decaying vegetation of stagnant waters. The males do not feed on blood. *Chrysops* are attracted by movement, light and smoke from wood fires, they bite in daylight and seem to prefer dark to white skins. They are commonly known as 'red-flies' or 'softly softly flies' from their quiet approach.

In man, all ages and both sexes are affected, although overt infection in young children is uncommon, probably due to the long incubation period of the filarial worm.

LABORATORY DIAGNOSIS

Microfilariae may be found in the peripheral blood taken preferably around midday and they can be differentiated on morphological grounds from other sheathed microfilariae. Concentration techniques are useful to detect scanty infections.

The adult worms may be seen wriggling under the conjunctiva. A high eosinophilia (60–80%) is usually present. The filarial complement fixation test gives the highest proportion of positive results with loaiasis, and is particularly useful in the early infections before microfilariae have appeared in the blood, or in unisexual infections when microfilariae are absent.

CONTROL

As in the case of Bancroft's filariasis, control measures are directed against the parasite in man and against the vector fly.

Reservoir

Diethylcarbamazine and Ivermectin clear microfilariae from the blood and kill the adult worm in recent infections, but they sometimes cause unpleasant reactions, especially in patients with high microfilarial counts (>3000/ml). DEC can be used as a chemoprophylactic at an adult dosage of 200 mg twice daily, for 3 successive days once a month.

Vector

The fly may be controlled by clearing shade vegetation at breeding sites or by applying residual insecticides to the mud in the breeding places. Personal protection against *Chrysops* can be effected by screening of houses, impregnated nets and wearing long trousers.

Onchocerciasis

Occurrence:	Focal distribution in Africa and Central America
Organism:	Onchocerca volvulus
Reservoir:	Humans
Transmission:	Simulium spp.
Control:	Vector control: Abate Chemotherapy with Ivermectin (African programme for onchocerciasis control: APOC)

This infection is caused by the nematode *Onchocerca volvulus* and is characterized by the development of skin changes, subcutaneous nodules and ocular lesions, lymphatic pathology and some systemic effects.

APPLIED BIOLOGY

The adult worms are found in subcutaneous nodules and tissue spaces. The females, which are ovoviviparous, measure about 30–80 cm in length while the males are only 3–5 cm long. Worms of both sexes are found coiled together in nodules and larvae are present in large numbers near the coiled gravid female. The developed larvae (microfilariae) vary greatly in size (250–300 μm) and are unsheathed. The life cycle is shown in Figure 7.17. The lifespan of *O. volvulus* is between 9 and 14 years.

EPIDEMIOLOGY

Onchocerciasis has a focal distribution in both Africa and Central America. It is endemic in West Africa, in equatorial and East Africa, and in the Sudan. One of the largest endemic areas occurs in the Volta River Basin area, which incorporates parts of Benin, Ghana, Ivory Coast, Mali, Niger, Togo and all of Upper Volta. This is the area of the Onchocerciasis Control Programme (OCP). In Latin America, endemic onchocerciasis occurs in Mexico, Guatemala, Colombia, Venezuela and Brazil. It is endemic in the southern part of Yemen, in and around Taiz and this focus may extend north into Saudi Arabia. It is endemic in 34 countries (Fig. 7.18).

The prepatent interval of *O. volvulus* in man varies between 3 and 15 months. A relationship between geographical forms of the parasite, which are genetically distinct, and patterns of blinding and non-blinding ocular disease, has been identified.

Although *O. volvulus* has been found in primates, in most endemic areas the infection is maintained by human to human transmission.

Vector

Simulium can breed at high altitudes (610 m or more) and the larvae and pupae are found attached to submerged vegetation and stones in highly oxygenated waters (Plate 93). They are also found at sea level along the banks of very large rivers such as the Niger. The larvae of *S. neavei* have been found adherent to the carapace of

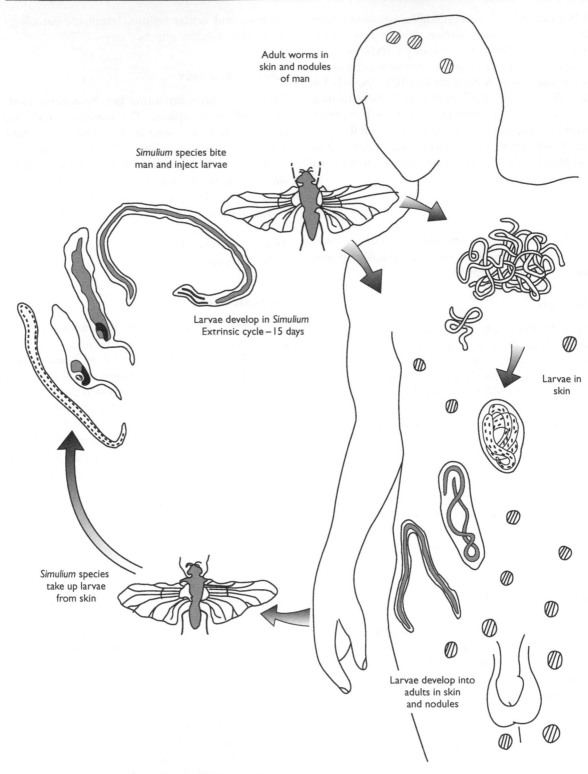

Adult worms in
skin and nodules
of man

Simulium species bite
man and inject larvae

Larvae develop in *Simulium*
Extrinsic cycle – 15 days

Larvae in
skin

Simulium species
take up larvae
from skin

Larvae develop into
adults in skin
and nodules

Figure 7.17: Life cycle of *Onchocerca volvulus*.

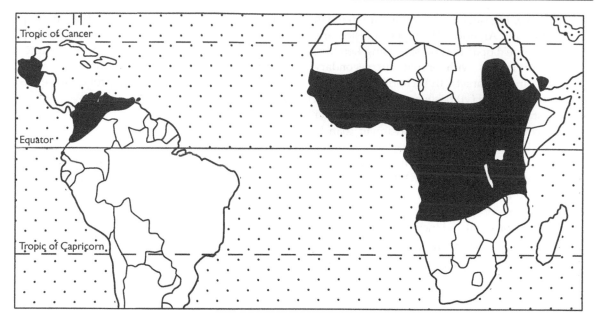

Figure 7.18: Distribution of *Onchocerca volvulus.*

aquatic crabs. Though some species of *Simulium* have a long flight range (400 km), the infection is mainly concentrated near the breeding sites, and thus tends to be focal. The period of greatest transmission is in the rainy season coinciding, as might be expected, with the period of maximal *Simulium* breeding. A clear relationship was found between vector infectivity and skin microfilarial load.

Host factors

The disease is widespread and males are infected more frequently than females, but this is an occupational hazard, for example fishermen. The incidence of infection increases with age: by middle age 75% of the population in an endemic area might be infected. In Central America infection is acquired at an early age and in the Cheapas State of Mexico 50% of children are infected by the age of 14 years. Both in Mexico and Guatemala *erysipela de la costa* is found in children and young persons and *mal morado* in the older age groups. Both these syndromes are associated with high microfilarial densities.

No clear relationship is necessarily found between the number of microfilariae in the skin and the extent or degree of the skin lesions. Comparisons between African and Central American onchocerciasis reveal certain epidemiological and clinical differences. Thus, in some parts of Africa there is a tendency for the microfilariae to be most numerous in the most dependent parts of the body; while in Guatemala microfilariae are abundant in the upper parts of the body. A relationship seems to exist between the site of biting of the vector and the localization of nodules. As would be expected, in Africa the majority of nodules are found in the lower parts of the body, whereas in Central America as many as 70% are found on the head. Bony lesions of the occipital region of the skull produced by these nodules are found in 5% of patients. The level of onchocerciasis endemicity can be adequately assessed by a method based on nodule palpation in 50 adult males – rapid epidemiological assessment (REA) – a rapid epidemiological mapping of onchocerciasis (REMO) has been developed. Under the REMO method, the distribution of onchocerciasis is estimated by extrapolation of the survey results for a sample of only 2–4% of all potential endemic villages.

OCULAR LESIONS

There is now no doubt that the lesions of the eye listed below are directly caused by infection with *O. volvulus*, and that their prevalence is related to the intensity of infection and particularly to the density of microfilariae found in the head region and in the eye. The same ocular lesions are found in Africa and Latin America. The types of lesion are: (i) 'fluffy' corneal opacities; (ii) sclerosing keratitis; (iii) anterior uveitis with or without secondary glaucoma and cataract; (iv) chorioido-retinitis; (v) optic neuritis; and (vi) postneuritic optic atrophy.

In West Africa the risk of blindness is higher amongst communities living in savannah than in rainforest. Elsewhere in Africa (e.g. Zaire – now Democratic Republic of the Congo) this is not invariably the case. The major differences in the epidemiology of the disease in the rainforest and savannah regions of Africa and in Latin America are probably multifactorial and include the following:

- distinct geographical strains of the parasite with differences in their vector infectivity and in their pathogenicity;
- social and behavioural patterns of the human host;
- the state of immunity of the individual;
- the intensity of transmission;
- unidentified nutritional factors;
- vector biting habits.

LABORATORY DIAGNOSIS

Identification

Microfilariae of *O. volvulus* are identified by examination of skin or conjunctival snips. They are most easily found in samples of skin taken from the region of the nodule. Alternatively, the skin snip is teased, immersed in saline, and the deposit examined after centrifugation. Excision of nodules for histological examination will reveal the adult worms, while aspiration of fluid from nodules will occasionally show microfilariae. Microfilariae may also be seen in the anterior chamber of the eye with an ophthalmoscope or slit lamp. A moderate eosinophilia is usually present. Ultrasonography has been used to detect impalpable nodules.

Serology

Various serological tests have been used with variable success in the diagnosis of onchocerciasis. These include: complement fixation, intradermal, precipitin, immunofluorescence, ELISA and a haemagglutination reaction.

Simple qualitative information is of little value. It is necessary to express the results quantitatively,

either as the number of microfilariae (m/f) per skin snip or, preferably as the number of m/f per milligram or per unit surface area, or volume of skin. Several quantitative techniques are available. Antigen detection and DNA probes have been developed.

CONTROL

Control is being carried out by attacking the *Simulium* fly and mass treatment with Ivermectin.

The vector

Control of the fly by attacking its breeding sites has to be continued for some 20 years before the disease can be expected to die out in the affected communities, because the lifespan of the adult female worm is around 14 years, and that of the microfilariae between 6 and 30 months.

Onchocerciasis Control Programme

This large control operation has been undertaken in the savannah area of the Volta River Basin in West Africa. It covers approximately 700 000 km^2 with about 10 million inhabitants. It was estimated that of these at least 70 000 were blind, mainly from onchocerciasis, while many more had serious visual impairment. The governments of the seven West African countries concerned recognized that onchocerciasis was the most important single deterrent to large-scale development of the potentially fertile river valleys in the area, which lay uninhabited and unproductive. Furthermore, the serious effects of drought in the Sahel for 6 successive years had gravely disturbed the delicate socioeconomic balance in the Volta River Basin area.

The Onchocerciasis Control Programme (OCP) is in its final quinquennial period. Because many of the breeding sites of S. *damnosum* are inaccessible by land the only feasible method of insecticide application is by aircraft. For large, open rivers, light fixed-wing planes can be used, but for narrow, twisting waterways and for those overhung by forest, helicopters are needed.

After years of research the insecticide finally selected for OCP was a biodegradable insecticide, temephos (Abate), which in suitable formulations combines high effectiveness against the blackfly larvae with very low toxicity for man, non-target fauna and plants. Monitoring of the effects of insecticide application to the large target area was shared with a specially created, independent ecological panel, which advised the programme director and the governments concerned on appropriate measures to ensure the satisfactory protection of the environment.

The control operations were being implemented progressively in three stages and, when the complete area was covered, approximately 14 000 km of river were under treatment. Helicopters and fixed-wing aircraft were used to apply the larvicide to the rivers weekly in amounts calculated to give an effective concentration of 0.05 mg/l for 10 minutes in the rainy season, and 0.1 mg/l for 10 minutes in the dry season. The insecticide was deposited in a single mass by means of a rapid release system specially designed for the programme. Drop points in the large rivers were approximately 30 km apart during the rainy season, when the riverine discharge is sufficient to transport the larvicide downstream. In the dry season applications were made just upstream from each breeding site.

The OCP programme has operated for 25 years using mass Ivermectin treatment to complement its entomological control since 1988. Twenty-five million hectares of fertile land – previously deserted – have become available for cultivation. When the programme comes to an end in 2002, 12 million children born since the beginning of control activities will have grown up without the risk of infection and the conquest of 'river blindness' will have been achieved (Plate 94). In anticipation of the termination of the OCP programme, the African Programme for Onchocerciasis Control (APOC) has been established based on the efficacy, safety and availability of Ivermectin. In parallel with APOC, the Programme for the Elimination of Onchocerciasis in the Americas (OEPA) is supporting the distribution of Ivermectin in the endemic countries of Central and South America. The APOC programme based on Ivermectin distribution now covers *all* the endemic areas of onchocerciasis in Africa.

The human reservoir

Chemotherapy

Ivermectin (Mectizan), a macrocyclic lactone, has been shown to be an effective microfilaricide which also has a temporary suppressive effect on the release of microfilariae for 6–12 months. Systemic reactions are less severe and less frequent than with diethylcarbamazine although qualitatively similar: fever, rash, lymph-node pain, limb swelling and hypotension. Ocular reactions have been minimal.

Annual treatment with Ivermectin is the cornerstone of the APOC and OEPA programmes. In Africa, it has been shown that community-directed treatment is feasible, effective and successful in a range of diverse settings. Distribution systems designed by communities achieved better coverage than programme-designed approaches, and the distribution performance was adequate in terms of coverage achieved, adherence to exclusion criteria and dosing level.

Dosage was determined using height measurements. A vertical wall in an appropriate place in the village or a stick, was calibrated to serve as the measuring instrument. Four dosage treatments which were indicated on the instrument were to be adhered to based on the following measurements:

Height (cm)	Dosage (tablets)
90–119	½
120–140	1
141–158	1½
159 or more	2

Mid-upper arm circumference (MUAC) has also been successfully used for community-based ivermectin treatment as follows: MUAC 13–15 cm, 0.5 tablet; 16–20 cm, 1 tablet; 21–27 cm, 1.5 tablets; >28 cm, 2 tablets.

Nodulectomy

Until recently the only community control of the human reservoir available was nodulectomy, which has been in operation in Guatemala for many years. The nodule carrier rate was found to decrease with time. No systematic nodulectomy campaigns have been initiated in Africa.

REMO and REA together with geographical information systems (GIS) are being used extensively for targeting control in APOC countries.

Other filarial infections

TETRAPETALONEMA PERSTANS

T. perstans has an extensive distribution throughout Africa, tropical America and the Caribbean. The adults have been reported in the liver, pleura, pericardium, mesentery, perirenal and retroperitoneal tissues. The microfilariae are non-periodic and are unsheathed. The intermediate vectors are *Culicoides austini* and *C. grahami* in Africa. The detailed epidemiology has not been studied, but it is known that many individuals in some African villages may harbour the parasite.

TETRAPETALONEMA STREPTOCERCA

This parasite lives both as an adult and as a microfilaria within the skin. In West Africa the vector is *C. grahami*. Both the adult worms and microfilariae are susceptible to diethylcarbamazine.

MANSONELLA OZZARDI

This filarial worm is confined to the New World and is found in South and Central America and in certain foci in the Caribbean. The adult worms are embedded in visceral adipose tissue. The vectors are *Culicoides* spp.

DIROFILARIASIS

Various species of *Dirofilaria* have been reported from the Mediterranean basin, the Balkans, South America, Turkey, Africa and the USA. They include *D. conjunctivae*, *D. repens*, *D. magalhaesi* and *D. louisanensis*. The life cycle of these parasites in man is not fully known and it seems probable that mosquitoes or fleas are the natural intermediate hosts. The adults do not develop normally in man.

Control

Control of *T. perstans*, *T. streptocerca* and *M. ozzardi*, which is dependent on controlling the vector species of *Culicoides*, has not been seriously attempted.

REFERENCES AND FURTHER READING

Abdulla S. *et al.* (2001) Impact on malaria morbidity of a programme supplying insecticide treated nets in children aged under 2 years in Tanzania. *British Medical Journal* 322: 270–273.

Chance M.L. & Evans D.A. (1999) The agent. In Gilles H.M. (Ed.) *Protozoal Diseases.* Arnold, London, p. 420.

Foege W.H. (1998) Mectizan and onchocerciasis: a decade of accomplishment and prospects for the future; the evolution of a drug into a development concept. *American Tropical Medicine & Parasitology* 92 (Suppl 1): 179.

Mekong Malaria (1999) *South East Asian Journal of Tropical Medicine and Public Health* 30 (Suppl 4): 101.

Mekong Malaria Forum (2000) Information exchange on malaria control in Southeast Asia. *Quarterly Bulletin European Commission* 6.

Mekong Malaria Forum (2001) Issue No. 8.

Porterfield J.S. (Ed.) (1995) *Exotic Viral Infections.* Chapman & Hall, London.

WHO Parasitic Diseases Programme (1988) *Guidelines for Leishmaniasis Control.* WHO/Leish/88.25.

WHO (1992) *Vector Resistance to Pesticides.* Technical Report Series No. 818. WHO, Geneva.

WHO (1993) *Implementation of the Global Malaria Strategy.* Technical Report Series No. 839. WHO, Geneva.

WHO (1993) *Implementation of the Global Malaria Strategy. Report of a WHO Study Group on the implementation of the Global Plan of Action for malaria control. 1993–2000.* WHO, Geneva.

WHO (1994) *Lymphatic filariasis infection and disease. Control Strategies.* TDR/CTD/Fil/Penang/94.1. WHO, Geneva.

WHO (1994) *The Onchocerciasis Control Programme in West Africa – An Example of Effective Public Health Management.* WHO, Geneva.

WHO (1995) *Vector Control for Malaria and Other Mosquito-borne Diseases.* Technical Report Series No. 857. WHO, Geneva.

WHO (1995) *Onchocerciasis and Its Control.* Technical Report Series No. 852. WHO, Geneva.

WHO (1996) *Community Directed Treatment with Ivermectin. Report of a Multicountry Study.* TDR/AFR/RP/96.1. WHO, Geneva.

WHO (1997) *Dengue Haemorrhagic Fever: Diagnosis, Treatment, Prevention and Control,* 2nd edn. WHO, Geneva.

WHO (1997) *Vector Control: Methods for Use by Individuals and Communities.* WHO, Geneva.

WHO (1998) *Control and Surveillance of African Trypanosomiasis.* Technical Report Series No. 881. WHO, Geneva.

WHO (1998) *Malaria Epidemics – Detection and Control. Forecasting and Prevention.* WHO/Mal./98.1084. WHO, Geneva.

WHO (1998) *TDR's Contribution to the Development of Ivermectin for Onchocerciasis.* TDR/ER/RD/98.3. WHO, Geneva.

WHO (1998) *Report of a WHO Informal Consultation on Epidemiological Approaches to Lymphatic filariasis elimination: Initial Assessment, Monitoring and Certification.* WHO, Geneva.

WHO (1999) *The Global Partnership to Roll Back Malaria – Initial Period Covered July 1998–December 2001.* Draft. 3.1B/July 1999. WHO, Geneva.

WHO (1999) *Roll Back Malaria. Proposed Strategy and Workplan (July 1998–December 2001).* WHO, Geneva.

WHO (2000) *WHO Expert Committee on Malaria.* 20th Report. Technical Report Series No. 892. WHO, Geneva.

WHO (2000) *Bulletin World Health Organization. Special Theme Malaria* 78: 1374–1491.

WHO (2000) *Malaria Diagnosis – New Perspectives.* WHO/CDS/RBM/2000.14. WHO, Geneva.

WHO (2000) Strengthening implementation of the Global strategy for Dengue Fever/Dengue Haemorrhagic Fever. Prevention and Control, WHO/CDS/(DEN)/IC/2000.1. WHO, Geneva.

(2001) Maladie du sommeil le renouveau. *Medicine Tropicale* 61(4–5): 1–448.

LATE ADDENDA

Malaria

The following drugs are available for the treatment of uncomplicated malaria (1) amodiaquine; (2) sulfadoxine-pyrimethamine; (3) mefloquine; (4) quinine; (5) atovaquone-proguanil (malarone); (6) chloroproguanil-dapsone (Lapdap); (7) artemisinin compounds; (8) artemisinin suppositories. Chloroquine can only be used in very limited areas of malarious countries except in Central America. Pre-packed single blisters aare now available e.g. artesunate (Plasmotrin®) and mefloquine (Mephaquin®) aimed at improving compliance. With the same objective and in order to delay the advent of resistance combination therapy (CT) must be accepted and made to work if malaria mortality is to fall. This is particularly crucial for Africa where most malaria deaths occur. It is hoped that artemisinin-containing combination therapy (ACT) will become affordable or available through support from the Global Fund to fight AIDS, Tuberculosis and Malaria or from some other donor international source.

CHAPTER EIGHT

NON-COMMUNICABLE DISEASE: HEALTH IN TRANSITION

- Chronic diseases
- Mental health
- Occupation: health and disease

- Genetics and health
- Heat disorders
- Further reading

In the past few decades, significant changes have occurred in the pattern of health and disease in many developing countries. These changes have resulted from the effects of social, economic and technological developments as well as from specific public health and population programmes:

EPIDEMIOLOGICAL TRANSITION

As communicable diseases, malnutrition and problems associated with pregnancy and childbirth come under control, chronic, non-communicable diseases replace them as the dominant public health problems (see Box 8.1 and Plate 95).

DEMOGRAPHIC TRANSITION

With reduction in fertility and child mortality, people in developing countries are living longer. Hence, the health problems of older people are assuming increasing importance.

CHANGES IN ECOLOGY AND LIFESTYLE

In addition to the demographic changes which bring the health problems of the elderly into prominence, ecological changes in developing

countries contribute to the changing pattern of disease. Industrialization, urbanization and the wider use of motor vehicles have increased the incidence of occupational diseases, respiratory problems associated with atmospheric pollution and road traffic accidents. Changes in diet, a more sedentary life, use of tobacco products, alcohol and other drugs have increased the risk of heart disease, stroke and other diseases associated with the altered lifestyle.

Box 8.1: Non-communicable diseases

Source: WHO: World Health Report (1999)

In 1998, an estimated 43% of all DALYs globally were attributable to non-communicable diseases. In low- and middle-income countries the figure was 39%, while in high-income countries it was 81%. Among these diseases, the following took a particularly heavy toll:

- neuropsychiatric conditions, accounting for 10% of the burden of disease measured in DALYs in low- and middle-income countries and 23% of DALYs in high-income countries;
- cardiovascular diseases, responsible for 10% of DALYs in low- and middle-income countries and 18% of DALYs in high-income countries;
- malignant neoplasms (cancers), which caused 5% of DALYs in low- and middle-income countries and 15% in high-income countries.

These changes have not occurred at the same rate in all developing countries. Furthermore, countries affected by the debt crisis have lost some of their earlier gains in the development of their services. The differences in the health situation between countries at varying stages of development is reflected in the wide range of under five mortality rates (U5MR). At one end of the spectrum, the U5MR is low (<50/1000 live births), comparable to some developed countries; but the rate remains very high (>150 per 1000 live births) in other countries. The massive pandemic of HIV/AIDS is eroding earlier gains in some communities especially in sub-Saharan Africa.

EPIDEMIOLOGICAL PATTERNS OF DISEASE

Developing countries can be classified into three broad groups on the basis of their health profiles.

Traditional epidemiological pattern

In these countries, parasitic and infectious diseases, acute respiratory-tract diseases and malnutrition occur frequently as major causes of morbidity and mortality; child and maternal mortality rates are high; fertility rate is high and expectation of life at birth is low.

Transitional pattern

These countries are undergoing rapid demographic and epidemiological change: infant, child and maternal mortality rates are declining, fertility rates are high but falling, life expectancy is rising; parasitic and infectious diseases are still prevalent but chronic degenerative diseases and non-communicable diseases associated with modern lifestyles and ageing populations are increasing. In some cases, countries carry a double burden: they are acquiring modern health problems whilst traditional ones persist.

Developed-country pattern

The more advanced developing countries have acquired the epidemiological pattern that is typical of the developed countries: fertility rates and infant, child and maternal mortality rates are low; life expectancy at birth is high; cancer, cardiovascular, neurological and mental disorders, degenerative diseases, and problems associated with the changed lifestyle and behaviour are common.

Earlier chapters in this book have focused largely on the problems affecting the developing countries which are still at the earliest stage of the development of their health services: problems of infection and malnutrition. As the countries evolve in this transitional process, health workers must increasingly pay attention to non-communicable diseases and other problems that commonly occur in developed countries. This chapter briefly discusses a few of such issues:

- chronic diseases – illustrative examples of current trends and risk factors;
- mental health;
- occupational health;
- genetics and health;
- heat disorders.

CHRONIC DISEASES

Non-infectious diseases take an enormous toll in lives and health worldwide. Nearly 60% of deaths globally are now due to heart disease, stroke, cancer and lung diseases. The growing problem of chronic diseases can be illustrated by a brief review of the rising trend in the prevalence of diabetes and by an examination of the tobacco problem as an important risk factor.

THE GLOBAL EPIDEMIC OF DIABETES

During the past 12 years, the World Health Organization has been collecting information on the prevalence of diabetes mellitus and impaired glucose tolerance (IGT) in adult communities worldwide. Within the age range 30–64 years, diabetes and IGT were found to be absent or rare in some traditional communities in Melanesia, East Africa and South America. In communities of European origin, the prevalences of diabetes and IGT were in the range of 3–10% and 3–15% respectively, but migrant Indian, Chinese and Hispanic American groups were at higher risk (15–20%).

The highest risk was found in the Pima Indians of Arizona and in the urbanized Micronesians of Nauru, where up to one-half of the population in the age range 30–64 years had diabetes (Table 8.1). The prevalence of diabetes showed a wide range between countries. Typically, variation within countries shows a higher prevalence in urban communities compared with relatively low frequency in rural communities, a pointer to modern lifestyles as risk factors for diabetes.

WHO drew three important conclusions from these findings:

- an apparent epidemic of diabetes has occurred – or is occurring – in adult people throughout the world;
- this trend appears to be strongly related to lifestyle and socio-economic change;
- it is the populations in developing countries, and the minority or disadvantaged communities in the industrialized countries, who now face the greatest risk.

WHO is following up these findings by promoting further monitoring of trends in various countries and encouraging governments to develop national programmes for the control of this disease. The

Table 8.1: Age-adjusted prevalence of diabetes in persons aged 30–64 years

Population	Male	Female
Australian Aborigines		
Bourke	24.0	20.9
Purfleet	14.0	21.9
Chile – Mapuches	0.0	1.4
Columbia – Bogota	7.0	8.7
Kirabati		
Rural (Tabiteuea)	4.4	4.6
Urban (Betio)	15.8	13.4
Malta	7.7	9.7
Nauru	41.2	41.5
New Caledonia		
Ouvea	0.0	3.3
Touho	3.0	2.3
Oman	13.9	14.4
Russia – Novisibirsk	1.8	3.6
Singapore	22.7	10.4
Tunisia	8.8	7.9
USA Pima Indians	49.4	51.1
Western Samoa		
Rural	2.1	5.9
Urban	10.7	10.4

long-term complications are steadily increasing the burden of disease in some communities. For example, diabetes is now the commonest cause of new cases of irreversible blindness. Apart from the direct complications of diabetes, the disease is a risk factor for cardiovascular diseases.

Control of diabetes

The explosive increase in the prevalence of diabetes has been in the adult form of the disease, the non-insulin-dependent diabetes mellitus (NIDDM). There is strong epidemiological evidence that this epidemic is related to the changing lifestyle: refined foods have replaced natural whole grain, high-fibre diets; and there is a lack of physical exercise. By adopting a healthier diet and increasing exercise, persons with impaired glucose tolerance can reduce the risk of progressing to frank diabetes.

TOBACCO – A MAJOR CAUSE OF AVOIDABLE BURDEN OF DISEASE

Over the past 50 years, sound scientific evidence has accumulated to show that prolonged smoking is an important cause of premature mortality and disability worldwide. WHO estimates that smoking causes about 4 million deaths annually worldwide (Table 8.2). There are about 1.15 billion smokers in the world today, consuming an average of 14 cigarettes each per day. Of these smokers, 82% live in low- and middle-income countries. Tobacco-related deaths will increase dramatically if current smoking patterns persist.

Trends in smoking

Tobacco consumption fell between 1981 and 1991 in most high-income countries (see Fig. 8.1). In the USA, the prevalence of smoking increased steadily from the 1930s and reached a peak in 1964 when more than 40% of all adult Americans, including 60% of men, smoked. Since then smoking prevalence has decreased, falling to 23% by 1997. By contrast, consumption is increasing in developing countries by about 3.4% per annum, having risen dramatically in some countries in recent years. Overall, smoking prevalence among men in developing countries is about 48%.

Table 8.2: Tobacco: cigarette consumption, mortality and disease burden by WHO region

WHO region	Annual cigarette consumption per capita estimates for around 1995	Mortality estimates for 1998 (000)	DALYs estimates for 1998 (000)
Africa	480	125	1900
The Americas	1530	772	8867
Eastern Mediterranean	890	182	2976
Europe	2080	1273	17 084
South East Asia	415	580	7439
Western Pacific	1945	1093	11 022
World total	**1325**	**4025**	**49 288**

These figures exclude other tobacco products and may significantly underestimate tobacco consumption. Because of a change in methodology, comparison with previous WHO estimates should be avoided. Based on data from the UN Department for Economic and Social Information and Policy Analysis, Industrial Statistics Section and the UN Comtrade database.

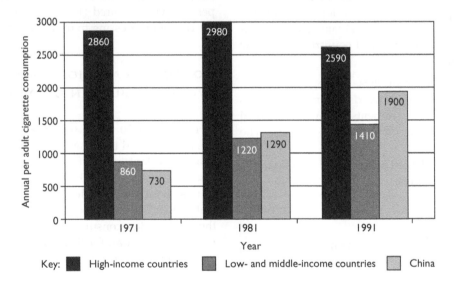

Key: ■ High-income countries   ■ Low- and middle-income countries   □ China

Data for China are also included in low- and middle-income countries

Source: Tobacco or health: A global status report Geneva, World Health Organization, 1997.

Figure 8.1: Trends in per capita cigarette consumption, 1971, 1981 and 1991.

The toll from tobacco smoking

In populations where cigarette smoking has been common for several decades, it accounts for:

■ 90% of lung cancer;
■ 15–20% of other cancers;
■ 75% of chronic bronchitis and emphysema;
■ 25% of deaths from cardiovascular disease at ages 35–69 years;
■ 16% of the total annual incidence of cancer cases;

■ 30% of cancer deaths in developed countries, and 10% in developing countries;
■ 12% of all tuberculosis deaths – this could be because a lung damaged by tobacco may offer a propitious environment for the infectious tuberculosis bacillus.

The pattern of smoking-related disease varies from country to country. In developed countries, cardiovascular disease, in particular ischaemic heart disease, is the most common smoking-related cause of death. But in China, smoking now causes far more deaths from chronic respiratory diseases than it does from cardiovascular disease.

Secondary smoking (i.e. exposure to other people's smoking) is associated with a somewhat higher risk of lung cancer, and with several other important health ailments in children such as sudden infant death syndrome, low birth weight, intrauterine growth retardation and children's respiratory disease.

Control of smoking

WHO recommends a four-pronged strategy:

1 Ban advertising and expand public health information:
   - Forbid all forms of advertising and promotional distribution of tobacco products and sponsorship of sporting events, etc.
   - Disseminate public health information – with special attention to youths, provide credible information about the health and other ill effects of smoking.
2 Use taxes and regulations to reduce consumption:
   - Increased taxation – this usually reduces demand for tobacco products.
   - Regulation to reduce public and workplace smoking – these bans reinforce the message that smoking is an undesirable activity.
3 Encourage cessation of tobacco use:
   - Promote the production and sale of less harmful and less expensive ways of delivering nicotine through patches, tablets, inhalers or other means. Since this type of substitute smoking product can satisfy the craving for the addictive drug nicotine, it offers the best practical approach to cessation for many current smokers.
   - Expand free and/or subsidized smoking cessation services and products.
   - Deregulate nicotine replacement products and increase access to smoking substitute products in developing countries.
4 Build anti-tobacco coalitions:
   - Use public revenues derived from tobacco taxes to fund groups and activities that support tobacco control.
   - Fund transition to other employment for tobacco farmers and others who would lose income as a result of tobacco control.

- Mobilize civil society and other groups to promote the message: 'Tobacco or Health'.

MENTAL HEALTH

Throughout the world there is an increasing awareness of mental disorder as a significant cause of morbidity. This awareness has increased with the steady decline of morbidity due to nutritional disorders, communicable diseases and other forms of physical illness. There is also a better understanding of certain behavioural and social problems which had previously not been properly recognized as manifestations of mental disorder. The role of the community both in the prevention of mental disorder and the care of the mentally handicapped has now been widely acknowledged and is regarded as the only appropriate basis for the development of mental health programmes.

DIMENSIONS OF THE PROBLEM

Mental and behavioural disorders are common, affecting more than 25% of all people at some time during their lives. They are also universal, affecting people of all countries and societies, individuals at all ages, women and men, the rich and the poor, from urban and rural environments. They have an economic impact on societies and on the quality of life of individuals and families. Mental and behavioural disorders are present at any point in time in about 10% of the adult population. Around 20% of all patients seen by primary health care professionals have one or more mental disorders. One in four families is likely to have at least one member with a behavioural or mental disorder.

Source: World Health Report, 2001

The importance of neuropsychiatric disorders was underestimated when health problems were ranked solely on their contribution to mortality rates. Now that the measurement of burden of disease includes calculation of the amount of disability, there is greater appreciation of the importance of neuropsychiatric disorders. In 1998, it was estimated that 11% of the global burden of disease was attributable to neuropsychiatric conditions. In high-income countries, one out of every four DALYs was lost to a neuropsychiatric conditions, while in low- and middle-income countries this group of conditions was responsible for one out of ten DALYs.

Of the ten leading causes of disease burden in young adults (in the 15–44 year age group) four were neuropsychiatric conditions. In 1998, alcohol dependence, unipolar major depression, bipolar disorder and schizophrenia were among the leading causes of disease burden in adults aged 15–44 years.

Psychiatric disorders are frequently a considerable drain on health resources as a consequence of being misunderstood, misdiagnosed or improperly treated. Mental health care, unlike many other areas of health, does not generally demand costly technology; rather, it requires the sensitive deployment of personnel who have been properly trained in the use of relatively inexpensive drugs and psychological support skills on an outpatient basis.

CLASSIFICATION OF MENTAL DISORDERS

Various forms of mental disorder are encountered:

- *Impaired intelligence.* Arrested or incomplete development of the mind.
- *Psychoses.* These include the manic–depressive psychoses and schizophrenia, and a variety of organic psychoses which are related to demonstrable lesions of the brain.
- *Psychoneuroses and psychosomatic disorders.*
- *Behavioural disorders.* These include maladjustment in childhood, juvenile delinquency, absenteeism, etc.
- *Psychopathic disorders.* These present as irresponsible, often aggressive antisocial acts, repeated in spite of appeals, warnings and sanctions.

Box 8.2 shows the classification of mental diseases as proposed in the 10th revision of the International Classification of Diseases (ICD-10).

OBJECTIVES OF A MENTAL HEALTH PROGRAMME

The main objective of a mental health programme is to ensure for each individual optimal development of mental abilities and a satisfactory

---

Box 8.2: The broad categories of mental and behavioural disorders covered in ICD-10

Source: WHO (1992)

- **Organic, including symptomatic, mental disorders**, e.g. dementia in Alzheimer's disease, delirium.
- **Mental and behavioural disorders due to psychoactive substance use**, e.g. harmful use of alcohol, opioid dependence syndrome.
- **Schizophrenia, schizotypal and delusional disorders**, e.g. paranoid schizophrenia, delusional disorders, acute and transient psychotic disorders.
- **Mood (affective) disorders**, e.g. bipolar affective disorder, depressive episode.
- **Neurotic, stress-related and somatoform disorders**, e.g. generalized anxiety disorders, obsessive-compulsive disorders.
- **Behavioural syndromes associated with physiological disturbances and physical factors**, e.g. eating disorders, non-organic sleep disorders.
- **Disorders of adult personality and behaviour**, e.g. paranoid personality disorder, trans-sexualism.
- **Mental retardation**, e.g. mild mental retardation.
- **Disorders of psychological development**, e.g. specific reading disorders, childhood autism.
- **Behavioural and emotional disorders with onset usually occurring in childhood and adolescence**, e.g. hyperkinetic disorders, conduct disorders, tic disorders.
- **Unspecified mental disorder**.

---

emotional adjustment to the community and the environment. Thus, the programme will include:

- promotion of mental health;
- prevention of mental disorder;
- provision of mental health care.

Promotion of mental health

The positive aspect of the mental health programme involves the design and creation of social and environmental situations in which mental health will grow and flourish. The factors that promote mental health are both physical and socio-cultural.

The physical aspect includes the promotion of the general fitness of the individual and the control of environmental stresses such as excessive noise. The socio-cultural factors include the consolidation of family life, the control of economic stresses, and the resolution of conflicts within the society.

The prevention of mental disorder

The prevention of mental disorder is to some extent limited because the aetiology of some of these disorders is not known. A number of underlying causes, predisposing or precipitating factors have been identified. The main aetiological groups are:

- genetic factors;
- organic brain damage;
- socio-cultural factors;
- idiopathic group.

GENETIC FACTORS

There has been a tendency to exaggerate the role of genetic factors in the aetiology of mental disorder. The familial occurrence of certain forms of mental disorder may be determined by social and environmental factors rather than by genetic factors. Thus, mental disorder in the child of alcoholic parents may have resulted from the stresses of an unsuitable home background rather than from genetic inheritance. There are, however, some clear examples of mental handicap resulting from genetic factors, for example Down's syndrome, which is determined by a demonstrable chromosomal abnormality. More subtle genetic factors that are manifested in the form of personality types, response to stresses and other behavioural patterns are recognized but are difficult to quantify. The role of genetic factors in the aetiology of the major psychoses (manic–depressive psychoses and schizophrenics) has not been clearly defined.

ORGANIC FACTORS

Organic brain damage may result from:

1 Trauma (including birth trauma).
2 Infections:
  - meningitis;
  - syphilis;
  - trypanosomiasis;
  - HIV infection;
  - kuru and other forms of encephalitis;
  - acute febrile illness;
  - hyperpyrexia.
3 Malnutrition:
  - vitamin deficiency, e.g. pellagra, beri-beri;
  - Korsakov's psychosis;
  - protein malnutrition – clinical and experimental studies suggest that severe protein malnutrition in childhood may result in permanent mental retardation.
4 Toxins:
  - alcohol;
  - lead;
  - opiates and other habit-forming drugs – amphetamines, cannabis, lysergic acid.
5 Degenerative lesions:
  - senile dementias including Alzheimer's disease – the increasing lifespan has brought the problems of old age into greater prominence;
  - specific degenerative diseases – Sydenham's chorea.

SOCIO-CULTURAL FACTORS

The social environment of the individual plays a prominent role in determining the state of his or her mental health. Social stresses can often be identified as initiating and precipitating factors of acute mental disorder. This association is most prominent in relation to behavioural problems in childhood which often reflect emotional problems within the family.

Although patterns of non-organic psychoses are similar in many communities, their manifestations are conditioned by cultural factors. Thus, the recognition of mental disorder depends on a careful evaluation of the norms, beliefs and customs within the particular culture. For example, a person who would not touch a particular object because they believe that it is inhabited by evil spirits may, in one culture, be manifesting signs of acute mental disorder, but in another culture, may be showing no more than reasonable caution.

IDIOPATHIC GROUP

Within this group are various psychotic and psycho-neurotic illnesses, psychopathic personality problems, and behavioural disorders. It seems likely that in most cases, each condition is not the result of a single aetiological agent, but that the occurrence of disease is determined by a chain or web of interrelated factors: a genetic predisposition, facilitating and inhibitory social, cultural and environmental factors, and the existence of various precipitating factors.

PROVISION OF MENTAL HEALTH CARE

In developing mental health services, priority should be given to four areas:

- psychiatric emergencies;
- chronic psychiatric disorders;
- mental health problems of patients attending clinics, health centres and other curative services particularly at the primary health-care level;
- psychiatric and emotional problems of high-risk groups.

THE ELEMENTS OF A COMMUNITY MENTAL HEALTH PROGRAMME

The basic ingredient of a community health programme is community concern for the patients and their families, and community acceptance of its responsibility for the prevention and care of mental handicap. It has been rightly said that 'Community care is possible only in a community which cares'. Community health education is therefore vital to the success of these programmes.

Education

ERADICATION OF SUPERSTITIOUS FEARS AND PREJUDICES

Traditional attitudes to mental disorder include superstitious fears that the ill patients are possessed by devils and evil spirits. Even in modern societies there are many social attitudes to mental disorder that are unfounded and illogical. These attitudes result in painful social stigma against the mentally handicapped and permanent prejudices against those who have fully recovered. Successful treatment and social rehabilitation of patients will be much enhanced by a tolerant and understanding attitude within the community.

DISSEMINATION OF KNOWLEDGE OF THE MANIFESTATIONS OF MENTAL DISORDER

It is particularly important that the early signs of mental disorder be recognized so that remedial action can be taken promptly. The early signs may be misinterpreted by relatives, friends and society as merely antisocial behaviour calling for punishment rather than treatment. The community should be taught that 'a person who is troublesome, may be a person in trouble'.

PARTICIPATION OF THE COMMUNITY IN THE CARE AND REHABILITATION OF THE MENTALLY HANDICAPPED

The attitude in many communities is to seek custodial care for the mentally handicapped where the patients can be isolated for indefinite periods. The modern concept is to treat the patients as far as possible within the community, thereby minimizing the effects of the disorder on patient and family, and also facilitating social rehabilitation.

PATTERNS OF CARE

Facilities are required for outpatient and inpatient care, follow-up services and general mental health promotion in the community.

Outpatient care

Outpatient care within the community would include psychiatric outpatient clinics, a variety of special clinics (child guidance, counselling) and day hospitals. The advantages of the day hospital are that it:

- conserves limited inpatient hospital resources for patients who require them;
- exploits the social dynamic forces of the community in the care of the mentally handicapped;
- avoids the disturbing effects of the unfamiliar and artificial environment of the hospital;
- assists in the rehabilitation of the patient within the home, the family and workplace.

PREVENTIVE MEASURES

The mental health problems of the community are stratified in terms of age and other social features.

The mental health programme would include measures to prevent mental disorder which are appropriate at each age group:

Prenatal

Good antenatal care and delivery services should:

- ensure normal fetal development;
- prevent congenital infections (e.g. syphilis);
- avoid intrapartum trauma.

Infancy

- Provide emotional security within the family circle.
- Care for abandoned children and children without families.
- Prevent malnutrition, communicable and other diseases.

School-age

- Provide a balanced programme of work and play to avoid excessive fatigue (physical and mental).
- Encourage positive use of leisure hours.
- Establish satisfactory social adjustment inside and outside the family.

Adolescence

- Prevent, identify and deal with emotional problems at puberty by health education (including sex education).

Young adult

- Assist adjustment to working life, especially where rural/urban, agrarian/industrial transfers are involved.

Adult

- Provide counselling service for family life and for resolving conflicts in relation to self, family and community.

Old age

- Provide substitute systems of care where traditional extended family systems are breaking down.

- Find alternative leadership roles for the elderly where they have been deprived of their traditional position of authority, e.g. provide ritual functions in the community.

It is clear from these examples that a successful mental care programme cannot be operated solely by professional psychiatrists and other specialist personnel, but it must include all medical and health workers, voluntary agencies and other community resources.

OCCUPATION: HEALTH AND DISEASE

Hippocrates in the introductory paragraph of 'Airs, Waters, Places' offered timeless advice on sound environmental medicine to physicians: 'to consider the effects of seasons, to observe how men live, what they like, what they eat and drink or whether they love their work or not'. But since manual work was not undertaken by the upper classes for which Hippocratic medicine catered, Hippocrates did not emphasize the importance of occupation as a factor in ill health. It was left to Bernando Rammazzini (1633–1714) to develop the Hippocratic teaching and to the questions recommended by Hippocrates he added one more: 'what is your occupation?' Since then, the associated physical and psychosocial hazards of work have continued to attract the attention of health professionals.

Occupational health has gone through many developments and has been variously defined. It was only in 1952 that a joint World Health Organization/International Labour Organization committee offered a definition of the aim of occupational health which was accepted by the World Community:

> the promotion and maintenance of the highest degree of physical, mental and social well-being of workers in all occupations; the prevention among workers of departures from health caused by their working conditions; the protection of workers in their employment from risks resulting from factors adverse to health; the placing and maintenance of the worker in an occupational environment adapted to his physiological equipment and, to summarize: the adaptation of work to man and of each man to his job.

MIXED BENEFITS OF INDUSTRIALIZATION

The vicious cycle of poverty and disease can only be broken by industrialization and economic progress. As the workers are the main support of economic and social progress, their health is an essential factor in development and represents an important human goal.

The problems associated with industrial progress may be summarized under five major headings:

1 The high prevalence of epidemic and endemic communicable diseases.
2 The high prevalence of occupational disease and injury because of inadequate identification and control.
3 Introduction of the hazards of modern agriculture.
4 Public health and social problems which arise from industrialization.
5 Problems of providing medical care, especially for small and widely scattered groups of workers.

Occupation and communicable disease

The range of communicable diseases found in the tropics has been covered in Chapters 4–7 of this book. However certain occupations constitute special risks by enhancing the spread of microbial infection. The sources of occupational exposure to infection are classified as follows:

1 Industrial:
   ■ contact with contaminated material, e.g. oils, coolants, dusts, aerosols, radioactive products.
2 Human:
   ■ direct, due to crowding, ventilation, air-conditioning;
   ■ indirect, e.g. laboratory infection.
3 Animal:
   ■ direct, by contact with living animals;
   ■ indirect from materials or products derived from animals.

Identification of an infection, which is prevalent in the population, as occupational depends on the awareness of the occupational health professionals and the care with which the cases can be investigated.

Occupational diseases

Occupation and health interact with one another. In *occupational diseases* there is a direct cause and effect relationship between hazard and diseases, for example silica dust and silicosis, lead fumes and lead poisoning. In *work-related diseases*, in contrast, the work environment and the nature of the job contribute significantly, but as only one of the factors, in the causation of a disease of multifactorial aetiology, for example ischaemic heart disease and musculoskeletal disorders. The insults from hazardous agents, whether direct or indirect, affect particular organs and systems of the body. Occupational diseases are usually classified according to the target organ systems: respiratory, cardiovascular, skin,

Table 8.3: Occupational diseases of the respiratory tract

Type of disease	Agents
Acute inflammation	Ammonia, chlorine, nitrous fumes, ozone, sulphur dioxide
Asthma	Cotton dust, epoxy resins, isocyanates, various metals, various woods
Extrinsic allergic alveolitis	■ Air-conditioner disease (bacteria, amoebae) ■ Bagassosis (sugar cane mould) ■ Bird fancier's disease (avian serum proteins) ■ Farmer's lung (*Microsporum faeni*, thermophyllic actinomyces from mouldy hay) ■ Animal handler's lung
Pneumoconiosis	Asbestos, coal dust, silica
Cancers	Asbestos, chrome, ionizing radiation, nickel, hydrocarbons (polycyclic)

genitourinary, nervous, liver, haemopoietic and endocrine.

OCCUPATIONAL LUNG DISORDERS

The lungs are the major route of entry of noxious gases and dust. The resulting disorders can be grouped into five categories:

- acute inflammation;
- asthma;
- extrinsic allergic alveolitis;
- pneumoconiosis;
- cancers.

Table 8.3 gives examples of agents that cause these various forms of respiratory disease.

OCCUPATIONAL SKIN DISEASES

The occurrence of a cluster of cases from the same work place should be highly suspicious. The occupational dermatoses and agents are shown in Table 8.4.

The major industries prone to cause occupationally related dermatoses are:

- agriculture and horticulture;
- building and construction;
- leather manufacture;
- catering and food processing;
- boat building and repair;
- hair dressing;
- wood working;
- chemical and electrical industries.

Table 8.5 gives examples of occupational diseases affecting other organs.

OCCUPATIONAL CANCER

Generally, cancers of occupational origin are not distinguishable by their clinical presentation from other cancers. Those agents that have been reported to have a high incidence of or mortality from cancer include:

- aromatic amines – high risk of cancer of the bladder (aniline, benzidine, l-naphthylamine and 2-naphthylamine);
- asbestos – significant increase in risk for cancer of lung, larynx, gastro-intestinal tract;
- benzene – acute myelogenous leukaemia;
- beryllium – increased risk of lung cancer;
- cadmium – increased risk of lung cancer;
- chromium – increased risk of nasal and respiratory cancer;
- nickel – increased risk of nasal cancer;

Table 8.4: Occupational skin diseases

Type of disease	Agents
Parasitic diseases	Animal fleas, scabies mites, cercariae
Physical conditions	Fibreglass, heat and cold damage, vibrations, chemical burns
Irritant contact dermatitis	Acids, detergents, alkalis, solvents
Allergic contact dermatitis	Dichromates, epoxy resins, dyes, formaldehyde
Cancers	Coal tar, mineral oil

Table 8.5: Occupational diseases of other organs

Organs affected	Agents
Peripheral nervous system	Arsenic, carbamate and organophosphate pesticides, triorthocresyl phosphate, inorganic lead and its compounds
Central nervous system	Arsenic, organic lead, inorganic mercury, trichloroethylene, chlorinated hydrocarbons, halothane
Liver	Carbon tetrachloride, chlorinated naphthylenes, trichloroethylene, halothane, aflatoxins
Haemopoietic system	Benzene, lead, trinitro-toluene
Genito-urinary system	Arsenic, cadmium, lead, mercury, carbon tetrachloride
Cardiovascular system	Cadmium, carbon disulphide, carbon monoxide, mercury

- polynuclear aromatic hydrocarbons – associated with cancers at all sites;
- vinyl chloride and polyvinyl chloride – cancers of liver, lung, brain;
- wood dust – nasopharyngeal carcinoma.

Hazards of modern agriculture

DEFINITIONS

Agriculture means all forms of activity connected with the growth, harvesting and primary processing of all types of crops; with the breeding, raising and care of animals; and tending market gardens and nurseries.

Agricultural worker means any person engaged either permanently or temporarily, irrespective of his or her legal status, in activities related to agriculture as defined above.

AETIOLOGICAL FACTORS

The diseases of agricultural workers relate to the socio-economic, cultural and environmental conditions in which they work and live. These include:

- geographic and ecological characteristics of the area;
- housing and environmental sanitation;
- inadequate medical and health services;
- occupational patterns of farming;
- association with plants and animals;
- association with chemicals and poisons;
- low income levels.

It is beyond the scope of this chapter to detail the diseases included in each category but certain examples can be given.

ACCIDENTS

Accidents are varied: those due to farm machinery such as tractors, harvesters and other mechanical equipment and those due to bad management around the farm or field.

OCCUPATIONAL DISEASES IN AGRICULTURE

These may result from:

- infections and parasitic diseases;
- poisoning;
- physical factors.

Infections and parasitic diseases

These can either be principally contracted through an agricultural occupation (e.g. anthrax, brucellosis, ankylostomiasis and schistosomiasis); or occasionally contracted through an agricultural occupation (e.g. rabies, hydatid disease and malaria).

Poisoning

The use of organophosphate and carbamate insecticides has increased greatly. Field workers may be exposed by:

- working in a recently sprayed field;
- handling sprayed crops;
- accidental spraying, and spraying without adequate protection;
- wind-borne spray from an adjoining field.

Safe use of pesticides and insecticides should be closely adhered to as outlined by WHO (1985).

Physical factors

Accidental injuries account for a lot of work-related illness. Poorly maintained equipment, failure to understand and observe safety instructions, poor supervision and other factors make such accidents common in developing countries. The climatic conditions such as temperature, humidity and radiation impose additional stress on the tropical worker. The different aspects of heat stress and disorders are discussed on page 253.

Public health and social problems

Rapid industrialization and development imply radical alterations in the society. This may lead to the health and social problems of:

- mass migration of whole communities from the rural areas to the towns;
- social disruption when migrant labourers leave home to work in neighbouring countries whilst family members remain at home;
- psycho-social problems and clashes of old and new values;
- occupational accidents and diseases;
- overcrowding and malnutrition.

However, if the development is well planned and properly implemented the benefits will be far greater than the disadvantages.

Problems of providing medical care

A comprehensive approach to the health problems of workers and the gainfully employed should be adopted when occupational health services are planned in developing countries.

POLICY ISSUES IN OCCUPATIONAL HEALTH

Thus far this chapter has outlined very general approaches to the recognition and prevention of occupational hazards as well as discussing some of the major health problems specific to developing countries. Another important area in the field of occupational health is the complex relationship between scientific public health issues and the development of healthy public policy. Policy develops through the interaction of workers, management, government and the scientific public health community, nationally and internationally. Countries throughout the world are members of the International Labour Organization (ILO), WHO and other agencies, adopting their recommendations and standards. The occupational health standards are varied, whether hygiene standards and recommended threshold limit values (TLVs) or notifiable industrial diseases or labour legislation.

Each country and each enterprise has to develop its own occupational health programme to deal with the full relationship between work and the total health of man.

The WHO Expert Committee on Environmental and Health monitoring in Occupational Health stated that occupational health programmes should have the following aims:

1   Control of hazards:
    - To identify and bring under control at the workplace all chemical, physical, mechanical, biological, and psycho-social agents that are known to be or suspected of being hazardous. Table 8.6 lists some suggestions on how to prevent occupational hazards.
2   Match suitable workers and jobs:
    - To ensure that the physical and mental demands imposed on people at work by their respective jobs are properly matched with their individual anatomical, physiological, and psychological capabilities, needs and limitations.

3   Provide protection:
    - To provide effective measures to protect those who are especially vulnerable to adverse working conditions and also to raise their level of resistance.
4   Improve the work environment:
    - To discover and improve work situations that may contribute to the overall ill health of workers in order to ensure that the burden of general illness in different occupational groups is not increased over the community level.
5   Implementation of health policies:
    - To educate management and workers to fulfil their responsibilities relevant to health protection and promotion.
6   Provision of occupational health:
    - To carry out comprehensive in-plant health programmes dealing with man's total health, which will assist public health authorities to raise the level of community health.

The above goals are in line with the 'Health For All by the Year 2000' policy which has been adopted by all countries of the world (WHO, 1978).

GENETICS AND HEALTH

The scientific basis of genetics has made tremendous strides in recent years culminating in the completion of the mapping of the human genome. Harnessing these new tools, biomedical scientists expect to make rapid, significant advances in many directions:

- diagnosis of hereditary disorders;
- identification of markers of disease susceptibility using molecular epidemiology;
- advances in biotechnology to develop diagnostic tools, prophylactic and therapeutic agents as well as novel vector control methods.

Interest in genetics was initially stimulated in the tropics and subtropics by the discovery that high gene frequencies for some genetic traits are maintained by providing protection to the carrier against falciparum malaria. The haemoglobin genetic markers vary in importance from one area to the other: while haemoglobin S is the most important abnormal haemoglobin in Africa, it is superseded by haemoglobin E and thalassaemia in

Table 8.6: General principles for preventing and controlling occupational hazards

Measures	Examples and comment
Educate the workers	Inform the workers of the hazards in the working environment and how they can protect themselves and other workers
Replace hazardous chemical	Use alternative safer compound as replacement for hazardous chemicals
Modify the process	Engineering and other modifications can make a process safer, e.g. wet drilling to reduce dust in mining
Eliminate toxic process at source	Remove the hazardous product to minimize contamination of the environment, e.g. use exhaust fans to remove dust at the point of drilling
Limit the number of workers exposed	Confine the hazardous process to a restricted area to which only essential workers have access; avoid unnecessary exposure of clerical workers. The use of remote action and in the most advanced processes, the use of robots may further reduce human exposure
Protect workers	Workers should use protective gowns, gloves, goggles and other protective equipment as required. Management should monitor the compliance of workers and if necessary impose sanctions on workers who fail to use prescribed protective gear
Monitor the environment	Measurement of environmental contamination, e.g. dust level, will indicate risks and impact of control measures
Monitor exposure of workers	Measure the degree to which individual workers are exposed, e.g. using film and thermoluminescent dosimeters (usually worn as badges) to measure individual exposure of radiographers and radiologists to ionizing radiation
Monitor the health of workers	Workers in hazardous employment should be monitored to look for early signs of adverse effects, e.g. blood tests in workers exposed to lead
Establish emergency and first aid services	Workers and health staff should be trained to deal with emergencies such as accidental spillage of hazardous chemicals or exposure of individuals. Appropriate first aid equipment should be easily accessible, e.g. emergency showers

South East Asia. Many other examples of the interplay between genetic factors and health are available (Table 8.7).

GENETIC MODIFICATION OF MALARIA

Several red cell inherited factors influence mortality from *Plasmodium falciparum* malaria. Substantial epidemiological, clinical, autopsy and culture evidence is now available to suggest that the following genetic red cell traits afford relative protection against death from malignant tertian malaria:

- haemoglobin S and E;

- α- and β-thalassaemia;
- ovalocytosis;
- G-6-PD deficiency;
- HLA-BW53;
- DRBI*1302-DQB1*0501.

Haemoglobin S

There is clear evidence that the heterozygote enjoys a selective advantage against the lethal effects of *P. falciparum* malaria:

- The sickle-cell gene is found in its highest prevalence in areas where *P. falciparum* malaria is, or was until recently, endemic (Fig. 8.2).

Table 8.7: Genetics and health: examples of relationships

Item	Comment
Genetic variations in response to drugs	▪ Glucose-6-phosphate dehydrogenase (G-6-PD) deficiency – common in some tropical countries; exposure to fava beans, primaquine and other agents may precipitate haemolysis; heterozygote confers some protection from malaria ▪ Variations in acetyltransferase enzyme are associated with marked differences in the blood level of isoniazid
Haptoglobins	Absence in a high proportion of Africans suggests operation of a selective process
Blood groups	Variations in risk of developing some cancers associated with blood group
Response of parasites and vectors	Drug resistance of falciparum malaria to antimalarial drugs, of bacteria to antibiotics and of mosquitos to insecticides are examples of genetic factors in diseases control

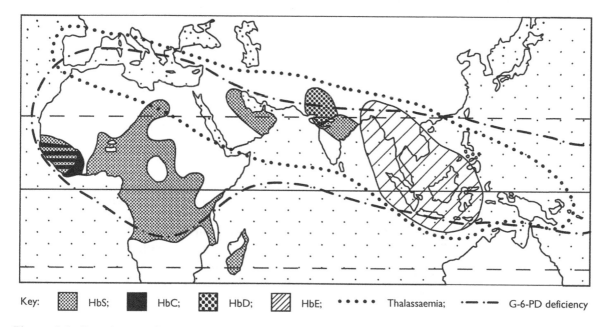

Key: ▓ HbS;   ■ HbC;   ▧ HbD;   ▨ HbE;   ••••• Thalassaemia;   •—•— G-6-PD deficiency

Figure 8.2: Distribution of abnormal red cell genes.

▪ In areas of stable malaria, high *P. falciparum* densities are significantly less commonly found in children with the sickle-cell trait (AS) than in normal children (AA).

▪ Post-mortem studies have revealed that death from cerebral malaria rarely occurs in the S. heterozygote (AS).

▪ The prevalence of the sickle-cell trait in a population increases with advancing years, suggesting a differential survival with a greater loss of normal genes (Fig. 8.3).

▪ Some studies showed that mothers with sickle-cell trait had a slightly higher fertility and lower stillbirth rate, and the birth weights of their children tended to be slightly higher than those of non-sickle cell mothers.

▪ Studies *in vitro* have demonstrated that *P. falciparum* parasites do not survive in cells with AS or SS haemoglobin when oxygen tension is decreased.

The S gene remained common in parts of the world (especially in Africa), despite the fact

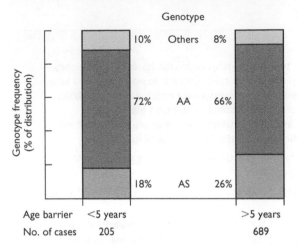

Figure 8.3: Haemoglobin genotype distribution in Akufo village, Nigeria ($\chi^2 = 6.3860$; $df = 2$; $0.02 < p < 0.05$).

homozygotes, SS, develop a severe anaemia from which most die in childhood. The selective advantage of the heterozygote, AS, compensates for the losses from the premature deaths of the homozygote. This phenomenon is termed 'balanced polymorphism': the persistence of a gene in the population is the resultant of losses and gains from homozygotes and heterozygotes respectively.

Haemoglobin C

Haemoglobin C is present in high frequencies in a localized part of West Africa, around Burkino Fasso and Ghana. Cells from the homozygote CC are refractory to parasite growth in culture; however AC cells support parasite growth normally.

In West Africa, where S gene frequencies are also very high, individuals carrying one S gene and one C gene (SC) are not uncommon and parasite growth is poor in SC cells. SC females have a reduced fertility and death from SC disease in pregnancy due to a severe haemolytic anaemia is not uncommon. Recent epidemiological studies have confirmed the protective effect of haemoglobin C homozygotes and, to a lesser extent, heterozygotes.

Haemoglobin F

It has been suggested that the presence of the 'F gene' for foetal haemoglobin might partially protect the bearer against the effects of *P. falciparum* malaria. An analysis of the results of various

observers who have examined infants living in malarious districts of Africa reveals a comparatively low level of malaria infection in infants under 3 months of age. An apparent relationship was found in Gambian infants between the disappearance of fetal haemoglobin and the onset of malaria infection, but no definite evidence exists from population studies that haemoglobin F (HbF) protects against the lethal effects of *P. falciparum*. However, recent *in vitro* studies have shown that parasite growth – as opposed to invasion – is impaired in HbF-containing red cells, regardless of their source.

Haemoglobin E

In vitro culture has demonstrated statistically significant reductions of *P. falciparum* growth in haemoglobin E (HbE)-containing red cells than in haemoglobin AA cells. The difference became even more pronounced at high oxygen concentrations. The oxygen effect was partially reversed by ascorbic acid. Moreover, 35% of South East Asian refugees with haemoglobin AE or haemoglobin EE had immunofluorescence antibody titres of 7200 compared with 13% with haemoglobin AA.

Thalassaemia

Epidemiological as well as *in vitro* evidence is now available that α- and β-thalassaemia heterozygotes enjoy a selective advantage in a malarious environment. However, recent evidence has shown that children with β-thalassaemia may experience more mild attacks of malaria in early life, suggesting that longer protection may stem from early immunization.

Glucose-6-phosphate dehydrogenase (G-6-PD) deficiency

G-6-PD deficiency renders its bearer vulnerable to haemolytic anaemia on exposure to primaquine, fava beans and other agents.

Confirmation of the malaria-protection hypothesis of the G-6-PD gene has been sought in various ways: (i) gene-frequency distribution studies in populations living in areas of different malarial endemicity; (ii) malaria parasite density surveys in G-6-PD normal and deficient children; (iii) induced falciparum malaria in human volunteers; and (iv) G-6-PD deficiency among patients with severe clinical falciparum malaria. Both heterozygote females and homozygote males are protected from severe malaria.

Ovalocytosis

This red cell shape abnormality commonly found in Papua New Guinea has been shown to protect against severe falciparum malaria.

HLA antigens

An HLA class 1 antigen, HLA-BW53 and an HLA class 11 haplotype, DRBI*1302-DQBI*0501 have been associated with reduced susceptibility to severe disease. Both these HLA antigens are common in African populations.

Rhesus-negative gene

A most interesting hypothesis has been put forward about the possible selection against the rhesus negative gene by malaria. The incidence of the rhesus (Rh) gene is generally low in areas in which malaria is, or was, endemic. It was suggested that a population, subject to a heavily malarious environment, might be superior antibody producers owing to selection by elimination of poor antibody producers. If this were so, haemolytic disease of the newborn should be more intense in malarious areas, and Rh-negative genes should be selectively eliminated if the frequency of the gene is or was below 0.50. Hence Rh-negative mothers in a malarious area should show a higher incidence of sensitization to a Rh-positive fetus than their counterparts in northern areas. In Ibadan, Nigeria, over 400 Rh-negative pregnant multiparae were studied and, apart from some who had received previous transfusions of Rh-positive blood, evidence of those sensitized by pregnancy was found in only 2.5% – a lower incidence than the figures recorded from Europe and elsewhere. This evidence does not, therefore, substantiate the above hypothesis.

CLINICAL SIGNIFICANCE OF GENETICS

Human genetics is one of the elements that can be used in the planning of co-ordinated attacks on disease, since it can sometimes differentiate those groups or individuals who are susceptible from those who are not.

Group susceptibility

Genetic factors often determine group susceptibility or resistance to disease, for example the racial immunity to vivax malaria of West African Negroes now shown to be related to the Duffy antigen. The recent advances in genetics have boosted interest in molecular epidemiology; that is, the study of genetic and environmental risk factors at the molecular level, to the aetiology, distribution and control of diseases in groups of populations.

Individual susceptibility

The role of genetic factors in individual susceptibility may be seen in twins that are sometimes more liable to certain morbid conditions; a comparison is made between monozygotic and dizygotic twins. In addition, immune deficiencies, whether cellular or humoral (e.g. agammaglobulinaemia), are consequent on genetic factors, and such genetic failure may be responsible for altered patterns of disease, for example defective cellular immunity in lepromatous leprosy. The clinical importance of the HLA genes in relation to transplantation and to possible abnormal immune response to some common chronic diseases has been recently emphasized, as has the remarkable association between HLS-B27 and ankylosing spondylitis and the possible association of *Schistosoma mansoni* hepatosplenomegaly and HLA-A$_1$ and B5.

Genetic counselling

Population genetic studies are a recent important expansion of the field of genetics and the knowledge thus acquired can be of practical value in preventive medicine, in the form commonly referred to as genetic counselling. This is particularly important in the situation, as it is at present in Africa, where sickle-cell anaemia has an incidence of nearly 2% in some countries and may be responsible for a childhood mortality of approximately 5 per 1000.

Implementing a programme

The ascertainment of follow-up of individuals in need of counselling and prenatal diagnosis should not be left to chance but should be achieved by the creation of a genetic register system.

Genetic counselling is essentially a process of communication and involves far more than the mere discussion of genetic risks. First, the nature of the disease has to be described, its prognosis given and the nature and efficacy of any treatment discussed. Feelings of guilt and recrimination may have to be dealt with. Second, the various options open to a couple will have to be considered: family limitation, sterilization, adoption, artificial insemination and prenatal diagnosis with elective abortion (see below). There is evidence that in coming to a decision, parents are influenced by the psychological, social and economic problems attendant on a serious genetic disorder.

ASSESSING THE RISK

Genetic risks are naturally assessed in terms of probabilities. They range from the big risk of 1 in 2 with a dominant gene (e.g. Huntington's disease) or 1 in 4 with a recessive gene (e.g. sickle-cell anaemia) through a spectrum of decreasing risks which ultimately reach very low values.

INTERVENTION

An increasing number of inherited conditions can be effectively treated if dealt with promptly, and in others treatment can at least reduce the degree of suffering. Where routine neonatal screening is possible but prenatal diagnosis not available, for example SS disease in some developing countries, there is a special obligation to make sure that early detection occurs. In some conditions, it is even possible to obtain a prenatal diagnosis of the foetus, for example spina bifida and β-thalassaemia. Indeed the recent advances in molecular biology have made prenatal diagnosis available for a greater number of genetically acquired diseases and at an earlier stage of pregnancy, making safer intervention possible if it is so desired (Table 8.8).

Table 8.8: Some genetic disorders in the tropics that can be diagnosed prenatally

Type	Examples
Disorders due to structural haemoglobin variants	■ Sickle-cell anaemia ■ Haemoglobin SC disease ■ Haemoglobin O Arab
Thalassaemias	■ $\alpha°$ thalassaemia (haemoglobin Bart's hydrops fetalis) ■ $\alpha°/\alpha^+$ thalassaemia (haemoglobin H disease) ■ $\beta°$ thalassaemia ⎫ (thalassaemia major, ■ β^+ thalassaemia ⎭ Cooley's anaemia) ■ $\delta°$ thalassaemia (thalassaemia intermedia)
Combinations of thalassaemia and structural haemoglobin variants	■ Sickle-cell thalassaemia ■ Haemoglobin E thalassaemia ■ Haemoglobin Lepore/β thalassaemia
Other genetic diseases	■ Phenylketonuria ■ Duchenne muscular dystrophy ■ Cystic fibrosis ■ Polycystic kidney disease ■ Retinoblastoma ■ Osteogenesis imperfecta ■ Haemophilia A and B ■ Al Antitrypsin deficiency ■ Lesch–Nyhan syndrome ■ Neurofibromatosis ■ Huntington's disease
Major chromosomal defects	■ Down's syndrome

HEAT DISORDERS

Heat-induced and heat-related disorders have been recorded since biblical time and are of particular importance in tropical countries.

PHYSIOLOGY

Human beings, like all mammals, produce heat as a result of metabolic activity. The metabolic heat is then lost to the environment in a controlled manner by peripheral vasodilation and sweating to maintain the body temperature at about 36.8°C.

Physical activity increases the demand for blood supply to several areas, particularly to the skin for heat transfer and to the muscles to allow for the increased metabolic activity. In hot climates, the circulatory demands are greatly increased with work, especially manual work, or with physical exercise.

HEAT EXCHANGE

The thermal environment which affects the human body can be exogenous and endogenous. The exogenous factors are:

- air temperature and speed;
- relative humidity;
- mean radiant temperature;
- duration of exposure;
- clothing.

The endogenous thermal load comprises:

- basal metabolism;
- physical activity (in a given environment, the heat generated depends on the energy expenditure).

If the skin temperature is lower than air temperature the body gains heat by convection. Mean radiant temperature, by far the major heat load, particularly in the tropics and subtropics, is the heat gained through radiation. It is estimated that the shortwave radiation from the sun may reach approximately $800 \, \text{W/m}^2$ at noon, 13 times greater than the average resting metabolic rate of $60 \, \text{W/m}^2$. The direct incidental radiation is supplemented by reflected radiation of as much as $400 \, \text{W/m}^2$. Moreover, long-wave radiation may increase the total radiant load to $2200 \, \text{W/m}^2$.

HEAT STRESS

Heat load generated from endogenous or exogenous sources must be dissipated if heat stress is to be avoided. Both climatic and non-climatic factors influence the outcome. The climatic factors are the exogenous factors (see above). The non-climatic factors affecting the outcome of heat stress are:

- *Clothing.* This may either reduce or increase heat exchange and in hot climates it acts as a barrier to solar radiation.
- *Ageing.* Men over age of 45 years are more vulnerable to thermoregulatory strain besides the fact that increasing age is associated with an increased disease factor.
- *Physique.* Obese persons are at a disadvantage in the heat over persons with slight build. This might be attributed to a greater ratio of body-weight to surface area in obese persons.
- *Sex.* Sweat glands in adult females have a lower threshold of response to thermal stimuli. Differences in distribution of subcutaneous fat can make dissipation of heat rather more difficult for the female.
- *Fever.* A febrile illness increases the vulnerability to heat stress.

The response to heat stress is modified by adaptations in cardiovascular, endocrine, exocrine and other systems that occur with prolonged exposure. This acclimatization requires 1–2 weeks to develop. The processes involved in thermoregulation and the outcome of heat stress are summarized in Figure 8.4.

HEAT DISORDERS

The WHO classification for heat illnesses or disorders is shown in Table 8.9. These heat disorders can be grouped into minor and major disorders. The minor comprise heat oedema, heat fatigue and heat exhaustion unspecified. The major, other than heat syncope, are often grouped in three clinical syndromes resulting from exposure to heat: namely,

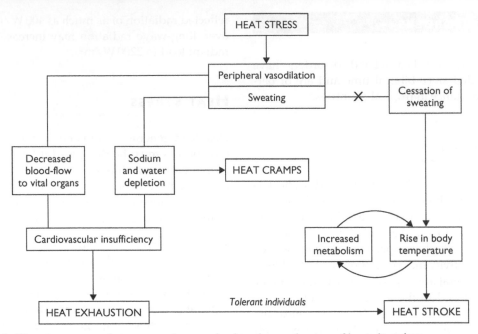

Figure 8.4: The responses to heat stress that may lead to the production of heat disorders.

Table 8.9: Heat disorders as classified by the World Health Organization. Source: WHO (1971)

- Heat stroke and sunstroke-heat apoplexy; heat pyrexia; ictus solaris; siriasis; thermoplegia
- Heat syncope-heat collapse
- Heat cramps
- Heat exhaustion, anhydrotic
- Heat prostration due to water depletion
- Heat exhaustion due to salt depletion
- Heat prostration due to salt (and water) depletion
- Heat exhaustion, unspecified
- Heat prostration NOS
- Heat fatigue, transient
- Heat oedema

Other heat effects
- Unspecified

heat cramps, heat exhaustion and heat stroke. This grouping facilitates diagnosis and treatment by identifying fairly distinctive signs and symptoms (Table 8.10).

Unfortunately the health professionals do not fully appreciate the extent and the size of the problem. Awareness must therefore be maintained for the debilitating effect in susceptible persons. The following section presents a core material with

which all physicians who are likely to encounter heat disorders should be acquainted.

Heat fatigue

This is a new term to designate the deterioration in skilled performance occasionally observed in an otherwise normal subject during short exposures to extreme heat. Recovery is prompt upon his or her return to a cool environment.

Heat syncope

This is a condition of sensation of giddiness and/or acute physical fatigue during exposure to heat, resulting from disturbance of the vasomotor tone, peripheral venous pooling and hypotension, occurring in the absence of observable water or salt depletion. Syncope can arise in a variety of hot conditions, and not necessarily in the presence of extreme heat. It is precipitated by long hours of standing, postural changes or physical activity in hot weather. Lack of acclimatization, poor physique and concomitant illness are also predisposing factors. Heat syncope has been described all over the world; among labourers in Saudi Arabia, road-builders in the Middle East, Egyptian agricultural

Table 8.10: Features of the major heat disorders

Disorder	Susceptible groups (water/salt intake)	Characteristic clinical features	Treatment and prevention
Heat cramps	Acclimatized, active (↑water/↓salt)	*Sweating*: profuse *Muscle cramps*: at the end of the working day	Increase sodium intake
Heat exhaustion Water-depletion	Those unable to indicate thirst, e.g. elderly, infirm, unconscious, infants (↓water) Active workers: in hot industries or in outdoor employment in a hot environment (↓water)	*Sweating*: present *Thirst*: present *Urine*: ↓ output, ↑ osmolarity *Serum Na*: ↑ *Temperature*: up to 38.9°C	Water replacement (oral or i.v.) Encourage drinking and rest periods
Salt-depletion	Large losses of thermal sweat, especially in those unacclimatized (adequate water, ↓salt)	*Sweating*: profuse *Muscle cramps*: may be present *Thirst*: classically absent *Urine*: normal output, ↓ Na *Serum Na*: ↓ *Temperature*: normal or ↓ *Vascular*: hypotension, tachycardia	i.v. normal saline or isotonic glucose Encourage adequate water and salt intake
Heat stroke	Classic: elderly Exertion-induced: active, young	*Sweating*: often absent *CNS disturbance* *Temperture*: >40°C	Anticipation Prompt recognition Rapid cooling

labourers, cane-cutters in East Africa, Indian and African miners and European servicemen.

SYMPTOMS AND SIGNS

The characteristic features include weakness, light headedness, restlessness, nausea, a sinking feeling and blurring of vision. Systolic blood pressure (BP) falls rapidly and markedly. Diastolic BP also falls but less rapidly. The pulse feels weak and slows in rate. Skin is moist and cold. Usually there is no clear rise in body temperature.

DIAGNOSIS

The condition is readily recognized from the circumstances of onset and the rapid recovery of consciousness. It is important to exclude other causes of collapse such as epilepsy or cardiac syncope (Stokes–Adams attack), anaemia and malaria in endemic countries. Fainting can be present as a sign in other heat exhaustion illnesses, but the presence of salt in urine will help to exclude salt

deficiency and a copious urine output will exclude water depletion.

TREATMENT AND PREVENTION

Heat syncope is a self-limiting condition. The patient should be allowed to rest in cool surroundings in the head low position. Simple beverages such as tea and soft drinks are indicated.

People not acclimitized to a hot environment should grade their physical activity gradually. For those acclimatized, strenuous activity should be modified if there is a sudden rise in environmental temperature or humidity. Pilgrims in a hot environment should minimize their physical activity, especially the old and diseased.

Heat cramps

The precise mechanism responsible for heat cramps has not been elucidated. Three factors are always present: hard physical work, environmental heat and sweating. The current view is that heat cramps are caused by water intoxication or by salt depletion, since large intakes of unsalted water precede the onset of cramps. There are three factors characteristic of individuals predisposed to heat cramps:

- they are acclimatized and hence produce sweat in large quantities in response to physical work;
- they consume adequate amounts of water to replace the sweat losses;
- they fail to replace sodium losses.

CLINICAL FEATURES AND DIAGNOSIS

Heat cramps tend to occur towards the end of the working day, while walking home or, having arrived, on relaxing or on taking a cool shower. Paroxysms of painful cramping tend to last no more than a few minutes and usually disappear spontaneously.

A word of warning – if any systemic symptoms coexist with muscular cramps, the disorder automatically falls into the category described as heat exhaustion (see below). Table 8.10 gives a comparison of the salient features of heat cramps, heat exhaustion and heat stroke.

TREATMENT AND PREVENTION

Most individuals who sustain heat cramps soon discover that ingestion of salt is successful in their prevention. In the event of severe, repeated, unrelenting cramps, oral or intravenous salt solutions rapidly relieve all symptoms.

Heat exhaustion

Heat exhaustion is the most common clinical disorder resulting from work or physical activity in a hot environment. It is used to describe a number of syndromes leading to collapse. The common feature of these syndromes is cardiovascular insufficiency – brought about predominantly by dehydration and insufficient drinking of water, or by salt depletion or a mixture of both when great losses of sweat have occurred. Heat exhaustion casualties are prevalent among civilian populations when exposed to heat waves. The condition is divided into two major forms: water-depletion and salt-depletion heat exhaustion.

WATER-DEPLETION HEAT EXHAUSTION

The condition is usually encountered amongst: (i) workers in hot industries, and workers in open air employment in hot climates (e.g. road building, construction work); (ii) amongst army recruits and soldiers during training in high environmental temperature; (iii) in long-distance athletes running in the heat; and (iv) in infants during exceptionally hot weather or when left in locked cars in a hot climate.

Voluntary under-drinking in heat leads to a mild degree of water deficiency which is known as voluntary dehydration. Even when drinking water is available, some individuals working or walking in hot environments never replace their sweat loss and are usually in mild negative water-balance. Moreover, the sensation of thirst is not strong enough to demand correction of the water losses. Voluntary dehydration increases with ambient temperature, work rate, temperature of the drinking water, the interval between meals and the palatability or flavour of the water available.

Clinical features and diagnosis

The earliest symptom of water-depletion heat exhaustion is thirst. The tongue and mouth become dry due to decreased salivation and appetite for solid food is lost. Coincidental with progressive water depletion is a fairly rapid fall in urine volume to approximately 500 ml/24 hours with a specific gravity in excess of 1.030. If this drop in output is insufficient to maintain fluid balance, there is a decrease in volume and increase in the osmolarity of the extracellular fluid.

Treatment and prevention

Treatment consists essentially of rest in a cool room. If the patient is conscious and able to take fluid by mouth, oral replacement of fluid is advocated. If the patient is unconscious intravenous fluid should be administered. An isotonic solution should be used if there is any serious doubt as to whether the unconscious patient is water- or salt-depleted. It is also important to avoid enthusiasm and not to overload the patient with fluids.

Prevention can be easily achieved by availability of an adequate supply of cool palatable drinking water. The most practical method is to encourage individuals to take sufficient water so as to ensure a minimum daily urine volume of approximately

1 litre. Programmed drinking in the absence of thirst and recurrent rest periods are key factors in prevention.

SALT-DEPLETION HEAT EXHAUSTION

This is a condition resulting from loss of large volumes of thermal sweat which are replaced by adequate water but no salt. It has been reported among workers in ship boiler rooms, amongst crews of oil tankers and workers in mines.

Clinical features

The condition is characterized by fatigue, severe frontal headache, giddiness, anorexia, nausea, vomiting, diarrhoea and skeletal muscle cramps and in the later stages by circulatory failure.

Diagnosis

The insidious onset, if taken together with the complaint of weakness and fatigue and the possible presence of muscle cramps, make the diagnosis less difficult. The laboratory investigations are very important to confirm diagnosis. The urine volume is within normal values but the amounts of sodium chloride are negligible. The plasma sodium and chloride are reduced. Also in contrast to water deficiency heat exhaustion, the body temperature usually remains normal or subnormal. Constipation is more common than diarrhoea. Headache, giddiness, syncope and peripheral vascular collapse are common. The resting pulse is of small volume with a rate of 80–90 beats per minute; the systolic blood pressure 100–110 mmHg is usually well maintained.

Treatment and prevention

Treatment of properly diagnosed cases of salt-deficiency heat exhaustion is fairly simple. It consists of administration of either normal saline or isotonic glucose solutions in accordance with the proportion of salt or water losses. Prevention can be achieved by adequate intake of salt when in hot surroundings.

MIXED HEAT EXHAUSTION

Patients usually present with a mixed clinical picture of both types of heat exhaustion. In a study of patients the common presenting symptoms were:

- high body temperature, mean 38.1 ± 0.5°C (43%);

- weakness (20%);
- giddiness and fatigue (15%);
- headache (6%);
- nausea and vomiting (6%);
- dry mouth and tongue (4.3%).

The early detection of heat exhaustion is of paramount importance in conditions of high ambient temperature. Heat exhaustion may be part of a series of events leading to heat stroke and it may indeed be regarded as incipient heat stroke. If so, then the more tolerant individuals become the victims of heat stroke while the less tolerant succumb to heat exhaustion.

Heat stroke

Heat stroke is a complex clinical condition in which an elevated body temperature, resulting from an overloading or failure of the normal thermoregulatory mechanism after exposure to hot environments, causes tissue damage.

CLINICAL FEATURES

It is usually diagnosed by the triad of:

- hyperthermia – core temperature of more than 40°C;
- central nervous system (CNS) disturbances;
- dry, hot skin.

The absence of one of these characteristics by no means excludes a diagnosis of heat stroke. For example, unless temperature is measured by thermometers that can be placed deep in the core and can read up to 45°C, unreliably low values may be recorded. Also, in cases of exertion-induced heat stroke, some patients might be sweating, especially in the early stages.

Heat stroke generally occurs in three forms:

- classical heat stroke (in the elderly);
- exertion-induced heat stroke (in young, healthy individuals);
- mixed heat stroke (seen during the Mecca pilgrimage).

Classical heat stroke is usually more common and occurs during heat waves. Advanced age and chronic illnesses are major risk factors especially when accompanied by dehydration and physical or emotional stress.

Exertion-induced heat stroke is a disorder of the young, healthy, probably inexperienced athlete or the military recruit during rigorous training in a hot environment or individuals performing heavy manual work, for example miners, construction workers. A history of intense physical activity is always present.

Heat stroke is a medical emergency: in all types of heat stroke, prompt, physiological and vigorous management is essential, otherwise the mortality can be very high, up to 70%.

DIAGNOSIS

The typical case of heat stroke is diagnosed easily, but heat stroke may be overlooked when there is no obvious history of excessive heat load. The following rule is practical: if a patient loses consciousness under conditions of heat stress, heat stroke should be suspected, and rectal temperature should be properly measured. If hyperthermia is present, it should be immediately treated and investigated for multiple system involvement and clotting disturbances. Proper rectal temperature measurement in the delirious hyperactive heat-stroke victim requires the application of an inlying thermistor with a scale reaching beyond the upper limit of 41°C of the standard clinical thermometer.

Differential diagnosis

Heat stroke, being essentially a systemic disease with a complex clinical picture, has a wide differential diagnosis. Conditions to be considered in differential diagnosis are heat collapse, encephalitis, meningococcal meningitis, tetanus, cerebral (particularly pontine) haemorrhage, infectious hepatitis, hysterical behaviour, cerebral malaria, epilepsy, and malignant hyperthermia. It is very important to examine the skull and surrounding soft tissues for signs of injury.

TREATMENT

The duration of hyperthermia is a crucial prognostic factor. The following steps should be closely adhered to:

First aid

At point of collapse, effective first aid is crucial. Remove the comatose patient to a shaded place,

strip off, place in semilateral position, spray with *tepid* (not cold) water and fan, either by electrical fan, if available, or by hand fan.

Transport urgently to hospital

Keep airway patent and keep patient in semilateral position so as not to inhale vomitus and suffocate. If facilities are available during transport, administer oxygen and intravenous fluid. Keep spraying and fanning.

Specific treatment

The corner stone for treatment of heat stroke is its early recognition, followed by rapid physiologically effective cooling and aggressive therapy similar to that for any other comatose or intensive care patient. The best cooling method is evaporative cooling from warm skin. The patient is sprayed with atomized spray which is evaporated by a flow of warm air. This is best achieved using the Mecca Body Cooling Unit, which is designed to enable cooling as well as the full treatment and handling of the heat stroke patient.

While cooling, monitor the vital signs and control convulsions by giving diazepam 10 mg intravenously. Correct hypovolaemia by i.v. fluids starting with normal saline as the fluid of choice. The precise amount and type of fluid depends on the response of each patient and the results of laboratory investigation. Acidosis is common and should be corrected according to the acid–base status.

PREVENTION

Preventive measures should be understood and applied by everyone, the physician, the nurse, the coach, the trainer, the athlete, the military recruit, the miner, the worker in a hot environment and the parents of children exercising in a hot climate.

FURTHER READING

CHRONIC DISEASES

Frenk J., Bobadilla J.-I., Sepulveda J. & Lopez-Cervantes M. (1989) Health transition in middle-income countries: new challenges for health case. *Health Policy and Planning* 4: 29–39.

King M.H. *et al.* (1991) Diabetes in adults is now a Third World problem. *Bulletin of WHO* 69(6): 643–648.

King M.H. & Brewers M. (1993) Global estimates for prevalence of diabetes mellitus and impaired glucose tolerance in adults. *Diabetes Care* 16: 157–177.

WHO (1997) *Tobacco or health: a global status report.* WHO, Geneva.

Occupation: disease and health

de Clanville H., Schilling R.S.F. and Wood C.H. (1979) *Occupational Health – A Manual for Health Workers in Developing Countries.* African Medical and Research Foundation, Nairobi.

Harrington M. & Gill F.S. (1983) *Occupational Health.* Blackwell Scientific Publications, Oxford.

Khogali M. (1982) A new approach for providing occupational health services in developing countries. *Scandinavian Journal of Work and Environmental Health* 8: 152–156.

London School of Hygiene and Tropical Medicine (1970) *Proceedings of the symposium on the Health Problem of Industrial Progress in Developing Countries.*

Raffle P.A.B. *et al.* (Eds) (1987) *Hunters Diseases of Occupations.* Hodder and Stoughton, London.

Symposium on Occupational Medicine (1978) *Annals of the Academy of Medicine of Singapore* 7(3).

WHO (1985) *Identification and Control of Work-related Diseases.* Technical Report Series No. 714. WHO, Geneva.

WHO (1985) *Safe Use of Pesticides.* Technical Report Series No. 720. WHO, Geneva.

WHO (1981) *Education and Training in Occupational Health, Safety and Ergonomics.* Technical Report Series No. 663. WHO, Geneva.

WHO (1988) *Health Promotion for Working Populations.* Technical Report Series No. 765. WHO, Geneva.

WHO (1988) *Training and Education in Occupational Health.* Technical Report Series No. 762. WHO, Geneva.

Mental health

WHO (1984) *Mental Health Care in Developing Countries.* Technical Report Series No. 698. WHO, Geneva.

WHO (1992) *The ICD-10 Classification of Mental and Behavioural Disorders: Clinical Descriptions and Diagnostic Guidelines.* WHO, Geneva.

The World Health Report (2001) *Mental Health: New Understanding; New Hope.* WHO, Geneva, Switzerland.

Genetics and health

Michel F. (1981) *Modern Genetic Concepts and Techniques in the Study of Parasites.* Schwabe, Basel.

WHO (1996) *Control of Hereditary Diseases.* Technical Report Series No. 865. WHO, Geneva.

Heat disorders

Hales J.R.S. (1983) *Thermal Physiology.* Raven Press, New York.

Khogali M. (1980) Heat Stroke. Report on 18 cases. *Lancet i:* 276–278.

Khogali M. & Hales J.R.S. (1983) *Heat Stroke and Temperature Regulation.* Academic Press, Sydney.

Unwin N., Setel F., Rashid S. *et al.* (2001) Non-communicable diseases in sub-Saharan Africa: where do they feature in the health research agenda. *Bulletin WHO* 79(10): 947–953.

Weiner J.S. & Khogali M. (1980) A physiological body cooling unit for treatment of heat stroke. *Lancet i:* 507–509.

CHAPTER NINE

NUTRITIONAL DISORDERS

A. Burgess

- Summary
- Introduction
- Multinutrient undernutrition
- Specific micronutrient deficiencies

- Obesity and related conditions
- Causes of undernutrition
- Control of nutrition disorders
- References and further reading/learning

SUMMARY

Malnutrition is an important public health problem that is caused by a deficient or excess intake of nutrients in relation to requirements. Undernutrition (nutrient deficiency) is the prevalent type of malnutrition in tropical developing countries. At most risk are the poor and disadvantaged, particularly women of reproductive age and young children. Undernutrition reduces immunity, physical activity and work productivity, and, in children, retards growth and psychological development. Undernourished women bear undernourished babies who often become stunted adults – thus perpetuating the undernutrition cycle.

Obesity (nutrient excess) and its comorbidities are less widespread in developing countries but rates are increasing.

Poor diets and disease (particularly HIV/AIDS) are the immediate causes of undernutrition. Underlying causes are food insecurity, inadequate care of women and children, unhealthy living conditions and poor health services. In turn, these result from lack of resources, the low status of women, environmental degradation and, sometimes, abnormal weather or conflict and violence.

The multicausal nature of malnutrition means many sectors (e.g. economics, agriculture, women's development, health) are involved in its control. Health-related strategies include: (i) distributing supplementary foods and nutrients; (ii) promoting breast-feeding and complementary feeding; (iii) controlling disease; (iv) checking food hygiene and safety; (v) monitoring nutrition and child growth; (vi) providing maternal health services and nutrition education; and (vii) facilitating community-based programmes.

INTRODUCTION

Nutrition disorders are a serious problem everywhere especially in tropical developing countries. They may be classified as:

1 Undernutrition, which occurs when there is an inadequate intake of one or more nutrients and/or when a disease, such as persistent diarrhoea or AIDS, disrupts intake and metabolism. Undernutrition is further subdivided into:
   - Multinutrient undernutrition in which the main signs are growth failure (in the foetus and child) and weight loss.
   - Specific micronutrient deficiencies, which cause specific clinical and biochemical conditions. For example, iron deficiency is an important cause of anaemia and affects cognitive development, vitamin A deficiency causes xerophthalmia as well as impaired immunity, and iodine deficiency causes mental retardation and goitre. Growth is not necessarily affected.

Both types of undernutrition often occur together.

Those at most risk of undernutrition are:

- Children aged 6–36 months and women of reproductive age from poor homes. Risk increases if households are headed by children or single, sick or old women.
- Children and adults who are abused, disabled, chronically sick (especially with HIV/AIDS), or who live alone, on the streets or in difficult circumstances (e.g. people living in areas of armed conflict, refugees and displacees, prisoners).

2   Obesity and related diseases such as cardiovascular disease, hypertension and diabetes.

Undernutrition is the most prevalent type of malnutrition in the developing world (Administrative Committee on Coordination, Sub-committee on Nutrition, 2000b) where:

- More than ⅙ of the population (~800 million) has insufficient food and are in energy deficit. Almost ⅔ of these people live in Asia and about ¼ in sub-Saharan Africa. Although the situation is improving overall, the rate of improvement is slow and uneven.
- Many adults are 'too thin'. In South Asia, the worst area, ⅓–½ of all adults are underweight.
- About 1 out of every 10 full-term babies has a low birth weight.
- More than ⅓ of young children are stunted. Rates of undernutrition among young children are declining in all regions except sub-Saharan Africa. However, it is estimated that ¼ of young children will still be undernourished in 2020, with the majority living in South Asia and Africa.
- It contributes to around ½ of all young child deaths.

Specific micronutrient deficiencies are significant causes of disease, disability and death. For example, iron deficiency and its anaemia:

- affects about ⅔ of people in developing countries, with women of reproductive age at most risk;
- contributes to nearly ¼ of all postpartum deaths in Africa and Asia;
- is common among many poor old people.

Over 200 million young children (or almost ½ of those in developing countries) have subclinical vitamin A deficiency and hence impaired immunity. Three million have xerophthalmia although the prevalence is decreasing (e.g. between 1985 and 1995 it decreased by 40%) and vitamin A deficiency is likely to be eliminated as a public health problem by 2020.

Iodine deficiency is widespread and is the leading cause of brain damage in the foetus and infant. In developing countries about 600 million people have goitre and around 40 million are brain damaged – of whom up to 11 million have cretinism. However, the increasing availability of iodized salt is significantly reducing iodine-deficiency disorders in many places.

Zinc deficiency is thought to be widespread among infants, children and pregnant and lactating women but currently there is no way to measure zinc status of communities. Deficiencies of folate and other B vitamins are important among some groups.

Obesity and related diseases (particularly diabetes) are less prevalent than undernutrition in developing countries (and so are covered only superficially here) but are increasing rapidly among some groups. However, there are few reliable data and rates vary widely. For example, 1% of adults in Ghana but 10% in Mauritius are obese. Prevalence is lower in children but is also increasing. In Bangkok the percentage of school-age children with obesity increased from 12 to 16% over just 2 years. The changes in diet (e.g. more fat, less carbohydrate) and reduced physical activity that are responsible for this type of malnutrition are one result of changes in lifestyle and of increased urbanization and income.

By 2020 the world's population may number 7.5 billion and agriculturists predict that food insecurity and hunger will remain a problem in many places. Around 1.2 billion people will be aged over 60 years, of whom ⅔ will live in developing countries, notably Asia. Almost half the population of these countries will live in urban areas. The increased proportion of the elderly and urbanized will require new strategies to deal with new patterns of malnutrition.

MULTINUTRIENT UNDERNUTRITION

Multinutrient undernutrition occurs when the body has insufficient energy and nutrients to grow or function normally. Previously, this condition in children was called 'protein energy malnutrition' but protein is not necessarily deficient while some micronutrients, such as zinc, often are. Multinutrient undernutrition is often accompanied by specific micronutrient deficiencies.

Young children

Multinutrient undernutrition is found when:

- a foetus is deprived of nutrients due to maternal undernutrition, or other maternal conditions such as malaria or smoking;
- a young child's diet is inadequate in quantity or quality and/or infection reduces nutrient intake and absorption, or increases needs (see Causes of undernutrition).

Significance

Between conception and around the age of 3 years there is rapid growth of the body including the brain, and rapid cognitive development. Multinutrient undernutrition often occurs within this crucial period.

Foetal undernutrition causes intrauterine growth retardation (IUGR) and a low birth weight for gestational age. It increases the risk of morbidity and of poorer cognitive and neurological development. IUGR seems to be associated with increased risk of diabetes and cardiovascular and other degenerative diseases in adult life.

Undernutrition in young children impairs immunity and increases morbidity and mortality from infectious disease. Psychological development is slower – partly because undernourished children are apathetic and so explore less and elicit less stimulation from carers. Chronic undernutrition results in stunting (low height for age) and acute undernutrition results in wasting (low weight

for height). Underweight (low weight for age) may be due to stunting and/or wasting (Table 9.1).

Recognition

The indicator of foetal undernutrition is a birth weight of <10th centile for gestational age or, more practically for full term babies, of <2500 g.

In children, poor growth is the best indicator of undernutrition and can be detected by:

- Monitoring weight gain using a growth chart (see Control of nutritional disorder).
- Comparing a child's weight or height to the median weight or height of a healthy reference population (reference values are given by WHO 1983 but new values are being prepared). This comparison is expressed as a percentage of median or a Z score. Z score is the number of standard deviations from the median.
- Measuring mid upper arm circumference (MUAC) which changes little between ages 12 and 60 months. Undernutrition is mild if MUAC is <13.5 cm, moderate if <12.5 cm and severe if <11 cm.
- Asking carers whether the child looks thinner or smaller than other children of the same age.

Severe undernutrition presents as marasmus in which the cardinal sign is severe muscle and fat wasting, or kwashiorkor in which there is bilateral pedal oedema accompanied by muscle wasting and often 'flaky paint' skin lesions and sparse pale hair.

Control

Adequate nutrient intake and control of infections prevent multinutrient undernutrition in young children. General feeding recommendations are:

- give girls and women a good diet before and during their reproductive years (see below);

Table 9.1: Indicators of type and severity of undernutrition. Source: WHO (1999)

Type of undernutrition	Indicator	Moderate and severe	Severe
Underweight	Weight for age	<(−2) Z scores or <80% of median	<(−3) Z scores or <70% of median
Stunting	Height for age	<(−2) Z scores or <90% of median	<(−3) Z scores or <85% of median
Wasting	Weight for height	<(−2) Z scores or <80% of median	<(−3) Z scores or <70% of median

- breast-feed children, exclusively until around 6 months of age and complement with other foods for at least 2 years;
- give children over 6 months energy/nutrient rich complementary foods 3–5 times/day;
- actively encourage young children to eat;
- give prescribed micronutrient supplements (see Specific micronutrient deficiencies).

'Control of nutritional disorders' explains how to promote breast-feeding and complementary feeding and describes other activities that address the underlying causes of undernutrition. Management of severe undernutrition requires inpatient treatment.

SCHOOL-AGE CHILDREN AND ADULTS

Severe multinutrient undernutrition is uncommon in older children and adults because nutrient needs per kilo body weight are lower, infections are less frequent and there is less dependency on carers for food. It is usually only seen in emergency situations or the very poor. However, stunting due to undernutrition in early life is common and mild/moderate undernutrition is often found among women of reproductive age and sometimes school-age children and old people. Pregnant adolescent girls are a high-risk group.

Immediate causes (see Causes of undernutrition) include a poor diet, adolescent or closely spaced pregnancies, and AIDS or other chronic or severe disease.

Significance

Undernutrition impairs immunity, reduces physical and mental activity and causes wasting. Among school-age children it retards school achievement and physical growth – resulting in stunting. Stunted people can do less physical work and stunted women have increased risk of obstructed labour. Undernutrition in fertile women increases the risk of problems associated with childbearing, including foetal undernutrition.

Recognition

The best sign is wasting, which, up to puberty, is detected by low weight for height. There is no

---

> **Box 9.1: Body mass index (BMI)**
>
> BMI = weight in kilograms/height in metres^2
> An adult is:
>
> - severely underweight if BMI <16;
> - underweight if BMI <18.5;
> - overweight if BMI is >25;
> - obese if BMI is >30.
>
> Ratios based on arm span instead of height are being developed for old people with kyphosis.

agreed indicator for adolescents. Body mass index (BMI) is used for adults (Box 9.1).

Other less reliable indicators are:

- In women – a weight of <45 kg or having a baby with IUGR.
- In adults – MUAC. Although there are no agreed cut off levels (due to ethnic differences in fat deposition), 21–22 cm is often used.

Control

Multinutrient undernutrition in older children and adults is prevented by:

- improving diets (see Box 9.2 and Control of nutritional disorders);
- avoiding closely spaced or adolescent pregnancies;
- reducing women's workloads, especially during pregnancy;
- controlling infection, especially HIV/AIDS;
- caring for the old and sick.

SPECIFIC MICRONUTRIENT DEFICIENCIES

More than one micronutrient deficiency may occur in the same person and multimicronutrient supplements are under investigation.

IRON DEFICIENCY AND ANAEMIA

Inadequate dietary iron results in decreased body iron stores, haemoglobin synthesis and finally

Box 9.2: Feeding guidelines for adults

- Eat 2–3 meals a day.
- Eat plenty of, and a variety of the following foods: staple foods (cereals, starchy roots and fruits), legumes, oilseeds, fruits and vegetables (particularly deep coloured ones), and flavouring foods (e.g. garlic, onions, herbs).
- Eat fish as often as possible.
- Eat iron-providing foods, such as meat and offal, when possible (see 'Specific micronutrient deficiencies').
- Obtain fat from plant oils or unrefined foods such as nuts, beans, fish; limit intake of fat from meat, milk products and fast/processed foods.
- Limit intake of alcohol and foods high in fat, sugar or salt.
- Limit intake of foods that are heavily preserved (e.g. pickled, salted).
- Use iodized salt and other fortified foods.
- Take micronutrient supplements if and as prescribed.

Food needs increase with pregnancy, lactation and activity.

Box 9.3: Iron availability in foods

Iron is present in foods as:

- Haem-iron, which is well absorbed. Sources are all types of flesh and offal (the redder the flesh/offal the more iron it contains) and blood.
- Non-haem iron that is found in plant foods, eggs and milk. Good sources are legumes and some green leaves (and unrefined cereals if eaten in large amounts). Non-haem iron is poorly absorbed but other foods and chemicals in the meal enhance or inhibit absorption:
  - Enhancers include meat, fish, poultry and foods rich in vitamin C. Milling and fermenting also improves absorption.
  - Inhibitors include phytates (in legumes and unrefined cereals) and tannins (in tea).

Iron needs and body stores also influence absorption. Iron in breast-milk is well absorbed.

haemoglobin concentration. Causes of iron deficiency are:

- Insufficient bioavailable iron in the diet to cover needs (which are highest for menstruating females and during pregnancy, infancy and puberty – see Table 9.8). Poor bioavailability is often due to an excess of absorption-inhibitors and a lack of absorption-enhancers in meals (Box 9.3).
- Blood loss – for example, due to heavy menstruation, childbirth or parasites such as hookworm.

Other factors that contribute to or cause anaemia include other micronutrient deficiencies such as folate, infections such as malaria and haemoglobinopathies.

Significance

Iron deficiency anaemia (IDA) leads to decreased attention spans, learning ability and work productivity. If severe, it increases mortality. In women it increases the risk of foetal undernutrition and

Table 9.2: Haemoglobin and haematocrit cut-off levels for anaemia. Source: Stoltzfus & Dreyfuss (1998)

Sex/Age	Haemoglobin below	Haematocrit below
	g/dl	%
6 month–5 years	11.0	33
5–11 years	11.5	34
12–13 years	12.0	36
Females >13 years		
Not pregnant	12.0	36
Pregnant	11.0	33
Males >13 years	13.0	39

postpartum maternal mortality (through haemorrhage and sepsis). In children aged 0–2 years IDA is associated with impaired cognitive development.

Recognition

Anaemia is best diagnosed by measuring haemoglobin or haematocrit. Table 9.2 shows the cut-off levels used to define anaemia at sea level (levels increase with altitude).

Pallor of the inferior conjunctiva, nail bed or palm indicates severe anaemia.

Control

Improving the iron status of populations or individuals is difficult. Strategies used are:

1   Modifying diets by:
    - increasing intake of haem iron-rich foods although this may be impractical where foods such as meat are expensive;
    - increasing intake of absorption enhancers (e.g. vitamin C-rich fruits and vegetables) and decreasing intake of absorption inhibitors (e.g. not drinking tea with meals);
    - fortifying foods. Wheat flour and condiments such as curry powder and fish sauce are fortified in some countries and fortification of salt and sugar are being investigated;
    - promoting exclusive breastfeeding which increases the period of maternal amenorrhea.
2   Plant breeding to increase iron and lower phytate content.
3   Giving supplements of iron, often with folic acid, to priority groups (i.e. women of reproductive age particularly pregnant and postpartum women, and young children especially low birth weight infants). Where IDA is common all women of reproductive age, children,

adolescents (especially girls) and vulnerable old people need supplements (Table 9.3) even where malaria is endemic. Recent research suggests that the benefits of oral iron usually outweigh the risk of increased malaria morbidity in most individuals. Other studies have shown that IDA responds more completely to iron therapy if vitamin A is also given.

Although supplementation programmes through antenatal clinics have existed for many years they are often not successful due to:

- poor compliance caused by women's non-perception of being anaemic, and inadequate counselling on the dangers of anaemia, the need for long-term medication and the side effects of iron supplements (e.g. constipation);
- low usage of antenatal clinics and unreliable supplies of supplements.

Weekly dosing may be a practical option for some groups.

New distribution and communication channels such as pharmacies, traditional birth attendants, schools and mass media are beginning to be used. For example, in parts of Indonesia women before

Table 9.3: Guidelines for iron and folic acid supplements. Source: Stoltzfus & Dreyfuss (1998)

Sex/Age	Prevalence of IDA in area	Dose/day		Duration	Comment
		Iron (mg)	Folic acid (μg)		
6–24 months	Low	12.5	50	From age 6–12 months	From age 2–24 month if low birth weight
	High	12.5	50	From age 6–24 months	
2–5 years	High	20–30	–	–	Weekly dosing is an option
6–11 years	High	30–60	–	–	Weekly dosing is an option
Adolescent boys and men	High	60	–	–	Weekly dosing is an option
Adolescent girls and women – not pregnant	High	60	400	–	Weekly dosing is an option
Pregnant girls and women	Low	60	400	6 months in pregnancy	If 6 months duration not possible double iron dose or continue postpartum
	High	60	400	6 months in pregnancy + 3 months postpartum	

– No guidelines.

marriage are required to learn about anaemia and are encouraged to buy iron tablets.

Other ways to prevent iron deficiency and iron deficiency anaemia are:

- delaying the first pregnancy until after adolescence, increasing birth spacing and reducing the number of pregnancies;
- controlling bleeding (e.g. during childbirth) and hookworm infection;
- in infants, delayed clamping of the umbilical cord.

Additional interventions are needed if there are other causes of anaemia such as malaria – see Chapters 5 and 7.

VITAMIN A DEFICIENCY DISORDERS

Vitamin A deficiency (VAD) occurs when there is insufficient vitamin A in body stores or the diet to cover needs. Factors affecting this balance are the quantity and bioavailability of vitamin A in the diet (Box 9.4) and the level of requirement. Requirements are relatively high for young children and pregnant and lactating women, and increase during infections such as measles.

VAD is found most frequently in areas where vitamin A-rich foods, particularly retinol-rich foods, are unavailable (e.g. arid areas) or where families are unable to afford them. Children may not receive these foods due to lack of information or food habits. The group at most risk is young children although there is increasing evidence of mild VAD among women of reproductive age and school age children.

VAD is classified as:

- subclinical when serum retinol levels are $<0.7\,\mu mol/l$ and immunity and other physiological processes are impaired;
- clinical when there are ocular signs collectively called xerophthalmia (Table 9.4).

Significance

VAD makes children vulnerable to, and worsens, many infections particularly diarrhoea and measles, and retards growth and development. Clinical VAD is the leading cause of blindness in young children. VAD probably contributes significantly to maternal morbidity and mortality and may play a role in the development of iron deficiency anaemia.

Recognition

At present there is no satisfactory field test to detect subclinical VAD. Serum retinol levels are

Box 9.4: Availability of vitamin A

Most vitamin A in food is in the form of:

- Retinol, which is absorbed efficiently and is the form used in the body. Enough retinol can be stored in the liver to last several months. Good sources are liver, milk fat, egg yolk and fortified foods (e.g. margarine).
- β-carotene whose bioavailability is lower than retinol and influenced by several factors; for example, cooking and fat in the meal increases it while gut helminths decrease it. Best sources are red palm oil and orange fleshy fruits (e.g. mango) and cooked vegetables (e.g. carrot, yellow sweet potato). The bioavailability of carotene in green leaves is generally lower than in orange foods.

Table 9.4: Signs and symptoms of xerophthalmia.
Source: McLaren & Frigg (2001)

Sign/symptom in usual order of appearance	Description
Night blindness	Inability to see in dim light
Conjunctival xerosis	Conjunctiva looks dry and rough
Bitot's spot	Small foamy whitish lesion on conjunctiva – not always present
Corneal xerosis	Cornea looks dry and lacks lustre
Corneal ulcers	May be small or large, often deep
Keratomalacia	Softening of cornea which progresses rapidly and may cause corneal deformation
Corneal scars	Healed sequelae of corneal disease – not vitamin A specific

used but are depressed by infection. The presence of any sign of xerophthalmia indicates clinical VAD. It is considered a public health problem when any of the following situations is present:

1 Among children aged under 6 years:
- 1% have night blindness; or
- 0.5% have Bitot's spots; or
- 0.01% have corneal xerosis and/or ulceration and/or keratomalacia; or
- 0.05% have xerophthalmia-related corneal scars.

A serum retinol of $<0.35\,\mu\mathrm{mol/l}$ among $>5\%$ of children supports the diagnosis.

2 5% of pregnant women are night blind.
3 The under five mortality rate is >70 per 1,000.

Control

Vitamin A deficiency disorders are prevented by:

1 Giving supplements of high-dose vitamin A (Table 9.5). The minimum period between doses is 1 month.

Supplements are given as capsules (cut open and squeezed on the tongue) or an oily solution. They have been distributed at national polio immunization days (e.g. in Mali and Cameroon), with regular immunizations (e.g. in Zambia and Yemen), at clinics, before seasons of special risk and at emergency feeding centres. Tanzania found that prior countrywide training of health workers and managers was essential to ensure good coverage through immunization programmes.

The priority age group is 6–36 months and high-risk children should be specifically targeted. These are children with severe undernutrition, measles, diarrhoea, respiratory disease, chickenpox and other severe infections, and those living with children with xerophthalmia (since VAD often occurs in clusters).

Children with measles (where prevalence of VAD is high) and xerophthalmia need three high doses: on day 1, day 2 and then at least 2 weeks later. Xerophthalmia requires urgent treatment. Only the first four signs in Table 9.4 are reversible and corneal xerosis can progress to ulceration, keratomalacia and impaired vision within hours.

There is some question as to whether the dose for post-delivery women and young infants is sufficient to prevent VAD and recommendations may change. Pregnant women should *not* be given high doses as there is a risk of teratogenicity. Pregnant women living in areas where VAD is common can take 10 000 IU a day or, 60 days after conception, 25 000 IU a week. This does not appear to affect viral loads or transmission rates in HIV+ women.

2 Improving diets by:
- feeding colostrum and breast-milk;
- increasing production and intake of vitamin A-rich foods such as orange-coloured fleshy fruits and vegetables and red palm oil. These foods may have more impact on retinol status than leafy vegetables. For example, in Indonesia orange fruits were twice as effective at raising serum retinol levels among school children than green leaves.

Table 9.5: Schedule for oral high doses of vitamin A to prevent VAD.
Source: McLaren & Frigg (2001) and personal communication

Group	Dose in International Units (IU)
Infants <6 months	
Not breast-fed	50 000 – one dose
Breast-fed but mothers received no supplements	50 000 – one dose
Infants 6–12 months	100 000 every 4–6 months
Children >12 months	200 000 every 4–6 months
Women	
Not lactating	200 000 within 4 weeks of delivery
Lactating but not menstruating	200 000 within 8 weeks of delivery

3 Increasing the vitamin A content of foods by plant breeding, biotechnology or fortification. For example, sweet potatoes with increased vitamin A content have been bred and successfully cultivated by women's groups in Kenya. Sugar is now fortified in Guatemala and some other countries. Emergency food aid rations such as dried milks and some oils, are routinely fortified.

Controlling measles and diarrhoea also helps to prevent VAD.

IODINE DEFICIENCY DISORDERS (IDD)

Iodine is needed to make thyroid hormones; so prolonged iodine deficiency impairs thyroid function resulting in lower metabolic rate, lethargy, growth retardation and brain damage. Goitre occurs when the thyroid gland enlarges in an effort to capture more iodine from the blood.

Diets in most places are low in iodine unless fortified foods or foods from the sea (which is rich in iodine) are commonly eaten. The iodine level of food is related to the level in the soil on which it is produced. So deficiency is often most severe in mountainous areas and flood plains where the soil has been leached. Where iodine deficiency exists, goitrogens (chemicals that reduce iodine uptake by the thyroid gland) make it worse. The toxin in 'bitter' cassava is a goitrogen and others occur in millet, cabbage and kale.

Significance

Iodine deficiency is the single most common cause of mental retardation. It has different effects (see Table 9.6) according to the severity of deficiency and stage of the life cycle:

- in 1st and 2nd trimesters of pregnancy it causes varying degrees of irreversible damage to the developing foetal brain and nervous system; if severe it results in neurological cretinism;
- in neonates it causes stillbirth, low birth weight and, occasionally, hypothyroid cretinism;
- in children and adults it causes goitre and hypothyroidism, which affects school achievement and work output.

Recognition

Iodine status of a community (Table 9.7) is assessed by measuring:

1 Thyroid volume. Goitres are detected by:
   - Inspection and palpation. A goitre is classified as:
   grade 1 – if palpable but not visible with neck in normal position;
   grade 2 – if visible with neck in normal position.

Table 9.6: Description of selected iodine-deficiency disorders

Disorder	Signs and symptoms
Hypothyroidism	Person feels cold easily, moves and thinks slowly, is lethargic, and may be sleepy, constipated or have a dry skin
Cretinism	
Neurological cretinism	Deafness and mutism, severe mental retardation, squint, spastic paralysis
Hypothyroid cretinism	Baby feeds poorly, grows slowly, feels cold, is sleepy, has a rough dry skin and hoarse cry and is mentally retarded

Table 9.7: Indicators and classification of IDD. Source: Savage King & Burgess (1992)

Indicator	Normal	Mild IDD	Moderate IDD	Severe IDD
Prevalence of goitre in school-age children (%)	<5	5–19	20–29	>30
Median urinary iodine in school-age children and adults (μg/l)	>100	50–99	20–49	<20

- Ultrasound which is more accurate especially where goitres are small.
2   Urinary iodine.

However, as IDD, particularly mild IDD, is widespread it may be better to use resources to control the condition (i.e. by iodizing salt) than to do surveys.

Control

Treatment with iodine can reverse hypothyroidism and reduce the size of some goitres. IDD is prevented by:

- Fortifying food. Iodization of salt is by far the most effective. In many countries it has significantly decreased prevalence of IDD and in some, such as Peru, IDD is virtually eliminated. However, even where iodized salt is available, rates of consumption can vary. For example, 95% of households in Nigeria but only 10% in Niger consume iodized salt.
- Fortifying water. Iodine has been added to borehole water in Mali and to containers of drinking water in schools in Thailand.
- Giving oral high doses of iodine where iodized salt is not available and IDD is a public health problem, for example, in remote parts of Tibet.

OTHER MICRONUTRIENT DEFICIENCIES

Zinc deficiency

Zinc promotes growth and helps maintain a healthy immune system. With vitamin A, it may play a role in determining resistance to malaria.

Severe zinc deficiency causes growth retardation, diarrhoea, skin lesions, loss of appetite and, in boys, slow sexual development. It is associated with impaired immune competence and complications during pregnancy. Zinc supplements have reduced respiratory and diarrhoea morbidity in deficient young children and reduced growth faltering during acute diarrhoea.

Zinc deficiency is controlled by:

- Increasing the intake of foods rich in bio-available zinc such as meat, fish and poultry.

Bioavailability of zinc in phytate-rich cereals (e.g. maize and sorghum) and legumes is low.
- Giving zinc supplements. Currently, there are no internationally recommended doses but most studies have given 20–25 mg of zinc/day to pregnant women. Care should be taken not to overdose malnourished children.

Folate deficiency

Folate deficiency is a cause of anaemia, especially among women, and may be a risk factor in cardiovascular disease and colon cancer; it is associated with neural tube defects in the foetus. It is controlled by increasing intake of folate-rich foods (e.g. liver, pulses, citrus fruit and green vegetables) and giving supplements of folic acid (see Table 9.3).

Less common micronutrient deficiencies

Scurvy, beriberi and pellagra caused by deficiencies of vitamin C, thiamine and niacin respectively are usually found only among very deprived groups such as refugees and prisoners. They are controlled by giving a more varied diet, supplements or fortified foods.

Calcium deficiency, one cause of osteoporosis, may become more significant as the elderly population increases. Rickets is still found in some places and calcium as well as vitamin D may be needed to treat it.

OBESITY AND RELATED CONDITIONS

OBESITY

Obesity is a condition in which excess body fat adversely affects health and increases the risk of other diseases. Obesity is caused by energy intake exceeding energy expenditure over a long period. After a certain time, weight usually stabilizes. There is considerable variation between populations and individuals in genetic susceptibility to weight gain, fat distribution and associated health consequences. Infants stunted in early life may be more prone to obesity later.

Obesity usually occurs when diets are high in fat (so there is increased energy density) and physical activity is low. For example, in India, middle income groups eat twice as much fat and have much more obesity than low-income groups. Underlying causes are environmental and social factors such as sedentary lifestyles, availability of transport and fat-rich fast meals.

Significance

In adults, obesity increases the risk of several chronic conditions including type 2 diabetes, cardiovascular diseases, gallbladder disease, osteoarthritis, back pain and some cancers. Abdominal obesity is an independent risk factor for diabetes, cardiovascular diseases and breast cancer. Obesity in children often leads to obesity later in life and, sometimes, psycho-social problems.

Recognition

Obesity is easy to see. Obesity in adults is identified by estimating body mass index (see 'Multinutrient undernutrition') although this does not assess abdominal fat. Indicators of abdominal obesity should be used with caution as health risks associated with a particular 'cut-off level' vary with ethnicity. A waist circumference of >94 cm in men and >80 cm in women has been used in industrialized countries.

For children, a weight for height of +2 Z scores is used and weight charts are being developed. There is no agreed classification of adolescent obesity. Increasing weight or waist circumference in a normal-weight adult are signs of potential obesity.

Control

Ways to prevent obesity are:

- advising at-risk people to eat diets low in fat and high in starch and fibre (i.e. cereals, roots, legumes, fruits and vegetables), take regular exercise and avoid too much sedentary activity;
- addressing underlying environmental and social causes, for example controlling inappropriate advertising, providing sports facilities

and encouraging activities such as cycling and walking.

Treating obesity is difficult. A weight loss of not more than 15% over a few months is usually more feasible than trying to reach an 'ideal weight'. Patients should:

- Reduce energy intake. Compliance is usually better if reduction is not more than 500 kcal/day. Crash diets are rarely successful.
- Increase physical activity. Many obese people prefer low intensity, prolonged, regular exercise.

Severe obesity may require more drastic action such as surgery. Obese patients need sympathetic continuous monitoring. Well-managed self-help or commercial weight loss groups can give useful support.

OBESITY-RELATED DISEASES

The risk of developing obesity comorbidities (see list above) is reduced by:

1 Controlling obesity.
2 Eating:
   - plenty of, and a variety of cereals, pulses, fish, fruits and vegetables. This ensures an adequate intake of protective micronutrients (e.g. folate, vitamins B6, B12, C and E, carotenes, selenium and zinc) and non-nutrient compounds called phytochemicals. Phytochemicals occur in some plant foods such as cereals, soybeans, onions, tomatoes and citrus fruits and appear to protect against cardiovascular disease and some cancers;
   - only moderate amounts of fatty animal foods, alcohol and salt (see feeding guidelines in 'Multinutrient undernutrition').
3 Taking regular aerobic and muscle-building exercise.

CAUSES OF UNDERNUTRITION

Undernutrition is a complex condition with complex causes that may be categorized as immediate, underlying and basic (Fig. 9.1). 'Obesity and related conditions' described causes of obesity.

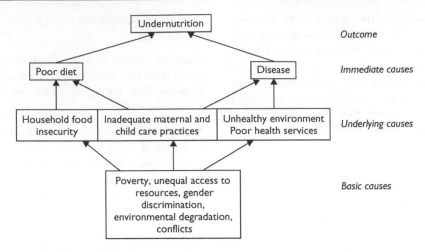

Figure 9.1: Causes of undernutrition.

IMMEDIATE CAUSES

These are a diet that lacks the nutrients required to cover needs and disease. An inadequate diet may be due to:

- insufficient quantity or variety of food;
- infrequent meals;
- insufficient breast-milk.

Maternal undernutrition is a common cause of foetal undernutrition.

Disease causes and worsens undernutrition because sick people may:

1 Eat less if:
   - they are anorexic, vomiting or have a sore mouth or throat;
   - carers give less or more watery food;
   - carers do not know how to persuade them to eat.
2 Absorb fewer nutrients (e.g. during persistent diarrhoea).
3 Lose nutrients when a disease (e.g. malaria) destroys blood or other tissues.
4 Use nutrients faster than normal (e.g. during fever).

The infections particularly associated with undernutrition are HIV/AIDS, measles, persistent and acute diarrhoea, respiratory infections, malaria, intestinal parasites and tuberculosis. Mild infections can cause undernutrition if they occur frequently.

UNDERLYING CAUSES

These are food insecurity, inadequate care of women and children, unhealthy living conditions and poor health services.

Household food shortages may be temporary, seasonal or persistent and have many causes including low income and low food production. Unhealthy living conditions (e.g. poor water supplies, poor sanitation, overcrowding) increase disease loads which are less likely to be controlled where health services are deficient. Even where food supplies are sufficient and the environment healthy, women and children may become undernourished if their care is inadequate. 'Care' encompasses behaviours affecting feeding (such as encouraging children to eat), women's workloads, household hygiene and care of the sick and old.

BASIC CAUSES

The basic causes of undernutrition are related to national and household poverty and powerlessness, unequal access to and distribution of resources, environmental degradation, abnormal weather, conflicts and violence, and gender discrimination especially in education. For example, women who have few legal rights or are poorly educated are less able to feed and care for their families and themselves than more advantaged women.

CONTROL OF NUTRITION DISORDERS

A variety of strategies are needed to deal with nutrition disorders and their causes. Many are not within the remit of the health sector, for example economic and political measures to improve family incomes, the environment and women's status and education. However, all health workers can try to influence development policies to ensure they result in improved nutrition of at-risk groups. Interventions that usually are the responsibility of health staff include those aiming to promote and improve:

- family food security;
- the feeding and empowering of women;
- breast-feeding and complementary feeding;
- the feeding of other family members;
- the control of infections;
- nutrition communication and education;
- nutrition surveillance and growth monitoring;
- community-based programmes.

FAMILY FOOD SECURITY

A family is 'food secure' if it has enough food to cover the nutrient needs of its members throughout the year. As well as economic measures (e.g. credit and income generating schemes), other ways to increase food security may be by:

1 Helping families improve:
  - food production and storage;
  - food budgeting and shopping.
2 Providing free rations or food-for-work for vulnerable groups such as young children or people living in difficult situations (e.g. refugees).
3 Increasing micronutrient content of family foods through fortification, plant breeding or biotechnology.

Family food security is a basic requirement for good nutrition but, by itself, is not enough. For each family member to be well nourished, food must be shared according to individual nutrient needs (Table 9.8).

Table 9.8: Approximate daily energy, protein and iron needs for different groups. Source: Savage King & Burgess (1992), WFP (2000)

Sex/Age (years)	Energy (kcal)	Protein (g)	Iron* (mg)
Both sexes			
0–	800	12	13
1–	1250	23	8
3–	1510	26	9
5–	1710	30	14
7–	1880	38	16
Girls			
10–	1925	52	26
12–	2040	62	27
14–	2135	69	32
16–	2150	66	32
Pregnant (latter half)	+200	+7	+60–120
Boys			
10–	2170	50	22
12–	2360	64	24
14–	2620	75	15
16–	2820	84	15
Women – active			
Menstruating	2140	48	32
Pregnant (latter half)	2240	55	+60–120
Lactating (1st 6 months if not menstruating)	2640	68	17
>60 years	1830	48	13
Men – active			
18– years	2944	57	15
>60 years	2060	57	15

*Assuming a diet low in haem–iron.

Action

Health workers can:

- support schemes to improve family production and access to food, particularly schemes for women – who produce 75% of family food supplies in Africa and 65% in Asia;
- give advice on budgeting, shopping and distributing food within the family according to need;
- encourage consumption of a wide variety of foods;
- plan, manage, monitor and evaluate feeding programmes.

FEEDING AND EMPOWERING WOMEN

Women who have equal status to men and who are well nourished and well educated are most likely to:

- provide for, feed and care well for their families;
- feel healthy and active;
- have well-spaced and healthy babies;
- avoid HIV/AIDS.

Action

Health workers should:

1 Encourage activities which help women to:
   - acquire education, knowledge, skills and self-confidence;
   - reduce workloads, especially when pregnant;
   - have better access to women's health-care services;
   - get their fair share of family nutrient-rich foods especially iron-providing foods (see 'Multinutrient undernutrition' and 'Specific micronutrient deficiencies').
2 Advise women to:
   - avoid pregnancy until after adolescence and until 6 months after breast-feeding a previous child;
   - eat more during pregnancy and lactation. Nutrient requirements increase during these periods, all except iron being greatest during lactation (see Table 9.8). Iron needs are very high during pregnancy, especially in the 3rd trimester and can rarely be supplied by diet alone;
   - take prescribed supplements of iron and other micronutrients before, during and after pregnancy and use iodized salt;
   - eat less fat and take more exercise if at risk of obesity (see 'Obesity and related conditions').
3 Help women avoid HIV/AIDS; support those who are HIV+ and explain how to reduce the risk of mother to child transmission (see below).

BREAST-FEEDING

Breast-feeding:

- provides all the nutrients needed for the first 6 months of life and up to a third of nutrient needs in the second year;

- promotes cognitive development and protects against infection and allergies in the child;
- reduces postpartum bleeding and delays menstruation in the mother and strengthens mother to child bonding.

The hazards of artificial feeding (i.e. with commercial or home-prepared formula) include greatly increased risks of infection and undernutrition – especially where lack of money, facilities and/or knowledge make it difficult to buy sufficient milk and prepare a safe feed.

Action

Health workers can promote breast-feeding by advising mothers to:

- start breast-feeding within an hour of birth;
- breast-feed exclusively on demand for about 6 months. Exclusive breast-feeding means giving only breast-milk (and micronutrients and medicines if prescribed but no water);
- then breast-feed on demand and give complementary foods until at least 2 years of age.

Health staff and traditional birth attendants should know how to help mothers start breast-feeding (and express milk or relactate if necessary) and deal with problems such as sore nipples, mastitis and worries about 'insufficient milk'. Many problems are avoided if the baby suckles in the correct position and is fed on demand.

Maternity units should introduce the 'Baby Friendly Hospital Initiative' (Box 9.5). Data from Brazil and elsewhere shows that this is most successful when all steps, including those giving information and encouraging support groups, are implemented. In the Gambia, village support groups which include traditional birth attendants and men and which target mothers and fathers have increased the rate of exclusive breastfeeding at four months from 1% to 99%.

HIV and infant feeding (UNICEF/UNAIDS/WHO 1998)

Infants of HIV+ women may become infected during pregnancy or delivery (about 20%) or through breast-feeding (about 15%). Risk factors for transmission during breast-feeding appear to include:

Box 9.5: Baby Friendly Hospital Initiative

A maternity unit is 'Baby Friendly' if it:

- has a written breast-feeding policy;
- trains staff to implement this policy;
- informs pregnant mothers of the benefits and management of breast-feeding;
- helps mothers to start breast-feeding. This is encouraged by putting newborns and mothers in skin contact within 30 minutes of birth for at least 30 minutes;
- shows mothers how to breast-feed and maintain lactation;
- gives babies no other food or drink unless medically indicated;
- keeps mothers and babies together;
- encourages breast-feeding on demand;
- gives no teats or pacifiers;
- encourages breast-feeding support groups.

- the mother has advanced AIDS or a high viral load;
- the mother becomes infected while she is breast-feeding;
- duration of breast-feeding;
- mixed breast and artificial feeding (even with water or dilute cereals);
- maternal mastitis or nipple fissure.

Giving antiretroviral drugs (e.g. Nevirapine) reduces the risk of transmission during delivery. There is evidence that *exclusive* breastfeeding for the first 6 months *only* also reduces the risk of transmission. However, if the infant is given any other foods or drinks, even water, the risk may be increased. In any case, artificial and mixed feeding of 0–6 month old infants always carry higher risks of mortality from other causes unless a family can afford enough milk and has the facilities and knowledge to make a safe feed.

Current guidelines to health workers (which may change) are (see Box 5.2, p.113):

1 If the mother's HIV is status unknown, advise exclusive breast-feeding for 6 months followed by continued breast-feeding for at least 2 years together with adequate complementary feeding.
2 If the mother is HIV+ help her make an informed choice. Her options may be:
   - feeding as recommended for infants of HIV− mothers;

- exclusive breast-feeding for 6 months and then an abrupt change to formula or other animal milk and complementary feeding;
- feeding commercial formula with a cup (which is easier than a spoon);
- cup feeding cow (or other animal) milk that has been modified at home together with supplementary micronutrients;
- feeding expressed and heat-treated breast-milk;
- wet nursing by an HIV− woman.

Feeding commercial formula may be the best option for HIV+ mothers if they can afford it and can prepare the feed safely, and if good health care is available. For mothers without these resources, breast-feeding exclusively, and for only 6 months, may be the best option. These women need help to:

- use a good breast-feeding technique;
- avoid cracked nipples and mastitis;
- feed their infants, when they reach the age of 6 months, good foods including foods from animals.

COMPLEMENTARY FEEDING

Complementary feeding means giving other foods in addition to breast-milk or a breast-milk substitute. It should start when the baby cannot get enough energy and nutrients from breast-milk alone – usually around the age of 6 months. However, unless the mother is HIV+, breast-milk should be the main food throughout the baby's first year, and an important food in the second year.

Complementary foods should not start before the age of around 6 months because these foods:

- are often watery porridges which fill the stomach but provide less nutrients than the displaced breast-milk;
- may carry infection and trigger allergies.

Action

Health workers should advise families:

1 To start complementary foods around 6 months of age but to continue breast-feeding as often as before.

2   To give a balanced mixture of nutrients. The following foods are nutrient rich and a variety of them, suitably prepared, should be given in addition to porridge or other staple foods:
- legumes (e.g. peas, beans, and groundnuts) and oil seeds (e.g. sesame seeds);
- flesh and offal from animals, fish and birds;
- eggs, and, as breast-milk eventually diminishes, milk and foods made from milk;
- all kinds of vegetables and fruits especially vitamin A-rich fruits and vegetables;
- oils and fats (to increase energy concentration). Sugar also increases energy concentration but sticky sugary foods (such as candy, lollies and bottled drinks) harm teeth.

3   That a small child has a small stomach. So to get enough nutrients:
- make porridges as thick as a child can eat;
- feed complementary foods frequently – three times/day at age 6–7 months increasing to five times/day by age 12 months.

4   That appetite is a good guide to the amount needed provided a child is healthy, fed frequently and encouraged to eat. If appetite decreases, something is wrong.

5   To actively encourage a child to eat. A young child often feeds slowly and is messy and easily distracted. A carer can ensure a child eats enough by:
- supervising meals;
- not hurrying the child who may eat a bit, play a bit, and then eat again;
- giving the child her own bowl of food;
- giving foods that the child can hold;
- not force feeding – this increases stress and decreases appetite;
- giving a drink if the child is thirsty.

When breast-feeding ends, children should continue eating nutrient-rich foods five times a day (e.g. three meals and two snacks).

FEEDING SCHOOL-AGE CHILDREN, YOUTHS, MEN AND OLD PEOPLE

Table 9.8 shows how nutrient needs vary with age. School-age children and youths are growing fast so have high needs and are often hungry. Iron requirements are especially high at puberty and remain so for girls due to menstruation. Men need large amounts of energy (due to their bigger muscle mass) but are unlikely to be undernourished because they often get the 'best' share of family meals and usually, having more control over money, eat outside the home more frequently.

Old people need less energy if activity decreases and postmenopausal women need less iron. However, old people are at risk of malnutrition if they:

- are ill, disabled, depressed or inactive;
- have difficulty eating, e.g. if they have few teeth;
- live alone and cannot shop, garden or cook;
- are poor or caring for several dependants such as orphaned grandchildren.

Action

Health workers can use the following guidelines to develop, with local people and colleagues, messages for feeding older children, men and old people:

- School-age children and youths need two to three meals a day plus snacks in order to grow, study and work well.
- Children and youths (especially girls) need meals rich in bioavailable iron.
- Men need two to three meals a day. Men at risk of obesity should eat little fat and take regular exercise.
- Families should use fortified foods such as iodized salt when available. People should take micronutrient supplements (e.g. iron tablets) if prescribed.
- Old people may need help procuring and preparing suitable meals and snacks, and must be encouraged to take exercise if possible.
- Households headed by disadvantaged women or by children need special help.

CONTROL OF INFECTIONS

Frequent infection is an immediate cause of undernutrition, especially in children. Other chapters describe common infections and their control. WHO/UNICEF's training modules on the Integrated Management of Childhood Illness are useful for diagnosing and treating children especially if adapted locally.

Action

Nutrition-related actions are:

1 Ensure public food safety and hygiene regulations are enforced.
2 Improve food and home hygiene. Important messages are:
   - wash hands thoroughly with soap before touching food, and after going to toilet, cleaning a baby or touching an animal;
   - use safe water especially for drinking;
   - keep surfaces and utensils used to prepare food clean;
   - protect food from insects, other pests and chemicals;
   - wash fruit and vegetables especially if eaten raw;
   - do not allow raw food, particularly poultry, to touch cooked foods;
   - cook food thoroughly;
   - eat cooked food immediately or store only until next meal unless refrigerated;
   - use a cup not a feeding bottle;
   - use toilets and keep them clean.
3 Give supplements of vitamin A and other micronutrients to improve immunity.
4 Feed during illness. Advise carers to:
   - frequently offer small amounts of food and encourage the sick person to eat;
   - give soft foods especially if the mouth or throat is sore;
   - if a child is breast-fed, increase the number of breast-feeds;
   - give extra fluids if the person has diarrhoea or fever;
   - feed when the person is alert and make the person comfortable before feeding, for example by clearing a stuffy nose.
5 Give extra food during convalescence to allow catch-up weight gain. Advise carers to:
   - feed (and breast-feed) more frequently and give bigger amounts at each meal;
   - give extra food until the person has regained lost weight or a child is growing well again.

NUTRITION COMMUNICATION AND EDUCATION

Good communication is essential in all nutrition activities, particularly those requiring voluntary behaviour change. Health staff may need to work with:

- policy-makers, government officials and local formal and informal leaders;
- staff in other sectors (e.g. government departments, non-government organizations, charities, businesses);
- mass media workers;
- community groups;
- school-age children and youth groups;
- malnourished families.

They may also need to train, supervise and support other health workers, especially community/village health workers.

When working with community groups and families, nutrition communication is most effective when:

- It is integrated with other interventions.
- It uses interactive learning methods which build self-confidence.
- Information and activities are based on local needs, perceptions, culture and resources.
- Only a few feasible, relevant messages are given and given frequently.
- A variety of channels and methods are used. For example, in a slum area of India, a limited number of messages on family and infant feeding were conveyed regularly for five years using mass media (pamphlets, posters, films, public announcements) and face to face communication (group meetings, discussions, exhibitions in schools, role playing, puppet shows, cooking competitions). This resulted in improved knowledge, attitudes, cooking practices and child nutrition.
- Both sexes are involved.
- All sectors give the same information.
- Activities are monitored and evaluated.

Action

Health workers may find it useful to work with the different groups in the following ways.

- Officials, leaders and staff in different sectors – explain nutrition problems and advocate feasible interventions, help secure political and financial backing and intersectorial co-operation. Politicians are often supportive if they think the intervention will enhance their popularity! Help to train and motivate health and other nutrition workers, and keep them updated.

- Mass media – give concise easy-to-understand information to convey through channels that reach target audiences (e.g. television, radio, video, internet and newspapers).
- Community groups – help members to assess, analyse and prioritize problems and decide on feasible effective action. If necessary, help to obtain outside advice and resources. Give pertinent nutrition information, for example on how to feed relatives with HIV/AIDS (Box 9.6). Women's groups are often effective agents of change as members support each other in implementing group decisions and increase each other's self confidence.
- School and youth groups – provide information for classroom lessons and school meals. Discuss with youth groups how to eat well and avoid malnutrition. For example, an informal school programme in Calcutta teaches students how to prevent VAD and in Sri Lanka similar education has lead to improved vitamin A status in adolescent girls.
- Malnourished or at risk families – try to visit the home and talk with household decision-makers and carers, being polite and sympathetic. Find out why a child or adult is malnourished, discuss ways to remove causes of the problem, obtain outside resources if needed and follow-up the family. In some situations, for example when

helping a new mother to breast-feed, it is better to counsel than advise. Counselling means listening carefully, not criticizing, encouraging a person to express her thoughts and feelings and helping the person to reach her own decisions.

NUTRITION SURVEILLANCE

The food and nutritional status of communities should be monitored to predict problems, check the progress and impact of interventions and plan future actions. The indicators collected depend on the situation; some examples are:

- predicted and actual crop yields and food supplies;
- incomes and food prices;
- consumption of key foods (e.g. iodized salt);
- indicators of micronutrient deficiencies (e.g. haemoglobin, nightblindness);
- anthropometric indicators such as BMI, birth weights and growth rates of young children;
- prevalence of HIV/AIDS, especially among those who are supporting children and other dependants.

Growth monitoring and promotion (GMP)

GMP means regularly weighing young children, plotting the weights on growth charts and comparing the weights and weight gains to those of reference healthy children (Fig. 9.2). This means parents and health workers can see how children are growing and take action to promote good growth; for example, if a child's growth falters the reason can be investigated and appropriate counselling or other help given to the family.

There are GMP programmes in most developing countries and the data can be used to assess the nutritional status of communities and monitor the impact of interventions.

GMP is resource intensive so some programmes target only the most vulnerable age group (e.g. 0–24 months) and weigh every 3 months. GMP is usually best done at community level so parents, local leaders and health workers are all closely involved. Often the time for individual counselling by medical staff is limited and community/village health workers or women's groups are trained to advise and help underweight children and their families.

Box 9.6: Feeding people with HIV/AIDS. Source: Piwoz & Preble (2000)

- Feeding extra energy and nutrient-rich foods can reduce weight loss in the early stages of HIV infection. Supplements of B vitamins and antioxidant micronutrients (e.g. β-carotene, vitamins C and E, and selenium) may be needed.
- Advise people with anorexia to eat small amounts of favourite non-spicy foods frequently and to eat extra food when they feel better.
- Some of the conditions associated with AIDS (e.g. sore mouth, nausea, bloating) are eased by avoiding coffee, alcohol, citrus fruits, very sweet or spicy foods and foods high in fat or fibre. Hygienic food preparation is especially important as people with AIDS are very susceptible to other infections.

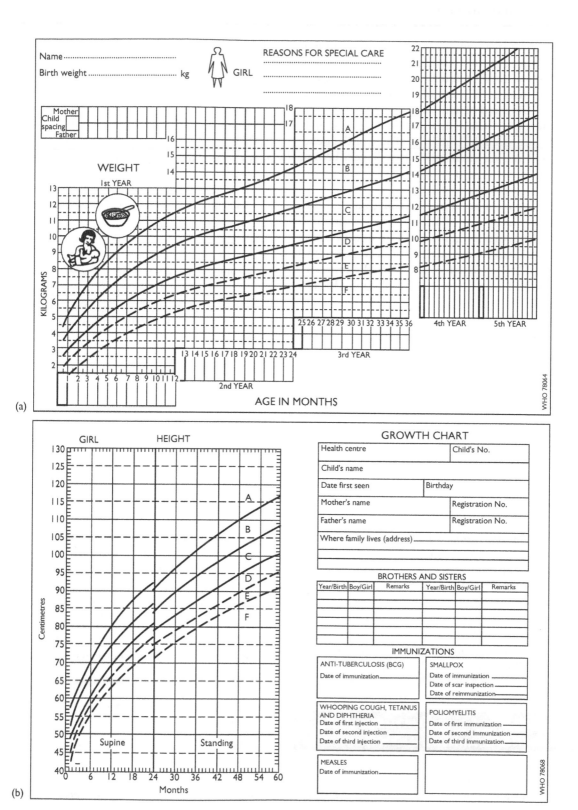

Figure 9.2: Example of a growth chart. (a) face; (b) reverse.

In Tanzania, a community weighing programme allowed parents and other villagers to assess the nutrition of their children and prompted them to find out why some were underweight. This information triggered community remedial activities that included increasing child feeding frequency, improving sanitation, training village birth attendants and raising small animals. Villagers became more resourceful and women emerged as leaders in initiating change.

To have most effect in controlling malnutrition, GMP should be part of an integrated programme. In Thailand, major improvements in nutrition have been achieved by a combination of activities that include GMP, provision of school lunches, rural job creation and increased small-scale food production.

COMMUNITY-BASED NUTRITION PROGRAMMES

Community-based programmes, like the one in Tanzania, are proving efficient and effective ways to improve nutrition. In these programmes all stake holders (e.g. families, local leaders, health and other development workers and, sometimes, outside donors) are actively involved in identifying nutrition problems, their causes and solutions, finding resources, implementing plans and monitoring and evaluating progress. This approach helps to increase the ability and will of communities to plan, monitor and sustain future interventions.

For example, in a programme in Kenya, several communities have assessed and prioritized health and nutrition problems, analysed their causes, and started remedial activities. These include community education through participatory theatre, training farmers in sustainable agriculture and teaching school children how to feed young children.

REFERENCES AND FURTHER READING/LEARNING

Administrative Committee on Coordination, Subcommittee on Nutrition (2000a) *Ending Malnutrition by 2020: An Agenda for Change in the Millennium.* ACCSCN, c/o WHO, Geneva. *accscn@who.ch*

Administrative Committee on Coordination, Subcommittee on Nutrition (2000b) *4th Report of the World Nutrition Situation.* ACCSCN, c/o WHO, Geneva. *accscn@who.ch*

Gillespie S. (1998) *Major Issues in the Control of Iron Deficiency.* Micronutrient Initiative/UNICEF, IDRC, PO Box 8500, Ottawa, Canada K1G 3H9. *mi@idrc.ca*

INACG (2000) *Safety of Iron Supplementation Programs in Malaria-Endemic Regions.* International Nutritional Anaemia Consultative Group, 1126 16th Street NW, Washington, DC 20036–4810, USA. *hni@ilsi.org*

Linkages (1999) *Recommended Feeding and Dietary Practices to Improve Infant and Maternal Nutrition.* Academy for Educational Development, 1255 23rd St NW, Washington, DC 20037, USA. *linkages@aed.org*

McLaren D.S. & Frigg M. (2001) *Sight and Life Guidebook on Vitamin A in Health and Disease*, 2nd edn. Task Force SIGHT & LIFE, Box 2116, 4002 Basel, Switzerland. *sight.life@roche.com*

Piwoz E. & Preble E. (2000) *HIV/AIDS and Nutrition: A Review of the Literature and Recommendations for Nutritional Care and Support in Sub-Saharan Africa.* SARA, Academy for Educational Development, 1825 Connecticut Ave, Washington, DC 20009, USA. *sara@aed.org*

Savage King F. & Burgess A. (1992) *Nutrition for Developing Countries.* Oxford University Press, Oxford.

Stoltzfus R.J. & Dreyfuss M.L. (1998) *Guidelines for the Use of Iron Supplements to Prevent and Treat Iron Deficiency Anaemia.* International Nutritional Anaemia Consultative Group, 1126 16th Street NW, Washington, DC, 20036–4810, USA. *hni@ilsi.org*

UNICEF/UNAIDS/WHO (1998) *HIV and Infant Feeding: Guidelines for Decision-makers.* WHO/FRH/NUT 98.2. WHO, Geneva. *publications@who.ch*

WFP (2000) *Food and Nutrition Handbook.* WFP, Via Cesare Guilio Viola 68/70, 00148 Rome, Italy. *anne.callanan@wfp.org*

WHO (1983) Reference data for the weight and height of children. In *Measuring Change in Nutritional Status.* WHO, Geneva. *publications@who.ch*

WHO (1999) Management of severe malnutrition. WHO, Geneva. *publications@who.ch*

WHO (2000) *Management of the Child with a Serious Infection or Severe Malnutrition: Guidelines for Care at the First Referral Level in Developing Countries.* WHO/FCH/CAH/00.1. WHO, Geneva. *cah@who.int*

WHO/UNICEF (1997) *Integrated Management of Childhood Illness*. WHO/CHD/97.3. WHO, Geneva. *publications@who.ch*

WHO (2000) *Nutrition for Health and Development*. WHO/NHD/ 006. WHO, Geneva.

LOW-COST NEWSLETTERS

Field Exchange. Emergency Nutrition Network, Dept Community Health & General Practice, 199 Pearse St, Trinity College, Dublin 2, Ireland. Fax +353 1 675 2391. *fiona@ennonline.net*

SCN News. ACC/Sub-Committee on Nutrition, c/o WHO, 1211 Geneva 27, Switzerland. Fax +41 22 798 8891. *accscn@who.ch www.unsystem.org/accscn/*

Sight & Life Newsletter. Task Force SIGHT & LIFE, PO Box 2116, 4002 Basel, Switzerland. Fax +41 61 688 1910. *sight.life@roche.com*

CD ROMS

Nutrition: Topics in International Health: 12 interactive tutorials on human malnutrition. CABI Publishing, Wallingford, OX10 8DE, UK. *publishing@cabi.org*

Integrating Vitamin A with Immunization: Information and training package. WHO, Geneva. *vaccines@who.int*

WHO (2000). *Turning the Tide of Malnutrition*: WHO/ NHD/007. WHO, Geneva.

ORGANIZATION OF HEALTH SERVICES

It is a painful irony that in parts of some developing countries, it is not uncommon for people to fall sick and die of diseases that can be easily prevented and treated. Many people in developing countries do not benefit fully from modern knowledge and technology that could have protected and restored their health. Some communities do not have access to simple remedies of proven efficacy or, where the services are provided, many people fail to make appropriate use of them. Individuals and communities often lack the essential knowledge on how to keep healthy, how to recognize dangerous signs in the individual and hazardous situations in the environment, and how to mobilize resources to solve health problems.

How can health services be organized to ensure that individuals, families and communities obtain the maximum benefit from current knowledge and available technology, for the promotion, maintenance and restoration of health? What can people do for themselves, what services do they require from government and other agencies, and how can they make the best use of such services? There is no simple stereotyped formula for the organization of health services. This chapter is intended to provide guidance through the examination of general principles and the use of illustrative examples. It looks at the tasks necessary for establishing

a health programme, its major components, and the levels at which health care can be delivered to the community.

THE CHALLENGE TO THE HEALTH SECTOR

Throughout the world, the health sector is in crisis. On the one hand, great advances in biomedical sciences have made available many new effective technologies for the prevention, diagnosis and treatment of diseases. On the other hand, even the most affluent developed countries cannot afford to make all these technologies available to all the people who need the various interventions. With annual spending of US $1000–3000 per head of population, the developed countries cannot afford to provide universal access to all modern health technologies. In some countries, rationing takes the form of long waiting lists, for example in the UK; in others, the services are rationed on the basis of ability to pay, for example in the USA. In developing countries, the poorest countries spending less than US $20 per head per annum, the situation is even more difficult. Painful choices have to be made. It is obvious that it would be inappropriate for poor developing countries to attempt to copy the pattern of health services in developed countries; such services can only be provided for a small proportion of the population.

Governments both in developed and developing countries have responded to this challenge by undertaking reform of the health sector. In this context, health reform means 'sustained purposeful change to improve efficiency, equity and effectiveness of the health sector'.

POLICY ISSUES

The Alma Ata Conference in 1978 set the philosophical basis for the global vision of health development on the basis of social justice. This goal was encapsulated in the slogan 'Health for All'. This historic declaration established the goal. It firmly established the principle that it is the responsibility of governments to ensure, for all their citizens, the highest level of health on the basis of available resources. Ideally, national health services should include the following features:

- *Equity* – fairness in the allocation of resources with particular attention to the needs of the poor.
- *Value for money* – carefully selecting the most cost-effective interventions and managing services efficiently.
- *Stewardship* – responding to the needs of the people with transparency and accountability.

EQUITY

The existing gross inequality in the health status of the people particularly between developed and developing countries as well as within countries is politically, socially and economically unacceptable and is, therefore, of common concern to all countries.

Alma Ata Declaration, WHO (1978)

Simply, equity in health means fairness and justice, but three different meanings are attached to the term:

- health status of families, communities and population groups;

- allocation of resources;
- access to and utilization of services.

HEALTH STATUS

Inequalities in health status reflect inequities in the health-care system. Differences in health status are strongly associated with the distribution of poverty; this strengthens the case in favour of programmes for the alleviation of poverty as a major foundation for health promotion.

ALLOCATION OF RESOURCES

Equity also relates to the allocation of resources to different sections of the population; allocative equity means that available resources are allocated in a fair manner. A simple formula would be to allocate equal amount of resources to each individual but this may perpetuate inequalities if large differences in health status already exist. There is thus an argument in favour of what is usually termed as 'vertical equity'; that is, to allocate resources from the more affluent sector of society to meet the needs of lower income individuals and families.

ACCESS AND UTILIZATION

Another view of equity is that everyone should have an equal opportunity to receive care. This so-called 'horizontal equity' proposes that individuals in like situations should be treated in like manner. Access is often defined in terms of the availability of services and its geographical coverage but experience has shown that the potential access, that is, the services that are within geographical range, does not necessarily correspond to real access as measured by the utilization of services. Marked disparities are often found in the geographical distribution of health facilities: between regions, between urban and rural areas, between rural areas and within urban areas. These disparities can be expressed in terms of the differential ratios of persons per facility – hospital beds, nurses and doctors. The distribution of health centres and other institutions in relation to the population – how far people have to travel to reach such facilities – is also used to indicate the uneven distribution of resources.

Promoting equity

Optimization of equity requires conscious attention to a number of important issues:

- political commitment;
- policy formulation;
- allocation of resources;
- intersectoral action;
- community involvement;
- information and research;
- monitoring of equity.

POLITICAL COMMITMENT

The political commitment of the government is the essential basis for promoting equity in health. It is easier to promote the concept of equity in welfare states that have the clear goal of providing universal coverage of comprehensive health care for the entire population 'from the womb to the tomb'; the question is how to achieve this goal in practice. It is more difficult where the political outlook is dominated by free market ideas, individual entrepreneurship and market forces. Political commitment is also required to correct the inequities that result from discrimination on the basis of gender, race, ethnic group and religion as well as policies that marginalize disadvantaged groups such as the indigenous communities in the Americas and Australasia.

POLICY FORMULATION

Every policy, both within the health sector and in other sectors should be critically examined as to its likely effect on equity in health. For example, the impact of macro-economic policies on health should be carefully assessed. For example, under pressure from the international finance agencies, some developing countries undertook structural adjustment programmes (SAP) and markedly reduced public investment in health and other social sectors. UNICEF and other agencies drew attention to damaging impact of SAP in the health of children. In future, careful analysis and relevant research should be used to design macro-economic policies that would not harm the health of vulnerable groups.

ALLOCATION OF RESOURCES

Government should aim to allocate financial resources fairly to the entire population taking note of the special needs of disadvantaged groups. Often, vociferous elite groups through powerful lobbies manage to acquire disproportionate shares of limited resources.

INTERSECTORAL ACTION

The profound effects of socio-economic circumstances on health have been widely recognized as they reflect the combined effects of income, education and culture.

Poverty

The association between poverty and poor health is a consistent finding. 'The poor die young' and their disease profile is largely dominated by communicable diseases, maternal and perinatal conditions, and nutritional deficiencies; not only are they at higher risk from the diseases of the poor but they also suffer more from the lifestyle health problems that are prominent in affluent communities – cancer, coronary heart disease, etc. Furthermore, with the increasing emphasis on free market economy, the gap between rich and poor is widening. Improved quantity and quality of health care is necessary but not sufficient to correct and prevent inequities in health status associated with poverty and social deprivation.

Gender

Discrimination against girls and women is a global phenomenon but it varies in its intensity in different parts of the world. It extends through the entire life cycle, ranging from selective abortion of female foetuses, discrimination in quality of health care for infants and children, access to education and salary differentials based on gender. Discriminatory practices have direct and indirect effects on the health of women. It is often an underlying or aggravating factor in the frequency, severity and outcome of some specific health problems. For example, poverty is a common cause of malnutrition in women in some parts of the world; not only does it predispose them to anaemia and other health problems but it also limits their access to health care. A common finding is the association between female education and various health indicators for themselves and their children.

The health sector must provide the leadership for mobilizing intersectoral action to achieve these three objectives:

- policies and programmes to alleviate poverty and social deprivation;
- creating an enabling environment for health by ensuring that people have the basic requirements for maintaining good health – food, safe and adequate water supply, sanitation, and housing;
- guaranteeing access to affordable health care.

COMMUNITY INVOLVEMENT (SEE CHAPTER 4)

Health services need to devise mechanisms for obtaining informed opinions from the whole community through credible representatives of civil society. The involvement of communities in decisions that affect their health care is widely recommended; it does not often work effectively in practice. Even in developed countries, the communities are often unable to participate effectively in decision-making because:

- authorities may not consult them;
- they lack relevant information;
- the civil society may not be well organized.

Lack of consultation

Health officials often make key decisions about health care and about priorities for allocation of resources without informed participation of the client communities.

Lack of information

The public often lacks information that would enable them to make informed judgements about health-care issues. Often this is because health officials do not present technical information in language that would inform the lay public nor do they clearly explain the significance of the specific issues. On occasions, there is deliberate suppression of information by government officials, for example there is a tendency to cover up information about outbreaks of infectious diseases – cholera, HIV/AIDS, etc. Some governments invoke the Official Secrets Acts and claims about sovereign rights and national security to justify their suppression of health information. Access to health information should be recognized as a human right.

Lack of effective organization of the civil society

Even in developed countries where the lay public is relatively sophisticated, the civil society is poorly organized with regard to health issues. Much of what goes for public opinion about health is stage managed by vociferous single-issue lobbyists and by sensational reports in the tabloid press. In modern societies, a variety of special groups maintain watching briefs on specific issues of interest to them – cruelty to animals or to children, protection of the environment, of wildlife, of birds, etc. Such groups collect and disseminate information, they lobby governments and engage in advocacy. Health care does not usually attract such strong lobbies from the lay public. The public response tends to be *ad hoc* and episodic rather than being well considered and systematic. Furthermore, there is usually no effective leadership and representation of the civil society to provide credible representation of the public. When consultations take place, the powerful elite, the politically influential and other privileged groups tend to dominate the debate, drowning the soft voices of the poor, the disadvantaged and marginalized groups.

INFORMATION SYSTEMS

In order to design services that are equitable and to monitor performance of health services, each health authority needs an appropriate management information system which must include measuring inequalities in health status and inequities in access to health care. The data collecting instruments must be designed to take note of groups and subgroups, especially vulnerable groups whose access to services is restricted by geographical, economic, social and cultural factors. It should include the usual demographic indicators (age, sex and marital status) as well as socio-economic indicators (race, ethnic origin, occupation, residence) and other social variables.

Special studies aimed at probing aspects of the operation of the health services with particular reference to the issue of equity, can usefully supplement routinely collected data. The studies should be designed not only to inform the debate on specific issues but also to provide clues about feasible solutions to the identified problems.

MONITORING EQUITY

The health system should include mechanisms for monitoring equity objectively. In the first instance, monitoring equity is the responsibility of health authorities at each level of care. They must build into their services sensitive indicators that would inform them of their performance with regard to equity and access to care.

In addition to such internal processes, it would be valuable to commission independent reviews of equity within the health system by groups outside the health departments. Another option would be to assign responsibility for a national equity watch to a local non-governmental organization.

In the past, policy-making was based largely on intuitive opinions of experts but was not always backed by sound knowledge and objective analysis. There is now increasing pressure to make decisions on the basis of sound scientific knowledge. Evidence-based decision-making requires that relevant information be collected and analysed, and that essential research be conducted to elucidate issues.

HEALTH RESEARCH

Developing countries are paying increasing attention to the role of research in policy-making. Following the report of an independent Commission on Health Research for Development (1990), developing countries are being encouraged to improve the management of health research in support of their health services. In its report, the Commission concluded that health research was the essential link to equity in development. The Commission recommended that each country should adopt the principles of essential national health research (ENHR) as a strategy for planning, prioritizing and managing national health research. The *goal* of ENHR is health development on the basis of social justice and equity; its *content* is the full range of biomedical and clinical research, as well as epidemiological, social, economic and types of studies (Table 10.1); and its *mode of operation* is inclusiveness, involving all stakeholders – research

Table 10.1: A simple classification of health research

Broad classification	Types of research	Goals	Disciplines involved include
COUNTRY SPECIFIC	1. Situation analysis	■ Define the distribution of health and disease ■ Identify determinants and risk factors	Epidemiology, statistics, sociology
	2. Health policy & systems research	■ To enhance the efficiency, effectiveness and cost-effectiveness of health interventions ■ To provide the basis for developing and testing health policies including equity issues	Management, economics, political science, communications science, other social sciences, etc.
GLOBAL	3. Developmental	■ To develop new and improved technologies for diagnosis, prevention and therapy	Biomedical sciences, clinical sciences, pathology, pharmacology, etc.
	4. Basic research	■ To advance knowledge of basic biology with particular reference to aspects that have a potential application in the tackling human disease ■ To expand understanding of human behaviour, poverty, dynamics of social organization, and aspects of individual as well as group behaviour	Biomedical sciences, behavioural and social sciences, comparative health policy and health systems research

scientists, policy-makers and programme managers and credible representatives of civil society.

Country specific research helps to define pattern and determinants of local health problems and to design more effective application of available technologies. It generates information that can be used to translate technologies into local programmes, and to improve the efficiency and cost-effectiveness of the services. It informs health workers about what is going on in the particular location and it helps to optimize the application of available technologies. Country-specific research is close to the point of application of health technologies and health-related interventions at the country level:

- it is multidisciplinary involving such disciplines as epidemiology, sociology, economics and political science;
- aspects of the methodology are universal but the research findings tend to be specific to the local site – a country or subgroups and communities within it;
- the situation analysis type of research is absolutely essential for assessing prevalence of disease and its determinants (biomedical, epidemiological, behavioural, etc.);
- health policy and health systems research are also intimately bound to local social, cultural and political characteristics.

Global research generates new technologies and expands basic knowledge of biology, behaviour and health systems. The expected products of global research are tools and knowledge that are generalizable and not bound to a specific country or location.

For example, the study of HIV/AIDS in the USA showed significant geographical variations in the epidemiological profiles: in one area, the most prominent feature was infection within the male homosexual lifestyle (California) and in another area, the picture was dominated by infection through contaminated needles (New York). These country-specific studies enabled the health authorities to design and adapt the control strategies taking note of these geographical variations. At the same time, global research on the virus, its structure, molecular biology, etc. generated new knowledge of value in the USA and in the rest of the world.

Research on problems affecting poor people in developing countries has been relatively neglected. According to the Global Forum for Health Research (1999), only 10% of $50–60 billion that is spent every year on health research is used for research on the health problems of 90% of the world's people – the so-called 10/90 disequilibrium.

PRIORITY SETTING FOR HEALTH RESEARCH

Table 10.2 shows a practical framework for setting research priorities.

The research priorities are also derived from an analysis of the relative share of the burden that can or cannot be averted with existing technologies. Table 10.3 illustrates the need for and type of research depending on the responsiveness of the health problem to currently available technologies.

Table 10.2: A practical framework for setting priorities in health research

Five steps in priority setting	Data and analytic requirements
I What is the burden of the disease/risk factor?	Health status Assessment of the burden of disease (DALYS, QUALYS, etc.)
II Why does the burden of disease (BoD) persist? What are the determinants?	Acquisition of knowledge about disease determinants
III What is the present level of knowledge?	What is known today about existing and new potential interventions? How cost-effective are they?
IV How cost-effective could future interventions be?	Is research likely to produce more cost-effective interventions than the present ones?
V What are the resource flows for that disease/risk factor?	Assessment of the public and private resource flows

Table 10.3: Relating research needs to efficacy of currently available technologies

Proportion of DALY	Recommendation
1. Averted with current mix of interventions and population coverage	Consolidate current control measures
2. Avertable with improved efficiency	Health systems research to improve efficiency and effectiveness
3. Avertable with existing but not cost-effective interventions	Biomedical research to develop new and improved tools – drugs, vaccines, diagnostic methods and vector control measures
4. Cannot be averted with existing interventions	

DALY, disability-adjusted life years (see p. 20).

In situations where more effective control of a disease can be achieved through efficient application of existing technologies, health systems research can provide useful answers. For example, although tetanus neonatorum can be prevented by a simple, affordable measure of toxoid immunization of pregnant women, about a quarter of a million children die each year from this preventable disease. Health services research would help to identify the underserved communities and develop strategies for ensuring that all pregnant women receive this simple and cost-effective intervention. On the other hand, for HIV/AIDS, there is an urgent need for biomedical research to discover and develop effective vaccines and new drugs to replace the current technologies that are crude, cumbersome and costly.

VALUE FOR MONEY

Severe resource constraint is a major issue in designing and managing the health services in developing countries. Since the available funds cannot meet all the health needs of the community, it is vital to ensure that the limited resources are wisely spent so as to achieve the maximum returns for minimum spending. A number of developing countries, notably Chile, Sri Lanka, China and Cuba have devised and managed highly successful health programmes with the limited resources available to them. Their models for achieving 'good health at low cost' have provided worthy examples for other countries to follow. There are relatively cost-effective interventions available against the diseases that account for most of disease, disability and death in developing countries and particularly to combat deaths and health losses among young

Box 10.1: Cost-effective packages recommended by the World Bank

The essential public health and clinical packages
The essential public health package proposed in the World Development Report (World Bank Report, 1993) includes the following:

- the expanded programme on immunization, including micronutrients (iron, vitamin A and iodine) supplementation;
- school health programmes to treat worm infections and micronutrients deficiencies and to promote health education;
- programmes to increase public knowledge about family planning and nutrition, about self-care or indications for seeking care, and about vector control and disease surveillance activities;
- programmes to reduce consumption of tobacco, alcohol, and other drugs and AIDS prevention programmes with a strong sexually transmitted disease component.

The essential clinical package recommended includes:

- prenatal and delivery care;
- family planning services;
- treatment of tuberculosis;
- case management of sexually transmitted disease.

children. Highly cost-effective interventions, costing less that US$100 per disability-adjusted life years (DALY) averted can deal effectively with the commonest causes of disease, disability and death in developing countries. In its 1993 World Development Report, the World Bank recommended cost-effective public health and clinical packages (Box 10.1).

PERFORMANCE OF HEALTH SERVICES

In its annual publication of 'The Progress of Nations', UNICEF compares the performance of countries using specific health indicators like the under 5 mortality rate. Making allowance for the national income, UNICEF compares the observed level of the specific health indicator with the rate predicted on the basis of the gross national product of the country. Some countries do better than predicted, others do worse than predicted; UNICEF calls the difference 'the national performance gap'. Figure 10.1 illustrates this point; although there is a broad relationship between national income and child mortality rates, there is a wide variation in the observed under 5 mortality rate at each level of national income. The WHO 2000 Report attempted a more comprehensive assessment and generated a ranking order for the overall performance of its 191 member states. Its methodology and findings have provoked extensive debate and discussion but the idea that is gaining ground is that the performance of national health should be scrutinized and compared with the achievements of states at a similar level of development.

STEWARDSHIP

WHO defines stewardship as a 'function of a government responsible for the welfare of the population, and concerned about the trust and legitimacy with which its activities are viewed by the citizenry'. As defined, stewardship is the essence of good government. It involves the performance of several key tasks:

- formulating health policy – defining the vision and direction;
- exerting influence – approaches to regulation;
- collecting and using intelligence.

HEALTH POLICY

In formally outlining the national health policy, the Ministry of Health aims at achieving the following objectives:

- to define a vision for the future, thereby establishing benchmarks for the short and medium term;
- to outline priorities and the expected roles of different groups;
- to build consensus and inform people, as an important function of governance.

Priority setting should take into account the:

- burden of illness;
- cost-effectiveness of available interventions;
- scale of existing action to address the problem;
- expressed preferences of the community regarding the value basis of priority setting.

REGULATION

This is an important function of the public sector to operate mechanisms that would ensure that services offered by public or private providers meet minimal standards.

PUBLIC INFORMATION

People have the right to know about health issues that can affect their lives especially in situations in which the government is making choices that affect their lives. Consultations with relevant groups in the formulation of the national health policy would help achieve the widest acceptance of the selected options. The consultations should include credible representatives of the following stakeholders:

- civil society – non-governmental organizations, etc.;
- health professionals – doctors, nurses, midwives, etc.;
- private health sector – including for profit health-care providers;
- other relevant partners, e.g. foreign donors, international agencies (WHO, UNICEF, etc.).

It is the duty of governments to provide timely, clear information that will enable people to take good care of their health. Governments, especially in developing countries, are sometimes tempted to hide or manipulate health information for fear of the adverse effect that news of a disease outbreak could have on trade and tourism. Thus, some governments refuse to admit the occurrence of epidemics such as cholera for fear of the repercussions on trade and commerce. The HIV/AIDS

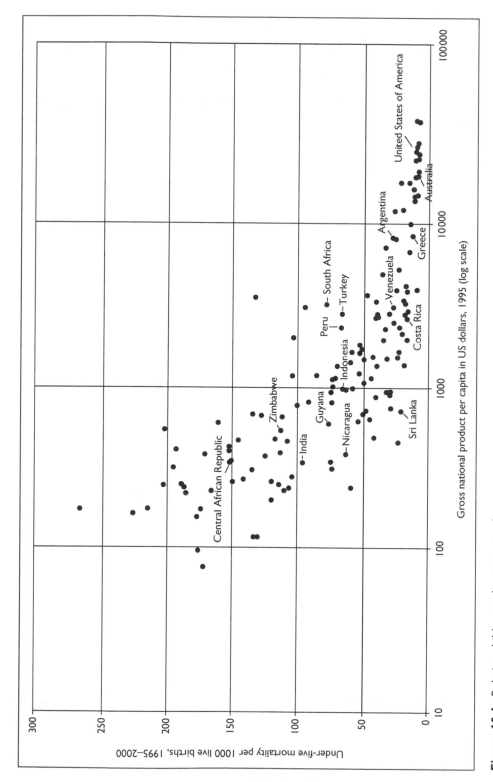

Figure 10.1: Relating child mortality to national income.

epidemic in Africa progressed unchecked for many years because some governments silenced researchers and public health workers. Instead of mounting a major programme of public awareness, the governments persisted in their policy of denial until the epidemic ravaged the continent.

TASKS FOR THE HEALTH SERVICES

In order to accomplish this process of translating knowledge into effective action, the health authorities need to perform five major tasks:

- measurement of needs;
- assessment and mobilization of resources;
- definition of goals;
- planning of programmes;
- delivery of services;
- monitoring and evaluation.

The relationships of these tasks in establishing effective health services are shown in Figure 10.2. Community participation in as many of these tasks as possible is highly desirable.

MEASUREMENT OF NEEDS

This includes all the activities aimed at gathering information about the health status of the community and identifying the factors which influence it. Such determinants include hereditary, environmental and cultural factors. The statistical evaluation of health services is described on page 296, and information on epidemiological methods used to study the health of communities is given in Chapter 3.

ASSESSMENT AND MOBILIZATION OF RESOURCES

There must be a realistic assessment of resources that are available or could be made available for improving the health of the community. These resources include money, manpower and materials that can be deployed for use in the health programme (see p. 293). Sources include:

- public funds generated from taxes;
- public insurance/social security;
- private insurance;
- out-of-pocket personal resources.

In addition to the resources that are available from government, other sources both internal (from self-help and community effort) and external (in the form of aid) must be explored. National health policy directly relates to the spending of public resources but it also gives guidance to the private sector in selecting the most beneficial, and most cost-effective interventions. There is increasing appreciation of the value of promoting public/private partnerships. National health policy guidelines can also guide individuals in making choices on how to use their personal resources.

DEFINITION OF GOALS

On the basis of information obtained about the health needs of the community and the available resources, it is necessary to set realistic targets in

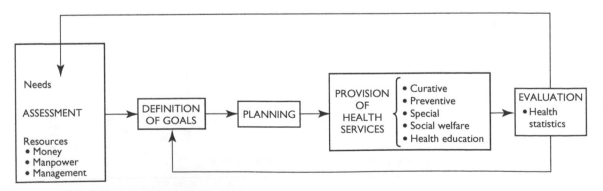

Figure 10.2: Processes involved in the organization of health services.

terms of measurable improvement in the health of the community. The matching of needs to resources requires a careful selection of priorities:

- What are the major problems?
- How can the problems be tackled?
- What is the expected impact of such interventions?

Setting priorities also involves making hard choices; with limited resources and relatively underdeveloped services and infrastructure, the health plan must selectively include the most cost-effective interventions.

PLANNING

Planning involves the specification of goals and the preparation of a strategy to achieve the goals.

Multisectoral approach

Although the health plan is first and foremost the responsibility of the health sector in the government, the important role of other sectors must not be overlooked – thus it is necessary to involve these other sectors:

- agriculture – from the point of view of nutrition as well as such issues as the use of pesticides;
- works – with regard to housing, drainage, community water supplies, and other aspects of environmental sanitation;
- education – with special reference to the health of school children, the school environment, and health education in schools;
- industry and labour – for the health of workers, and problems of environmental pollution.

This multisectoral approach should not be regarded as being solely for the benefit of the health sector but should be perceived as a collaborative effort of mutual advantage. Thus, healthier workers may be more productive, school children that are freed from disease and disability should perform better in their academic work, and the safe use of pesticides would protect the health of farmers and the community.

Community participation

The value of the involvement of the community in devising the health plan cannot be over-emphasized.

The people must be consulted, they must be persuaded and they must be given responsibility in decision-making under the technical and professional guidance of health workers. The plan must not be imposed but at every step the people must participate in devising the strategies which are most compatible with their needs and resources (see pp. 354 for a fuller discussion).

MONITORING AND EVALUATION OF HEALTH PROGRAMMES

Did the intervention occur as planned and did it have the desired effect? This process of monitoring and evaluation must be built into the health programme and should be an essential feature of each health unit no matter how small. Without it, things could go far wrong for a long time without coming to the notice of the health authorities. Failure to include mechanisms for monitoring and evaluation is one of the commonest causes of waste in health services. Using objective indicators, baseline data must be collected, the planned interventions must be monitored and the impact of the activities must be studied. The collection and analysis of health statistics is described on page 27.

RESOURCES FOR THE HEALTH SERVICES

The resources required by the health services include money, manpower, materials and management.

MONEY

The financing of the health services takes many different forms. In some countries, health care is provided as a welfare service which is paid for almost exclusively from government revenue or compulsory insurance schemes. At the other extreme, government provides some general public health services, but individuals and communities must pay for other items of health care. In most communities there is a mixture, with some services being subsidized by the government and other services paid for by individuals either directly or through voluntary insurance schemes.

In developing countries, the funds available for the health sector are very limited and inadequate to provide all the services that are desired by the community. Affluent countries spend US $1000–3000 per head on health care whereas the poorer developing countries spend less than US $20 per head. Difficult and painful choices have to be made in allocating these scarce resources. Ideally such judgements should be made objectively, giving highest priority to the most cost-effective way of achieving the desired goals and distributing the resources with a sense of social justice, ensuring that the most needy are well served. The community should be encouraged to participate in making these difficult decisions and when appropriate they should be encouraged to make additional contributions from their own resources.

Cost recovery schemes and user fees

Many countries that previously offered health services at no cost or at highly subsidized rates are now imposing fees on users at the point of delivery of health care. The aim is to generate additional income for use by the public sector, to enable the public sector to redistribute resources in favour of the poor and to achieve increasing self-reliance for sustainable community health programmes. The main objective of user fees is to generate resources that can be used to expand the quantity and improve the quality of health services. These schemes are designed not only to recover some of the costs involved in providing the services but also to focus public resources on top priorities. In favour of user fees is the observation that free health services selectively subsidize the more affluent members of society. This is particularly true for curative services in hospitals. Hospital services take up a substantial proportion – 40–80% – of the recurrent expenditure of the national health budget but only a small minority of the population benefits from the services.

User charges enable the public sector to reallocate the resources by withdrawing subsidies from those who can afford to pay and redirecting the savings to expand cost-effective public health services to the poor. User fees have also been designed to promote self-reliance and make community health

programmes sustainable. At the primary health care level, the so-called 'Bamako Initiative', charges for medications with a small profit margin that can be used to support local health services.

The imposition of user fees remains a controversial issue. The advocates of this policy claim that it promotes equity; the public sector generates additional revenue from clients who are willing and are able to pay. The additional income can be used to improve the quality of services and to subsidize poor people who are exempted from payment. Noting the sharp decline in the utilization of services when user fees are introduced, other public health practitioners have criticized such schemes for further widening the gap between the rich and the poor. Some of the concerns about equity can be met by carefully designed exemptions for persons and for specific services.

MANPOWER (HUMAN RESOURCES)

Several questions need to be answered with regard to the provision of health personnel. How many are required and can be employed? What is the role of each category of staff and what tasks are they expected to perform? What training do they require to enable them to fulfil their respective roles? For a fuller discussion of these questions, see 'Health personnel'.

MATERIALS

It is necessary to determine what buildings and capital equipment are required for the efficient delivery of health care, and what funds are required for drugs, vaccines, and other consumables. A difficult issue to resolve is the correct balance between expenditure for buildings and capital equipment on the one hand and the running costs of the services on the other hand. In many developing countries, there is a tendency to invest too heavily in lofty buildings and expensive equipment, often poorly maintained, whilst relatively few funds are left for the purchase of drugs, vaccines and other essentials.

Careful planning is also required in the purchase, storage and distribution of drugs and vaccines. Each health authority should produce a basic list of essential drugs which would meet the

---

Box 10.2: National drug policy: essential drug programme

Pharmaceuticals represent a substantial component of the costs of health services. In most countries, next to staff salaries, the highest expenditure is for the purchase of drugs. Until WHO introduced the concept and practice of 'Essential Drugs' (now referred to as 'Essential Medicines') some 25 years ago, this massive expenditure was poorly managed in most countries. There was little attention paid to important issues relating to the acquisition and use of medications:

- analysing needs for medication in relation to the most important health problems;
- procuring the most effective medications at an affordable price;
- assessing the quality of drugs, to detect and eliminate fake medicines;
- managing of storage and distribution of drugs;
- ensuring universal access to basic medication;
- training of doctors, nurses and health personnel on the rational use of drugs;
- involving communities in making decisions especially about the hard choices that need to be made to contain costs.

WHO defined *'essential drugs as those that satisfy the health care needs of the majority of the population; they should therefore be available at all times in adequate amounts and in the appropriate dosage forms, and at a price that individuals and the community can afford'*. WHO introduced the essential drug programme in 1975 to focus 'on those drugs that represent the best balance of quality, safety, efficacy and cost for a given health setting'. The aim is to provide the best of modern, evidenced-based and cost-effective health care.

WHO has stimulated each country to design and implement its national drug policy. A key element of the policy is the Essential Drug list which forms the basis of procurement, staff training, reimbursement and other drug activities. In 1977, WHO published an initial model list of about 200 items; every 2 years, it convenes an expert panel to review and update the list. The expert panels base their recommendations on sound and adequate data on efficacy and safety from clinical studies and on consideration of many factors in countries such as pattern of prevalent diseases, treatment facilities, training and experience of available personnel, financial resources and genetic, demographic and environmental factors. WHO encourages each country to adapt the list to develop and update the national list of essential drugs on the basis of its own needs and circumstances.

---

most important needs of the service, concentrating initially on simple, safe remedies of proven value at reasonable cost. Box 10.2 summarizes WHO's programme on essential drugs which aims at promoting improved management of drug programmes within national health services.

MANAGEMENT

The resources available to the health authorities should be skilfully managed at all levels, from the most peripheral unit to the central office at the headquarters of the Ministry of Health. Training in management is essential for health workers, especially those who are placed in positions of authority and supervision. In small units, the health workers would need to devote some of their time to dealing with administrative and other managerial issues. In large units such as large tertiary hospitals, trained administrators can make

a useful contribution to the management of the services.

HEALTH PERSONNEL

The terminology used in classifying health personnel is wide and varied, reflecting differences in local practices and in organization. Often, different titles are given to personnel who perform essentially the same function and in other cases the same title is used for workers who perform different functions. Terms such as medical personnel, health personnel, professionals, paramedical personnel, subprofessionals and auxiliaries have been subject to varied interpretations. However, important general principles can be widely applied:

- What *tasks* need to be performed?
- What *types* or *categories* of personnel should perform the tasks?

- What *training* and *supervision* do they require to function effectively?

Tasks

The tasks to be performed include:

- *leadership* in health matters;
- *health promotion* within the community;
- *education* of the public;
- *specific interventions* especially those requiring knowledge and skill, e.g. prophylaxis, diagnosis, treatment including surgery and rehabilitation;
- *monitoring and evaluation* to assess performance of the services, outcomes and eventually, impact.

There is a tendency to overlook the first three tasks and to think of the function of the health personnel solely in terms of the performance of technical interventions.

Types of health personnel

Each component of the health services requires a team of personnel with different skills who are working together in pursuance of common goals. Some members of the team are usually described as professionals. whilst others are variously described as subprofessional or auxiliary personnel. It is not possible to provide rigid criteria for separating these categories.

At one end of the spectrum, the auxiliary health worker is trained to perform a number of specific tasks, of limited scope under supervision. This may either be as a monovalent worker in a special programme, for example a vaccinator, a yaws scout, etc., or as a multipurpose health auxiliary who can perform a list of specific tasks in accordance with clearly defined guidelines. At the other extreme, the professional worker is expected to have acquired sufficient basic knowledge and skills to be able to identify and analyse problems and arrive at independent judgements of situations, for example doctors, dentists, nurses, midwives, and so on. Regardless of the nomenclature and classification, the important issue is to recognize the need for team effort with allocation of tasks on the basis of skill and experience.

In order to meet special needs, some health practitioners take bold innovative uses of health personnel. For example, in some remote communities, where no doctors are available, nurses have been trained to perform emergency caesarean sections and other life-saving obstetric procedures.

Supervision

One important aspect of the management of health services is the appropriate supervision of staff. This is an essential function to be performed by the leader of each group or subgroup. To be effective, the leader must know what tasks need to be performed and what skills the workers under supervision possess.

Experience has shown that the best results are obtained if feedback is positive, not only blaming when things go wrong but also praising and rewarding good performance. The supervisor's role also includes teaching colleagues as well as learning from them. Spot checks of performance should be carried out regularly to prevent slackness in procedures.

MONITORING AND EVALUATION: HEALTH STATISTICS

Statistics are essential for the proper management and evaluation of the health services. They serve to provide essential information about:

- *needs* of the population;
- *demand and utilization* of services;
- *effectiveness and cost* of services.

Much information is usually collected in the course of the operation of health services. Such data should be obtained and processed in such a way as to provide suitable guidance for the management of the health programmes (see Chapter 2 for a full account of the type of data, methods of collection and analysis).

DATA COLLECTION

The information collected should be selective, concentrating on the data which can be used for making decisions. Forms for collecting information should be reviewed, pruned and simplified: items should be limited to the essential information that can be and will be used; the wording and layout of the forms should make them simple to complete and it should be easy to extract data from them.

ANALYSIS

The data should be analysed in a relevant manner relating events to the population at risk. For example, it is common to count the number of visits by pregnant women to antenatal services. The information is of little value when it is presented in this form. It is preferable to relate the number of pregnant women using the antenatal services to the number of pregnant women in the area. This ratio is a meaningful indicator of the coverage of the services; it provides a means of comparing the performance of the services from one area to the other and also to monitor changes over time.

Simple indicators of this type should be used to monitor each component of the health services. For example:

- What proportion of children who die have been treated by the health services in the course of their last illness or within the 48 hours prior to dying?
- What proportion of newborn children are vaccinated against the common infectious diseases of childhood?
- What proportion of the population has access to a safe potable water supply and how much is available per head of population?
- What proportion of households have hygienic latrines?
- What proportion of pregnant women are immunized with tetanus toxoid?
- What proportion of women in the childbearing age group accepts family planning devices and what proportion continues to use them?

For each important health activity, appropriate indicators should be selected with regard to the *input* (i.e. the services offered); the *output* (i.e. the actual uptake of the services provided); the *outcome* (i.e. the impact on the health of the population); and the *equity* of access (i.e. the percentage of the population in need of a specific service that obtains it, noting in particular groups that are underserved).

DELIVERY OF HEALTH CARE

THE MAJOR COMPONENTS OF HEALTH SERVICES

It is convenient to group the elements within each health service into five major components:

- *curative* – providing care for the sick;
- *preventive* – for the protection of the health of the population;
- *special services* – dealing with specific problems (e.g. malnutrition) or special groups (e.g. pregnant women);
- *social welfare* – providing support services for disadvantaged groups (e.g. chronic sick, mentally and physically handicapped, orphans, etc.);
- *health education* – giving the people essential information to modify their behaviour in matters affecting their health.

This classification can be used as a simple checklist for reviewing the health services in any community regardless of the details of the organization. These components must not be regarded as existing in watertight compartments but they should be seen as interrelated elements. Public health laws may give legal support in implementing and setting minimum standards in some or all of these components.

CURATIVE SERVICES

Allocating resources

Curative services deal with the care of the sick members of the population. There is a tendency to regard them as the most important element of the health services – they are usually in greatest demand by the public and in the planning of health services there is a tendency to commit an unduly high proportion of resources to them. On the other hand, there is less spontaneous demand for preventive services, especially those aspects that are aimed at the protection of people who feel well. The demand for the treatment of the sick must be met and the curative services should be designed in such a way as to give maximum benefit to the population.

Estimating disease priority

The highest priority must be given for the most common and the most severe diseases, especially those conditions that can be significantly improved by appropriate intervention. In selecting priorities the concept of *public health significance* can provide useful guidance. The public health significance of a disease depends on two factors:

- *Frequency* – how many people are affected and what is the potential for spread?
- *Severity* – how much disease, disability, and death does it cause?

The concept can be represented by this formula:

$$\text{Public health significance} = \text{frequency} \times \text{severity}.$$

One limitation of this approach is that it does not specifically include consideration of the age of the affected persons. Obviously, a disease with high morbidity and mortality in childhood and adolescence is a more serious public health problem than one that has a similar effect on elderly persons, say over the age of 80 years. An alternative approach is to compute the *impact* of the disease by calculating the number of useful years lost. In addition to allowing for the age of onset of the disease, this approach can also take account of partial disability.

BURDEN OF DISEASE

New tools have been developed for measuring the impact of individual diseases and risk factors, as well as their amenability to control. These measurements of the burden of disease are increasingly being used to make objective decisions when setting priorities. They attempt to summarize the impact of specific health problems in terms of disease, disability, and premature death. The disability-adjusted life years (DALYs), combines losses from death and disability, but also makes allowance for:

- a discount rate, so that future years of healthy life are valued at progressively lower levels;
- age weights, so that years lost at different ages are given different values.

The DALY can therefore be used to compare the losses from childhood infections like measles that cause premature death with chronic diseases like diabetes or stroke that involve many years of disability.

Curative measures

Even without making such detailed calculations, it should be possible to identify the most commonly occurring diseases. The curative services must be equipped to deal with them.

TREATMENT

Simple, cheap, symptomatic relief must be provided for benign self-healing conditions.

EARLY INTERVENTION

Early and appropriate interventions must be available to deal with serious, life-threatening disease. Such conditions must be detected as early as possible, preferably before irreversible damage has occurred and in the case of communicable diseases, before the infection has spread to affect others.

EDUCATION

In order to ensure early detection it is important to educate the public to make people aware of danger signals that could indicate serious illness and to encourage them to seek help whenever these occur, for example chronic cough, abnormal bleeding, lump in the breast.

DETECTION

Facilities must be provided for the detection of diseases of local importance, for example staining of sputum to identify acid-fast bacilli; simple microscopy of urine, blood and other specimens to detect parasites; serological tests for common infectious diseases. In some cases, a special survey may be indicated for the active detection of cases. The survey method may include history taking (e.g. haematuria), physical examination (e.g. hypopigmented hypoaesthetic patches and thickened nerves indicative of leprosy) or special investigations (e.g. chest X-ray, serology, cervical smear).

FACILITIES

Staff should be trained to recognize and treat the most commonly occurring diseases in the population, and they should be equipped to do so either in the local health unit or at referral centres.

PREVENTIVE SERVICES

Preventive services are designed to maintain and protect the health of the population. They include:

- personal protection (e.g. immunization);
- environmental sanitation (e.g. water supply, waste disposal – see Chapter 13);
- specific disease control (e.g. infectious: typhoid, tapeworm; non-infectious: goitre).

Education

Unlike the curative services which are provided for the sick, the preventive services are directed at the entire population. Whereas people generally appreciate the value of curative services, it is often difficult to persuade them of the value of preventive services. Furthermore, whereas sick persons, especially those experiencing uncomfortable symptoms, will readily seek medical care, it is not always easy to persuade healthy persons to take precautionary measures for their own protection. It is an important duty of the health personnel to educate individuals and the community on the value of preventive services, to persuade the community to make appropriate investments in environmental sanitation or susceptible individuals to accept immunizations.

SPECIAL SERVICES

Apart from the components of the health programme that are made available to all members of the community, special services are designed to cope with the needs of specific groups and to deal with problems that deserve particular attention. Services for special groups include those for:

- mothers and children (see Chapter 12);
- workers (e.g. migrant labourers);
- the elderly;
- the handicapped.

Services may be provided to deal with special problems like:

- tuberculosis;
- leprosy;
- malnutrition;
- mental illness (see Chapter 8);
- blindness;
- sexually transmitted disease.

Through such special services the specific needs of sections of the population can be more adequately met and difficult problems can be more effectively tackled.

Organization of special services

At the national level, special services may be provided and monitored by a Division within the Ministry of Health, for example a malaria service. The special Division may have its own central organization and peripheral units. In a small unit such as a rural health centre, special services can be provided by setting apart a particular time and place for dealing with the group or the specific problem. It is common to find that such health centres run general clinics on most working days but schedule special clinics (nutrition, family planning, etc.) for specific days.

SOCIAL WELFARE

Departments of social welfare in the tropics provide a variable range of welfare services for the community. In some countries, for example in middle-income developing countries, a wide range of social services is available while in others, for example those of tropical Africa, social welfare services barely exist. The aim is to provide welfare and protection to needy groups, for example children and young persons; women and young girls; and to provide probation and aftercare services for young offenders, endeavouring to place them in employment whenever possible. Public assistance schemes provide financial assistance to the aged, the chronic sick, the physically and mentally handicapped, the widows and orphans and the unemployed. Institutional care may be provided for special cases.

Voluntary organizations continue to play an important role in welfare work, usually complementing government programmes. In some developing countries the only welfare work available is that provided by major voluntary organizations, for example the care of handicapped children.

HEALTH EDUCATION

The aim of health education is to encourage people to value health as a worthwhile asset and to let them know what they can do as individuals and communities to promote their own health. In effect health education is designed to alter attitudes and behaviour in matters concerning health. The more people know about their own health, the better they are able to take appropriate measures in such personal matters as diet, exercise, use of alcohol, and hygiene. They are also enabled to make the most appropriate use of the health services and to participate in making rational decisions about the operations of the health services within their community.

The variety of methods used in health education is described in more detail in Chapter 14. No single method can be wholly successful and because of the wide range of response from place to place, methods must be tested and evaluated within the local setting. Above all, the example set by health personnel is of great importance especially in such matters as personal hygiene and social habits.

PUBLIC HEALTH LAWS

Public health laws are enacted in order to protect and promote individual and community health. The extent to which public health laws are used varies from country to country and is dependent on the legal system of individual countries. They may cover such topics as:

- registration of births and deaths;
- quarantine and prevention of disease;
- sales of food and drugs;
- control of disease-bearing insects including the control of breeding sites in households;
- registration of medical personnel;
- registration of schools;
- environmental health.

The application and enforcement of these laws is a function of health officers, public health inspectors and the medical officers of health. They are usually given power to enter into premises and to take action to prevent the propagation of disease.

LEVELS OF CARE

It is convenient to classify the health services available to the community into three levels (Fig. 10.3).

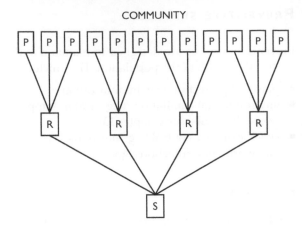

Figure 10.3: The relationship between the community and the health care services. P, primary health care unit; R, referral services; S, specialist services.

Primary

This refers to the point at which the individual normally makes the first contact with the health services. In a rural area, it may be a health centre, a dispensary or a health post. In an urban area it could be a general medical practitioner's clinic, a polyclinic or health centre or even the outpatient department of a hospital. The eight elements of primary health care are illustrated in Figure 10.4.

Referral

The primary health care services can deal effectively with most of the problems that present at this level but more difficult cases will be referred for more detailed evaluation and for more skilled care.

Specialist

Specialist services, often backed by high technology, are provided for dealing with the most difficult problems. For example, the majority of pregnant women can be cared for at the primary level including the community-based services and the referral hospital that can deliver emergency obstetric care; high-risk groups, for example

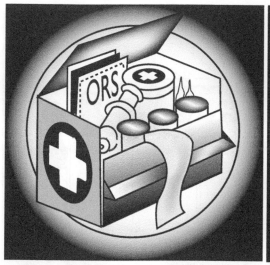

ILLNESS AND INJURY

Adequate provision of curative services for common
ailments and injuries should be made within the community

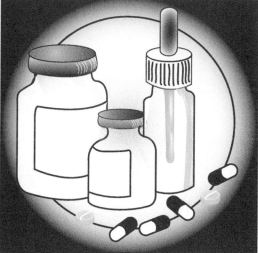

ESSENTIAL DRUGS

The most vital drugs should be available and
affordable by all

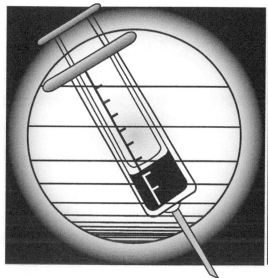

IMMUNIZATION

An increasing number of infectious diseases
can be prevented by vaccination

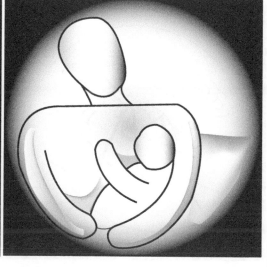

MATERNAL AND CHILD CARE

Services should be targeted to those groups most in
need and where they can produce maximum benefit

Figure 10.4: The eight elements of primary care.

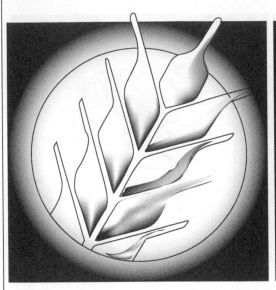

FOOD AND NUTRITION

The family's food should be adequate, affordable and balanced in nutrients

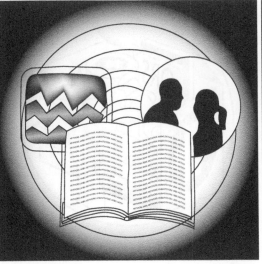

EDUCATION

The community should be informed of health problems and methods of prevention and control

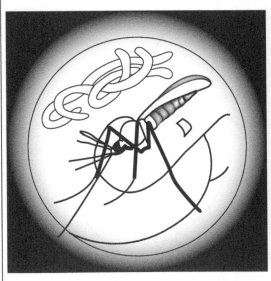

VECTORS AND RESERVOIRS

Endemic infectious disease can be regulated through the control or eradication of vectors and animal reservoirs

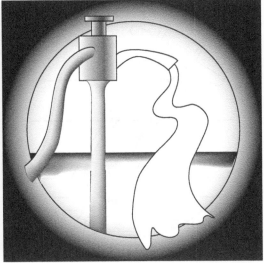

WATER AND SANITATION

A safe water supply and the clean disposal of wastes are vital for health

Figure 10.4: (Continued)

primigravidae and grand multigravidae, may go directly to the referral unit; difficult cases, including those presenting with serious complications, may need specialist services.

DISTRICT HEALTH SERVICES

WHO strongly recommends integrated health care at the district level, involving all health-care providers, both public and private, and all health systems – modern and traditional, orthodox and non-orthodox.

WHO's model defines the district as the smallest planning unit for health care, involving community-based services through health centres and other institutions providing ambulatory care as well as the referral hospital. The model is inclusive and involves collaboration of all stakeholders: the public sector represented by the local government, the private sector, both for profit and the not for profit, and credible representatives of civil society. The hope is that the consensus that emerges from the interaction of these stakeholders would lead to the development of realistic health programmes that are culturally sensitive, sustainable and capable of growth and expansion as the community develops. A District Health Management Team, consisting of various cadres of staff, manage the programmes at the district level. Some critics felt that WHO's approach was too broad and therefore unrealistic. They proposed instead 'Selective Primary Health Care' a strategy that aims at delivering a limited number of interventions of proven efficacy and cost-effectiveness, for example immunization and mass chemotherapy of some endemic infections. Rather that grant the local authorities the right to define local priorities and strategies, they would be required to conform to a centrally determined national programme, which is made up of a limited list of well-defined, cost-effective interventions. There is some danger that selective primary health care would merely

recreate vertical programmes in which practitioners in the field would be required to implement prepackaged interventions blindly. An acceptable compromise would be to use UNICEF's GOBI-FFF[1] and the World Bank's clinical and public health packages as building blocks of primary health care.

PRIMARY HEALTH CARE

In recent years, there has been increasing recognition of the pivotal role of primary health care. The definition of this role culminated in the Alma-Ata declaration in 1978 which is reproduced here in full as it represents a global consensus among governments on this important issue (Box 10.3). As defined, primary health care includes seven important features (Table 10.4). The salient features are highlighted below:

- The primary health care concept is not intended to represent second best medicine acceptable only to the rural poor or the dwellers of urban slums. Rather, it is essential care for all based on practical, scientifically sound and socially acceptable methods and technology.
- It is not a stopgap solution to be replaced by something better at a later stage. Rather, the primary health care approach is intended to be a permanent feature of all health services; the quality of care should steadily improve, and at all times it should be appropriate to the resources and the needs of the community.
- Primary health care is not intended to function in isolation but in collaboration with the referral and specialist services. These various services should be mutually supportive. Without good primary health care, the referral services would be overwhelmed by problems which could have been dealt with efficiently at the primary level. Many of these would be advanced cases with complications which could have been prevented by early detection and prompt care at the primary unit. On the other hand, primary health care requires the support of the referral services to cope with problems which are beyond the scope of the peripheral units.

---

[1]Growth monitoring, oral dehydration, breast feeding, immunization, family planning, female education and supplementary feeding of pregnant women.

The International Conference on Primary Health Care, meeting in Alma Ata this twelfth day of September in the year Nineteen hundred and seventy-eight, expressing the need for urgent action by all governments, all health and development workers, and the world community to protect and promote the health of all the people of the world, hereby makes the following Declaration:

I

The Conference strongly reaffirms that health, which is a state of complete physical, mental and social wellbeing, and not merely the absence of disease or infirmity, is a fundamental human right and that the attainment of the highest possible level of health is a most important worldwide social goal whose realization requires the action of many other social and economic sectors in addition to the health sector.

II

The existing gross inequality in the health status of the people particularly between developed and developing countries as well as within countries is politically, socially and economically unacceptable and is, therefore, of common concern to all countries.

III

Economic and social development, based on a New International Economic Order, is of basic importance to the fullest attainment of health for all and to the reduction of the gap between the health status of the developing and developed countries. The promotion and protection of the health of the people is essential to sustained economic and social development and contributes to a better quality of life and to world peace.

IV

The people have the right and duty to participate individually and collectively in the planning and implementation of their health care.

V

Governments have a responsibility for the health of their people which can be fulfilled only by the provision of adequate health and social measures. A main social target of governments, international organizations and the whole world community in the coming decades should be the attainment, by all peoples of the world by the year 2000, of a level of health that will permit them to lead a socially and economically productive life. Primary health care is the key to attaining this target as part of development in the spirit of social justice.

VI

Primary health care is essential health care based on practical, scientifically sound and socially acceptable methods and technology made universally accessible to individuals and families in the community through their full participation, and at a cost that the community and country can afford to maintain at every stage of their development in the spirit of self-reliance and self-determination. It forms an integral part both of the country's health system, of which it is the central function and main focus, and of the overall social and economic development of the community. It is the first level of contact of individuals, the family and community with the national health system bringing health care as close as possible to where people live and work, and constitutes the first element of a continuing health care process.

VII

Primary health care:

1 reflects and evolves from the economic conditions and sociocultural and political characteristics of the country and its communities and is based on the application of the relevant results of social, biomedical and health services research and public health experience;

(Continued)

2 addresses the main health problems in the community, providing promotive, preventive, curative and rehabilitative services accordingly;

3 includes at least: education concerning prevailing health problems and the methods of preventing and controlling them; promotion of food supply and proper nutrition; an adequate supply of safe water and basic sanitation; maternal and child health care, including family planning; immunization against the major infectious diseases; prevention and control of locally endemic diseases; appropriate treatment of common diseases and injuries; and provision of essential drugs;

4 involves, in addition to the health sector, all related sectors and aspects of national and community development, in particular agriculture, animal husbandry, food, industry, education, housing, public works, communications and other sectors; and demands the co-ordinated efforts of all those sectors;

5 requires and promotes maximum community and individual self-reliance and participation in the planning, organization, operation and control of primary health care, making fullest use of local, national and other available resources; and to this end develops through appropriate education the ability of communities to participate;

6 should be sustained by integrated, functional and mutually-supportive referral systems, leading to the progressive improvement of comprehensive health care for all, and giving priority to those most in need;

7 relies at local and referral levels, on health workers, including physicians, nurses, midwives, auxiliaries and community workers as applicable, as well as traditional practitioners as needed, suitably trained socially and technically to work as a health team and to respond to the expressed health needs of the community.

VIII

All governments should formulate national policies, strategies and plans of action to launch and sustain primary health care as part of a comprehensive national health system and in co-ordination with other sectors. To this end, it will be necessary to exercise political will, to mobilize the country's resources and to use available external resources rationally.

IX

All countries should co-operate in a spirit of partnership and service to ensure primary health care for all people, since the attainment of health by people in any one country directly concerns and benefits every other country. In this context the joint WHO/UNICEF report on primary health care constitutes a solid basis for the further development and operation of primary health care throughout the world.

X

An acceptable level of health for all the people of the world by the year 2000, can be attained through a fuller and better use of the world's resources, a considerable part of which is now spent on armaments and military conflicts. A genuine policy of independence, peace, détente and disarmament could and should release additional resources that could well be devoted to peaceful aims and in particular to the acceleration of social and economic development, of which primary health care, as an essential part, should be allotted its proper share.

The International Conference on Primary Health Care calls for urgent and effective national and international action to develop and implement primary health care throughout the world and particularly in developing countries in a spirit of technical Cupertino and in keeping with a New International Economic Order. It urges governments, WHO and UNICEF, and other international organizations, as well as multilateral and bilateral agencies, non-governmental organizations, funding agencies, all health workers and the whole world community to support national and international commitment to primary health care and to channel increased technical and financial support to it, particularly in developing countries. The Conference calls on all the aforementioned to collaborate in introducing, developing and maintaining primary health care in accordance with the spirit and content of this Declaration.

Table 10.4: Seven features of primary health care (PHC)

No.	Features of PHC	Quotation from Alma Ata declaration
1.	An element of the health system	*Primary* health care... It forms an integral part both of the country's health system... It is the first level of contact of individuals, the family and community with the national health system bringing health care as close as possible to where people live and work, and constitutes the first element of a continuing health care process
2.	Focus on priorities	... essential health care ...
3.	Scientific basis	... based on scientifically sound ...
4.	Culture sensitivity	... socially acceptable methods and technology ...
5.	Equity	... made universally accessible to individuals & families in the community ...
6.	Community participation	... through their full participation ...
7.	Sustainability and self-reliance	... at a cost that the community and the country can afford to maintain at every stage of their development in the spirit of self-reliance and self-determination

CONCLUSION

The contents of this chapter are meant to provide general guidance about the nature and organization of health services. In conclusion, seven points need emphasis:

- Explicit and unequivocal commitment to *equity* as the goal of health development.
- *Science-based and knowledge-based decision-making* at all levels of the health system.
- *The need for planning.* This involves a careful assessment of needs and resources, a definition of goals and a strategy for achieving them.
- *The coverage of the population.* Coverage should be measured in terms of the actual services delivered to the people rather than in terms of buildings, staff and other resources provided.
- *Evaluation.* The performance of the health services should be kept under review, and appropriate adjustments should be made to render them more efficient and more effective in achieving the desired goals.
- *Primary health care.* The pivotal role this plays is the delivery of health services to the community.
- *Community involvement.* This is essential for achieving maximum participation in the planning, organization and implementation of health services.

REFERENCES AND FURTHER READING

Barnum H. & Kutzin J. (1993) *Public Hospitals in Developing Countries: Resource Use, Cost, and Financing.* The Johns Hopkins University Press, Baltimore, MD.

Commission on Health Research for Development (1990) *Health Research: Essential Link to Equity in Development.* Oxford University Press, New York.

Creese A.L. (1991) User charges for health care: a review of recent experience. *Health Policy and Planning* 6(4): 309–319.

Evans T., Whitehead M., Diderichsen F. *et al.* (Eds) (2001) *Challenging Inequities in Health: From Ethics to Action.* Oxford University Press, New York.

Global Forum for Health Research (1999) *The 10/90 Report on Health Research.* Geneva.

Griffiths A. & Bankowolli Z. (Eds) (1980) *Economics and Health Policy.* WHO proceedings of the 13th CIOMS Round Table Conference.

Lucas A.O. (1992) *Public Access to Health Information as a Human Right.* Proceedings of the International Symposium on Public Health Surveillance. *Morbidity & Mortality Weekly Report* 41: 77–78.

McMahon R. (1980) *On Being in Charge. A Guide for Middle-management in Primary Health Care.* WHO, Geneva.

Mejia A. (1980) World trends in health manpower development. A review. *World Health Statistics Quarterly* 33(2).

Montoya-Aguilar C. & Marin-Lira M.A. (1986) Intranational equity in coverage of primary health care: examples from developing countries. *World Health Statistics Quarterly* 39: 336–344.

Murray C.J. (1994) Cost-effectiveness analysis and policy choices: investing in health systems. *Bulletin of the World Health Organization* 72: 663–74.

Murray C.J. (1994) Quantifying the burden of disease: the technical basis for disability-adjusted life years. *Bulletin World Health Organization* 72: 429–445.

Shaw R.P. & Griffin C.P. (1995) *Financing Health Care in Sub-Saharan Africa through User Fees and Insurance.* The World Bank, Washington, DC.

Task Force on Health Research for Development (1991) *Essential National Health Research. A Strategy for Action in Health and Human Development.* United Nations Development Programme, Geneva.

Walsh J.A. & Warren K.S. (1979) Selective primary health care: an interim strategy for disease control in developing countries. *New England Journal of Medicine* 301: 967–974.

WHO (1985) *Health Manpower Requirements for the Achievement of Health for All by Year 2000.* Technical Report Series No. 717. WHO, Geneva.

WHO (1986) *Regulatory Mechanisms for Nursing Training and Practice Meeting Primary Health Needs.* Technical Report Series No. 738. WHO, Geneva.

WHO (1989) *Strengthening the Performance of Community Health Workers in Primary Health Care.* Technical Report Series No. 780. WHO, Geneva.

WHO (1989) *Management of Human Resources for Health.* Technical Report Series No. 783. WHO, Geneva.

WHO (2000) *The Use of Essential Drugs. Ninth Report of the WHO Expert Committee (November 1999). Geneva.* Technical Report Series No. 895. WHO, Geneva.

WHO (2000) *The World Health Report 2000 Health Systems: Improving Performance.* WHO, Geneva.

World Bank (1993) *World Development Report 1993: Investing in Health.* Oxford University Press, New York.

World Bank (1994) *Better Health in Africa: Experience and Lessons Learnt.* The World Bank, Washington, DC.

CHAPTER ELEVEN

APPROACHES TO ECONOMIC EVALUATION

S. Forsythe

- Cost analysis
- Cost-effectiveness analysis (CEA)
- Cost-utility analysis (CUA)

- Cost-benefit analysis (CBA)
- Conclusion
- References and further reading

There is an array of different economic approaches which can be used to evaluate health interventions. The most common approaches are cost analysis, cost-effectiveness analysis (CEA), cost-utility analysis (CUA) and cost-benefit analysis (CBA). Each of these four approaches serves a different purpose. None of these four approaches is right for every situation or for every audience. However, it is important to know when it is appropriate to use each approach, as well as understanding the pitfalls of each.

Both economists and non-economists frequently confuse the different approaches and misuse the corresponding terminology. Therefore this chapter is designed to define and differentiate the various forms of economic analysis, as well as to identify the problems associated with each approach.

As shown in Figure 11.1, cost analysis, CEA, CUA and CBA can be viewed as a continuum of economic evaluations.

Each of these four different forms of economic evaluation have their own advantages and disadvantages, in terms of the resources required to perform the study and the utility of the information to the policy-makers. These four types of economic evaluation are described in greater detail below.

COST ANALYSIS

A cost analysis is the simplest form of economic evaluation, as it involves evaluating costs but does not require estimating the effectiveness of the output produced. Cost analyses are particularly useful for evaluating budgetary requirements or for determining if an intervention is affordable. A cost analysis can also provide a breakdown of costs to describe the current and future cost requirements.

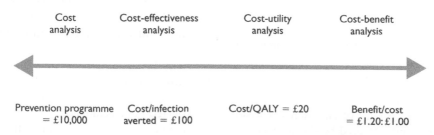

Cost analysis	Cost-effectiveness analysis	Cost-utility analysis	Cost-benefit analysis
Prevention programme = £10,000	Cost/infection averted = £100	Cost/QALY = £20	Benefit/cost = £1.20:£1.00

Figure 11.1: Continuum of economic evaluation.

Cost analyses are most successful when they begin by calculating all the costs used in any way to carry out the intervention. This includes identifying recurrent and capital costs, direct and indirect costs, and fixed and variable costs.

RECURRENT VS CAPITAL COSTS

Recurrent costs refer to any item with a life expectancy of 1 year or less. A capital cost refers to any item that has a life expectancy of more than 1 year. Recurrent items usually include disposable materials, labour, utilities, etc. Equipment, vehicles, furniture and buildings are all considered capital items.

The distinction between recurrent and capital costs is important because it is necessary to spread the cost of a capital item over its expected lifetime in order to combine capital with recurrent costs. It can also be important because some donors will pay for capital costs but will not pay for recurrent costs.

In order to perform an annualization of capital costs, it is necessary to identify each capital item and estimate its replacement value and its remaining life expectancy. It is also necessary to determine an appropriate discount rate that can be used to annualize capital costs.[1] The cost of the capital equipment is then annualized over its expected remaining lifetime using an annualization table.

DIRECT VS INDIRECT COSTS

A direct cost refers to any item that is exclusively used to carry out a particular intervention. Conversely, indirect costs refer to resources which are shared with a variety of other interventions.

If one were to perform a cost analysis of a family-planning unit within a health centre, the family-planning commodities, the direct labour, etc. would all be considered to be direct costs. However, the health centre maintenance staff and receptionist, as well as the overhead costs, would be considered to be indirect costs. These indirect costs should be allocated to the intervention using one of a number of techniques.

---

[1]Determining the appropriate discount rate can be a highly complex technical issue. When in doubt, it is best to identify the discount rate used by similar interventions and to vary this rate in a sensitivity analysis.

While it is often easy to omit indirect costs, it is important to include these costs in the initial data collection. This is particularly the case when it is necessary to evaluate or to recover the full cost of the intervention. It can be difficult to determine the portion of the indirect costs that should be assigned to a particular intervention. For example, what portion of the maintenance staff's time should be allocated to the family-planning service within a health centre? Indirect costs are most often allocated based on the throughput of clients (i.e. when allocating a receptionist's salary) or physical space (i.e. when allocating utility costs).

FIXED VS VARIABLE COSTS

Economists also differentiate between fixed and variable costs when performing cost analyses. The differentiation is made so that projections can be made of how costs will rise with an increase in the amount of health service provided. Fixed costs do not change with small increments in the output produced, while variable costs do. For example, a variable cost would increase as a health centre increased the number of clients that it sees, while the fixed costs will remain the same. Within a health centre, fixed costs generally include equipment, overheads and labour. Variable costs include such items as disposable materials and medication.

Ultimately, cost analyses are most useful when it is only necessary to define how much an intervention costs, now or in the future. A simple cost analysis does not address questions such as 'does this intervention produce good value for money?'

COST-EFFECTIVENESS ANALYSIS (CEA)

An explanation of CEA should begin with a definition of the numerator and the denominator used. The numerator is defined as the cost and should include any cost savings that are expected as a result of the intervention. The denominator, or the measure of effectiveness, can be any measure of output that accurately reflects the totality of what is expected to be achieved.

Cost-effectiveness is a term that is used to compare interventions that have similar goals.

An intervention can only be 'cost-effective' relative to other interventions.

One advantage of the CEA approach is that it can be relatively easy for policy-makers to comprehend (i.e. for every £1000 invested in malaria control, an average of 20 illnesses can be averted). Another advantage to this approach is that the denominator (effectiveness) does not have to be converted into monetary terms. Therefore an economist can avoid the 'political pitfalls' associated with making any direct judgement regarding the value of the life that has been saved.

However, there are various reasons why CEA is problematic.[2] First, in order to compare interventions, it is necessary that all services have the same measure of effectiveness. However, all health services do not necessarily produce one common output. The effectiveness of a hepatitis vaccine might be measured in terms of illnesses averted. The measure of effectiveness for hepatitis care might be the number of patients successfully treated. Thus these two interventions, designed to address the same illness, would not be easily comparable using CEA.

Next, prevention programmes are often extremely difficult to associate with a specific number of illnesses averted (Rowley & Anderson, 1994). In the case of HIV/AIDS, this is due in part to a lack of knowledge about such basic inputs as the probability of transmission for any particular sex act. This problem is confounded by the lack of data regarding the impact that interventions have on 'downstream infections' (i.e. a medicine might cure a case of TB, but it also is likely to subsequently prevent TB infections among the people that the patient would have infected if the patient hadn't been treated). As a result, most models designed to measure the effectiveness of preventing infectious diseases have been unable to reliably estimate the number of infections averted as a result of any particular intervention.

Another problem arises when trying to develop one measure of effectiveness for any one particular service. Unless the measure of effectiveness truly reflects all the benefits of a particular service, it inevitably will underestimate its value. A good example of this would be voluntary counselling and testing (VCT) for HIV, which has been evaluated using CEA (Sweat, 1998). The problem is that the benefits of VCT are much broader than simply the number of infections that are averted. VCT has value because it prevents new infections, but it also has value because it: (i) informs clients; (ii) improves treatment for those who are infected; and (iii) increases discussion and 'normalization' of the epidemic. Thus, narrowly defining the gains of VCT in terms of only HIV infections averted severely underestimates the true value of the service and CEA will not reflect the real value for money invested in the provision of this service.

CEA is also problematic in that it assumes that an intervention has succeeded in preventing or treating an illness for an indefinite period of time. However, as noted by Rehle *et al.* (1998), 'Model estimates on HIV infections averted should be interpreted cautiously, especially in populations with high risk behaviors where the observed behavior changes suggest that the interventions may only postpone the timing of infections rather than prevent infections indefinitely'.

Finally, a CEA does not necessarily reflect the utility of the service from the perspective of the community. In CEAs, the value of each HIV infection averted is of equal value. However, in reality society may not view all lives in equal terms. For example, an intervention that prevents a healthy adult from becoming infected would be determined by the economist performing a CEA to be of equal value to preventing the transmission of HIV from an infected mother to her child. The society, however, may put a very different value on preventing the infection of a child who will be orphaned to the prevention of an adult infection. Thus the health economist is placing a judgement on society that may not reflect that society's valuation.

COST-UTILITY ANALYSIS (CUA)

CUA[3] usually states the denominator of an economic evaluation in terms of quality-adjusted life years saved (QALYS), disability-adjusted life years saved (DALYS), or healthy years equivalent (HYE) rather than illness averted or treated. This approach has been shown to reflect the effectiveness of the

---

[2]For a more detailed assessment of the problems with cost-effectiveness and cost-utility as applied to HIV/AIDS interventions, see Forsythe (1999).

[3]Some economists categorize CUA as a subset of CEA, while others identify CUA as a separate form of evaluation.

intervention in more comprehensive terms since it combines both gains in morbidity and mortality in one measure.

CUA also places interventions in a context of years of life saved rather than simply counting the number of lives saved. For example, a project may succeed in preventing an infection. However, that individual may be at such high risk that they could become infected the following week. A CEA would only indicate that the intervention prevented an infection, while a CUA would reveal that there was only one week's delay in the individual's morbidity.

As illustrated in Figure 11.2, an individual's health can be measured on a scale from 1 (perfectly healthy) to 0 (dead) (tools for measuring quality of life include Euroqol, SF36, SF12, etc.) (Table 11.1 provides an example of the types of questions that are asked to determine a person's quality of life). In this example, this person's health will decline and eventually the person will die without a medical intervention. However, with a medical intervention the person's quality of life will improve and their death will be postponed for a number of years. The difference between the quantity and quality of life with and without the intervention can be measured in terms of QALYS. Programmes that produce the greatest number of QALYS for a given investment of funds are considered to be cost-effective.

In the 1993 World Development Report, the World Bank developed a list of diseases and estimated the average number of DALYS produced by each disease. The diseases with the largest health impact were: (i) respiratory; (ii) diarrhoea; (iii) perinatal causes; (iv) neuropsychiatric diseases; and (v) cancer.

Like CEA, CUA requires a comparison among interventions (however, unlike CEAs, CUAs can be used to compare interventions that deal with different diseases). Ideally, an intervention should be compared to a 'league table' of health interventions measured in terms of their cost/QALY (or DALY or HYE) saved. One problem with this approach is that few countries have such league tables and therefore policy-makers have difficulty determining if an intervention is truly a good investment of limited resources. Policy-makers are left wondering if a CUA represents a comparatively good or poor investment, since they lack the data necessary to compare interventions.

Another problem with this approach is that CUAs fail to have much meaning to most policy-makers or their constituents. A policy-maker who is presented with the 'good news' that their wise investment in health has produced 10 000 QALYS is usually either unimpressed or unable to translate this accomplishment to their constituents. As a result, CUAs are often unsuccessful in convincing policy-makers how they should invest their limited health resources (or the wisdom of public investments already taken).

CUA is also problematic because people not only place value on health outcomes, but also the type of procedure used. As shown in various studies (Berwick & Weinstein, 1985; Grimes, 1988; Ryan, 1996), information has value even if it does not change the eventual treatment proposed. This may be particularly the case of VCT when knowledge of HIV status is likely to have significant value even in the absence of treatment. Thus CUA, like CEA, may seriously underestimate the value of VCT.

Finally, like CEAs, CUAs do not necessarily reflect the utility of the services to the community. Using the example of mother to child transmission of HIV, a CUA might conclude that saving the life of the child would have greater value than saving the life of the mother, since the new-born would have a greater number of future healthy years than the mother. However, as already indicated, the community may place a much greater value on the life of the mother (although it is possible to adjust the discount rate to reflect the value of life to the community, most CUAs instead use a standard discount rate that does not necessarily reflect a

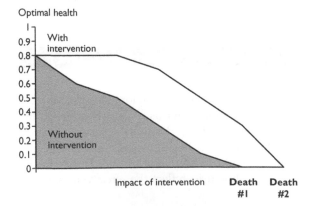

Figure 11.2: Quality-adjusted life years saved (QALYS).

Table 11.1: SF-12 health survey scoring

1. In general, would you say your health is:

Excellent	Very Good	Good	Fair	Poor

The following questions are about activities you might do during a typical day. Does your health now limit you in these activities? If so, how much?

2. Moderate activities, such as moving a table, pushing a vacuum cleaner, bowling, or playing golf

Yes, limited a lot	Yes, limited a little	No, not limited at all

3. Climbing several flights of stairs

Yes, limited a lot	Yes, limited a little	No, not limited at all

During the past 4 weeks, have you had any of the following problems with your work or other regular daily activities as a result of your physical health?

4. Accomplished less than you would like

Yes	No

5. Were limited in the kind of work or other activities

Yes	No

During the past 4 weeks, have you had any of the following problems with your work or other regular daily activities as a result of any emotional problems (such as feeling depressed or anxious)?

6. Accomplished less than you would like

Yes	No

7. Didn't do work or other activities as carefully as usual

Yes	No

8. During the past 4 weeks, how much did pain interfere with your normal work (including both work outside the home and housework)?

Not at all	A little bit	Moderately	Quite a bit	Extremely

These questions are about how you feel and how things have been with you during the past 4 weeks. For each question, please give the one answer that comes closest to the way you have been feeling.
How much of the time during the past 4 weeks…

9. Have you felt calm and peaceful?

All of the Time	Most of the time	A good bit of the time	Some of the time	A little of the time	None of the time

10. Did you have a lot of energy

All of the Time	Most of the time	A good bit of the time	Some of the time	A little of the time	None of the time

11. Have you felt downhearted and blue?

All of the Time	Most of the time	A good bit of the time	Some of the time	A little of the time	None of the time

12. During the past 4 weeks, how much of the time has your physical health or emotional problems interfered with your social activities (like visiting friends, relatives, etc.)?

All of the time	Most of the time	Some of the time	A little of the time	None of the time

community's value). Therefore CUAs do not necessarily reflect the judgement of society regarding the value of different lives saved and therefore may not produce a welfare-maximizing recommendation.

> One weakness of cost-effectiveness analysis is that its theoretical foundation in economic welfare theory is unclear. The classical tool of economic evaluation based on welfare economic theory is cost-benefit analysis, where both costs and health effects are measured in the same units.
>
> (Johannesson, 1995)

Cost-benefit analysis (CBA)

As already mentioned, a CBA puts a monetary value on both the cost of the programme and its output. This produces information that is often more appealing to policy-makers, especially those concerned about assuring value for money. CBA gains from the fact that any intervention can be evaluated on its own merit, rather than requiring a comparison of interventions. CBA also allows programmes which have very different objectives to be compared (i.e. should the government invest in new roads or malaria control?).

> A cost-effectiveness analysis gives the most narrow options for comparison. It may only facilitate comparisons between different ways to treat a specific disease. Cost-utility analysis has been developed to facilitate comparisons between different medical specialties. Cost-benefit analysis offers a direct comparison between costs and outcomes, since both are expressed in monetary terms.
>
> (Johannesson et al., 1996)

While CBA is a theoretically and politically appealing tool, it also faces tremendous obstacles in implementation. The greatest problem with this approach is that it is very difficult and controversial to assign a monetary value to changes in a person's health. For example, should the value of someone's life in a developing country be worth less than the life of someone living in a developed country?

There are currently two primary economic methods of measuring benefits within a CBA: (i) the cost of illness (COI) approach; and (ii) the contingent valuation (CV) approach. Both of these methods are described below.

Cost of illness (COI)

The COI approach involves the measurement of benefits by using two components. The first component, averting direct costs, values the benefit of treating or preventing a disease by the change in the net cost of health care associated with its treatment. The second component in the COI approach is the aversion of indirect costs. The indirect cost of an illness is equated to the value of lost earnings attributable to that illness (Rice, 1966).

For example, assume a case of cancer costs £10 000 to treat and that the patient loses £50 000 in discounted earnings due to the morbidity and premature mortality caused by the illness. Therefore the benefit of averting that illness could be equated to £60 000. A public programme to prevent a case of cancer would be recommended if it cost less than £60 000 per case averted, but would be considered too expensive if it cost more than £60 000.

One of the first studies on the economic impact of HIV/AIDS on developing countries was published using this COI methodology in Tanzania and Zaire (Over et al., 1988). COI was subsequently used in a variety of other developing countries, including Kenya (Forsythe et al., 1992; Leighton, 1993), Malawi (Forsythe, 1993), Mexico (Tapia & Martin, 1990), Honduras (Nuñez et al., 1995) and Thailand (Leighton, 1993). The COI approach has the advantage of being relatively simple for economists to calculate and for policy-makers to understand.

However, for a number of reasons, the COI approach has been viewed as a theoretically inadequate methodology for evaluating the benefits of preventing or treating diseases and has been widely rejected by most economists (Byford et al., 2000).

Some of the problems associated with the COI approach include:

- Direct cost analyses generally ignore the fact that the cost of care does not reflect the full benefits of care to the patient. For example, patients might put a high value on a life-saving drug, but its price would not necessarily reflect that value. In this case, the cost of the treatment does not reflect its benefit to the patient.

- Because it is so influenced by direct costs, COI may inaccurately recommend that life-prolonging treatment should never be pursued, since allowing a patient to die is frequently the least expensive treatment alternative. Thus, even when society puts a high value on treatment strategies, COI will frequently suggest that such treatment is not cost-beneficial.
- Indirect costs are a poor measure of a human being's value, especially of work that is not compensated (i.e. education, home-making, child rearing, etc.). As a result, the value of saving or extending a woman's life, particularly when she is not formally employed, is often underestimated or completely ignored.
- A methodology for determining indirect costs has never clearly been defined (i.e. it remains unclear if the indirect costs should reflect the fact that individuals consume as well as earn. If so, then should an elderly person who consumes but has no potential earnings be considered of negative value?).
- COI assigns a monetary value to an individual's life, and therefore makes some implicit assumptions about the differing values associated with different people's lives (typically it has been assumed in CBA that a wealthier individual's life has greater value than a poor person's, because the loss of a wealthy person would result in greater monetary losses in terms of productivity). Similarly, human life is implicitly assumed to have more value in developed countries than in developing countries when performing COI studies.
- COI does not permit an adequate comparison between diseases. The fact that one disease creates a greater impact than another does not necessarily mean that public funds should be invested in the disease with the greater impact. Instead society may favour equity in health care over reducing the overall impact of disease.
- COI lacks any basis in economic theory. Since any measure of benefits should be capable of satisfying the *pareto criterion*,[4] and future earnings are not necessarily related to such an

improvement, the COI technique does not necessarily reflect the value associated with a change in health (Kenkel, 1994).

...valuing benefits in terms of rates of pay neglects the health benefits that accrue to people who are not employed – for example, non-working wives and retired people. It also ignores the non-financial costs of pain, suffering, and grief that are often associated with illness. But from an economist's perspective, the main criticism of the approach is that it is not based on an individual person's valuations of benefits. Indeed, a third party view is taken about people's 'worth' to society in terms of their productive potential. This viewpoint is inconsistent with the prevailing view among economists that the individual person is the best judge of his or her own welfare.

(Robinson, 1993)

As a result of these and other significant problems with the COI approach, economists have begun to focus their attention on alternative methodologies of evaluating benefits as a part of a CBA.

CONTINGENT VALUATION (CV)

One methodology that has developed as an alternative to the COI approach is CV. CV allows the user of the service (and in some cases the community as a whole) to indicate for themselves how they value a particular service by asking people's willingness to pay (WTP) to obtain that service (or, less commonly, their willingness to accept (WTA) the lack of the health service). The approach resolves some of the problems associated with the COI approach, although it does not resolve all of them.

CV was originally developed as a tool for valuing the environment. However, the technique was subsequently refined to address issues of health care (for a review of the CV technique as applied to health, see Tolley *et al.*, 1994). The CV approach involves creating a hypothetical market for good or services which otherwise could not be readily exchanged.

Some criticize the CV approach on philosophical grounds, arguing that the desires of individuals should not be the major determining factor in

---

[4]An allocation of resources is only 'pareto efficient' if it is impossible to make one person better off without making someone else worse off.

choosing to publicly subsidize a good or service. In other words, policy-makers may prefer to finance public goods based on grounds of paternalism rather than economic demand (Sagoff, 1990).

Another criticism of the CV technique concerns its hypothetical nature (i.e. it's easy to say you would be willing to pay substantial sums to obtain a service, but when actually asked to pay that amount, many people will not). CV is also criticized on logistical grounds, since carrying out surveys of sufficient size is also expensive and extremely complicated (it's less expensive for an economist to value life from his or her desk rather than to get out in the field and actually derive it from the community).

> The advantage of WTP over QALYs stems from the fact that the latter permits the valuation of health gains only. It could be argued that, although health gain is the main attribute of health care, there are other important attributes which QALYs and other health indices do not account for. Such attributes include the 'process of care' which often means more to patient than does clinical outcomes.
>
> (Donaldson & Shackley, 1997)

CONCLUSION

This chapter has attempted to identify some of the advantages and disadvantages of various forms of economic evaluation. It is clear that there is not one technique that is useful for all purposes. Cost analyses are most useful when making simple evaluations or projections, but where it is not necessary to develop a measure of output produced. CEA is most useful when comparing interventions that have a similar output and where it is important to have results that are easy for policy-makers to understand. CUA is most effective when evaluating or comparing health interventions that have an impact on morbidity, mortality, and quality of life. COI is useful when a cost-benefit analysis is required and the measure of benefit needs to be simple and easy to understand. Finally, CV is most useful when a theoretically sound approach to evaluating benefits is required, and where respondents have a clear and realistic understanding of the intervention being described.

REFERENCES AND FURTHER READING

Berwick D. & Weinstein M.C. (1985) What do patients value? Willingness to pay for ultrasound in normal pregnancy. *Medical Care* 23(7): 881–893.

Byford S., Torgerson D.J. & Raftery J. (2000) Cost of illness studies. *British Medical Journal* 320: 1335.

Donaldson C. & Shackley P. (1997) Does 'process utility' exist? A case study of willingness to pay for laparoscopic cholecystectomy. *Social Science and Medicine* 44(5): 699–707.

Forsythe S. (1993) *Economic Impact of HIV and AIDS in Malawi.* AIDSTECH/Family Health International, Durham, NC.

Forsythe S. (1999) The cost-effectiveness of HIV/AIDS interventions: why aren't the policymakers listening? *SafAIDS News* 7(3): 10–15.

Forsythe S., Sokal D., Lux L. et al. (1992) *Assessment of the Economic Impact of AIDS in Kenya.* AIDSTECH/Family Health International, Research Triangle Park, NC.

Grimes D.S. (1988) Value of a negative cervical smear. *British Medical Journal* 296: 1363.

Johannesson M., Jönsson B. & Karlsson G. (1996) Outcome measurement in economic evaluation. *Health Economics* 5: 279–296.

Kenkel D. (1994) *Cost of illness approach.* In: Tolley G., Kenkel D. & Fabian R. (Eds) *Valuing Health for Policy: An Economic Approach.* The University of Chicago Press, Chicago.

Leighton C. (1993) Economic Impacts of the HIV/AIDS Epidemic in African and Asian Settings: Case Studies of Kenya and Thailand. Abt Associates, Inc.

Moses S., Plummer F.A., Ngugi E.N. et al. (1991) Controlling HIV in Africa: effectiveness and cost of an intervention in a high-frequency STD transmitter core group. *AIDS* 5(4): 407–411.

Nuñez C., Flores M., Forsythe S. et al. (1995) El Impacto Socioeconómico del VIH/SIDA en Tegucigalpa y San Pedro Sula, Honduras. Ministerio de Salud Publica de Honduras and AIDSCAP/Family Health International, Tegucigalpa, Honduras and Arlington VA.

Over M., Bertozzi S., Chin J. et al. (1988) The direct and indirect cost of HIV infection in developing countries: The cases of Zaire and Tanzania. In: Fleming A., Carbalo M., FitzSimmons D.W. et al. (Eds) *The Global Impact of AIDS.* Alan R. Liss, New York, pp. 123–125.

Rehle T.M., Saidel T.J., Hassig S.E. et al. (1998) AVERT: a user-friendly model to estimate the impact of

HIV/sexually transmitted disease prevention interventions on HIV transmission. *AIDS* 12(Suppl 2): S27–S35.

Rice D.P. (1966) Estimating the Cost of Illness. US Department of Health, Education and Welfare. Health Economics Series, No. 6. DHEW Pub No. (PHS) 947–6. Rockville, MD.

Robinson R. (1993) Cost-benefit analysis. *British Medical Journal* 307: 924–926.

Rowley J.T. & Anderson R.M. (1994) Modeling the impact and cost-effectiveness of HIV prevention efforts. *AIDS* 8(4): 539–548.

Ryan M. (1996) Using willingness to pay to assess the benefits of assisted reproductive techniques. *Health Economics* 5: 543–558.

Sagoff M. (1990) *The Economy of the Earth: Philosophy, Law and The Environment*. Cambridge University Press, Cambridge.

Sweat M. (1998) The *Cost-Effectiveness of HIV Counseling and Testing*, AIDSCAP/Family Health International, Arlington, Virginia.

Tapia R. & Martin A. (1990) Direct *Cost of AIDS: Current and Projected Resource Requirements in Mexico*. CONASIDA and Family Health International, Mexico City and Durham, NC.

Tolley G. *et al.* (Ed.) (1994) *Valuing Health for Policy: An Economic Approach*. University of Chicago Press, Chicago.

CHAPTER TWELVE

FAMILY HEALTH

- Special health services for women and children
- Maternal health
- Child health
- Integrated management of childhood illness (IMCI)

- Family planning
- Organization of family health services
- School health programme
- References and further reading

This chapter deals with the maternal and child health (MCH) services that are designed to meet the special health needs of women and children. Family health services usually include three components:

- maternal health;
- child health;
- family planning.

SPECIAL HEALTH SERVICES FOR WOMEN AND CHILDREN

The very high level of mortality and morbidity in pregnant women and children in developing countries places them in a high-risk group. Various statistical indicators like infant and child mortality rates, and maternal mortality ratio show the serious health problems that affect this group in developing countries. Box 12.1 summarizes the reasons for the combined services for women and children.

MATERNAL HEALTH

OBJECTIVES OF MATERNAL HEALTH SERVICES

The objectives of the maternal services are to ensure that, as far as possible, pregnant women should:

- remain healthy throughout pregnancy;
- have healthy babies;

- recover fully from the physiological changes that take place during pregnancy and delivery.

In many developing countries, complications of pregnancy and childbirth are the leading causes of death among women of reproductive age. In 1996, WHO and UNICEF estimated that 585 000 women die each year from problems associated with

> **Box 12.1: Family health services – linked risks and joint opportunities**
>
> Why special services for women and children?
>
> - *High-risk groups* – maternal and perinatal conditions together with childhood diseases make a substantial contribution to burden of disease.
> - *Interrelated problems* – the health of the mother and that of the unborn baby are intimately related.
> - *Opportunities for prophylaxis* – some specific health interventions jointly protect pregnant women and their babies, e.g. nutritional supplement during pregnancy, tetanus toxoid immunization.
> - *Early diagnosis* – for both mother and child, early detection and treatment of complications is an important approach for preventing serious complications and death.
> - *Critical care at delivery* – because both the mother and the baby are at high risk during childbirth, it is essential for the delivery to be managed by a skilled person.
> - *Operational convenience* – family health services can provide continuity of care of the child from the womb, jointly with the care of the mother.

Table 12.1: Measures of maternal mortality

Maternal mortality ratio	Maternal mortality rate	Lifetime risk of maternal death
Represents the risk associated with each pregnancy, i.e. the obstetric risk. It is calculated as the number of maternal deaths during a given year per 100 000 live births during the same period. Although the measure has traditionally been referred to as a rate it is actually a ratio and is now usually called such by health practitioners	Measures both the obstetric risk and the frequency with which women are exposed to this risk. It is calculated as the number of maternal deaths in a given period per 100 000 women of reproductive age (usually 15–49 years)	Takes into account both the probability of becoming pregnant and the probability of dying as a result of the pregnancy cumulated across a woman's reproductive years

Table 12.2: Women's risk of dying from pregnancy and childbirth

Region	Risk of dying
All developing countries	1 in 48
Africa	1 in 16
Asia	1 in 65
Latin America & Caribbean	1 in 130
All developed countries	1 in 1800
Europe	1 in 1400
North America	1 in 3700

Box 12.2: What is a maternal death?

A maternal death is the death of a woman while pregnant or within 42 days of termination of pregnancy, regardless of the site or duration of pregnancy, from any cause related to or aggravated by the pregnancy or its management. Maternal deaths are subdivided into direct and indirect obstetric deaths. Direct obstetric deaths result from obstetric complications of pregnancy, labour, or the postpartum period. They are usually due to one of five major causes – haemorrhage (usually occurring postpartum), sepsis, eclampsia, obstructed labour, and complications of unsafe abortion – as well as interventions, omissions, incorrect treatment, or events resulting from any of these. Indirect obstetric deaths result from previously existing diseases or from diseases arising during pregnancy (but without direct obstetric causes), which were aggravated by the physiological effects of pregnancy; examples of such diseases include malaria, anaemia, HIV/AIDS and cardiovascular disease.

pregnancy and childbirth. These deaths occur mainly in developing countries where maternal mortality ratios per 100 000 range from 50 in East Asia to 640 in Africa; whereas they are 20 or less in developed countries. Less than 1% of these deaths occur in developed countries, demonstrating that they could be avoided if resources and services were available. Many of the survivors suffer long-term disabilities such as vesico-vaginal fistulae. The lifetime risk of dying from pregnancy-related disease is 1 in 16 in Africa but only 1 in 4000 in some developed countries (Tables 12.1 and 12.2).

The main causes of these deaths are well known: haemorrhage obstructed labour, sepsis, eclampsia and abortion (Box 12.2 and Fig. 12.1). Technologies for the prevention of these deaths are available and affordable. The challenge is to organize the services to achieve universal coverage with good quality care.

At least 40% of women experience complications during pregnancy, childbirth and the period after delivery. An estimated 15% of these women develop potentially life-threatening problems. Long-term complications can include chronic pain, impaired mobility, damage to the reproductive system and infertility.

MATERNAL HEALTH SERVICES

Ideally, every pregnant woman should have access to a minimal module of maternal health services consisting of three elements:

- community-based services (primary health care);
- essential obstetric care at a first referral centre to deal with complications;

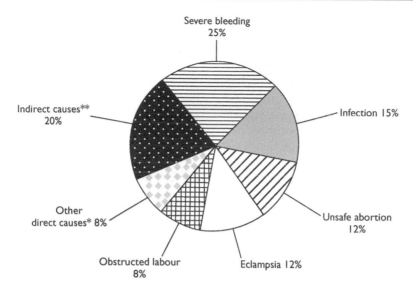

Figure 12.1: Causes of maternal mortality.

- effective communication and transportation between the community-based services and the first referral centre.

The module should link to family planning service and specialist obstetric services at the tertiary level.

Components

The services provided in each community to each community include:

- antenatal care;
- delivery services;
- postnatal care.

ANTENATAL CARE

Previously, a major feature of maternal care was the assessment of risk of each pregnancy based on the woman's previous obstetric history and health status. Special services were offered to high-risk pregnancies including closer supervision during delivery. It has, however, become increasingly clear that complications cannot be accurately predicted nor prevented. Many maternal deaths occur in women whose pregnancies were judged to be low risk. These observations and analyses led to a reformulation of the goals of antenatal care and its content (Box 12.3).

> **Box 12.3: Functions of antenatal care service**
>
> - Preparing the pregnant woman and her family for delivery.
> - Educating the pregnant woman, her family and the community.
> - Assessing and monitoring the health status of the woman and the progress of the pregnancy.
> - Providing appropriate preventive measures – nutritional supplements (iron, folic acid), tetanus immunization, malaria prophylaxis/treatment as indicated.
> - Diagnosis and treatment of complications.

Preparing for delivery

In consultation with the patient and her family, the staff should work out a plan for the delivery of the baby. Where will the birth take place? If, at home, who will be in attendance? Should the situation demand it, how can the woman be transported to a referral centre to deal with complications? This plan should be reviewed and updated during pregnancy.

Education

The visits to the antenatal clinic provide a valuable opportunity for the education of the pregnant woman on how to look after herself during pregnancy, what to expect during labour, and also how to prepare for the care of her new baby. Because of their anxiety to have healthy babies, pregnant women are very attentive and receptive to health education. Health-care providers should take advantage of this interest to engage the women in discussions about relevant issues: nutrition, personal hygiene, and environmental sanitation. They should learn how to obtain a balanced diet using locally available foodstuffs. They should become aware of the dangers associated with dirt, and should appreciate the value of personal hygiene and good environmental sanitation. Apart from lectures and demonstrations at the clinics, where feasible, the community nurse or other health personnel should visit the pregnant woman at home. In this way, she can be guided to use the resources available to her in improving the sanitary condition of her home and in making other preparations for the arrival of the baby.

The pregnant woman should also learn about the normal changes that occur during pregnancy as well as danger signals of serious complications (Box 12.4). The messages about danger signals should be given not only to the pregnant woman but also to her family and influential members of the community. They should all learn to recognize danger signals that call for emergency action. Broad awareness of these facts within the community would facilitate decision making within families.

Preventive measures

Many of the serious ailments occurring in pregnancy are best approached by prophylaxis and/or by early diagnosis and treatment. For example, detecting pre-eclamptic toxaemia at an early stage

---

Box 12.4: Danger signals during pregnancy and childbirth

- Swelling of woman's feet and hands.
- Severe headache or fits.
- Fever.
- Smelly vaginal discharge.
- Vaginal bleeding before labour.
- Any part of the baby showing other than the head.
- Heavy bleeding during or after labour.
- Labour lasting more than one nightfall to one sunrise or vice versa.

---

and taking appropriate action best controls eclampsia. Puerperal and neonatal tetanus are controlled by immunization with tetanus toxoid and ensuring hygienic conditions during delivery and the puerperium. Pregnant women are particularly susceptible to certain infections and diseases. Depending on the local health problems, specific prophylactic measures may be indicated. For example, in an area endemic for malaria, chemoprophylaxis or presumptive treatment (p. 206) may be of vital importance. Active immunization of the pregnant woman with tetanus toxoid is highly effective in preventing neonatal tetanus, a disease that still occurs in communities where the health services are poorly developed. To reduce the incidence of anaemia of pregnancy, supplementary iron and folic acid are usually prescribed. Other prophylactic measures may be indicated by the local situation. The important principle is to do everything possible to improve the general health of the pregnant woman and to anticipate as far as possible any factor that may cause a deterioration in her condition.

Monitoring

Antenatal care provides the opportunity of monitoring the progress of the pregnancy so that any deviations from normal can be detected at an early stage before serious complications occur. The woman is encouraged to note and describe any symptoms or signs that she has observed since her last visit to the clinic and she can be reassured when these do not signify any serious abnormality. Simple indicators have been devised for monitoring pregnancy including measurement of body weight, haemoglobin and blood pressure, examination of urine for protein and sugar, and physical examination including specific obstetric observations.

Where resources exist, more sophisticated investigations (e.g. ultrasound) can be used to follow the development of the foetus and to detect abnormalities. For example, because of the higher risk of Down's syndrome in women over the age of 35 years, obstetricians in developed countries recommend that amniocentesis be done in such cases to offer the possibility of therapeutic abortion if this is acceptable.

DELIVERY SERVICES

The modern trend is for an increasing proportion of births to take place in maternity centres, hospitals and similar institutions. Home delivery may be appropriate for a normal delivery, provided that the person attending the delivery is suitably trained and equipped and that referral to a higher level of care is available in case of complications. Home delivery could be considered after the first pregnancy if the pregnant woman has a clear history of uncomplicated delivery and there are no contrary indications with the current pregnancy.

Since the situation can alter dramatically in the course of delivery, emergency services providing skilled intervention should always be available regardless of the initial estimate of the risk or place of delivery.

Skilled attendant at every birth

A skilled attendant is a doctor, midwife or nurse who has learnt the skills necessary to manage normal deliveries and diagnose or refer obstetric complications. The skilled attendant must be able to manage normal labour and delivery, recognize the onset of complications, perform essential interventions, start treatment, and supervise the referral of mother and baby for interventions that are beyond their competence or not possible in the particular setting. Other health-care providers, such as auxiliary nurse/midwives, community midwives, village midwives, and health visitors, may acquire appropriate skills if they have been specially trained. These individuals frequently form the backbone of maternity services at the periphery, and pregnancy and labour outcomes can be improved by making use of their services, especially if they are supervised by well-trained midwives. All staff who are involved in delivery must receive regular in-service training to ensure that they maintain a high level of performance.

Traditional birth attendants (TBAs)

In many developing countries, traditional birth attendants play an important role in the delivery of pregnant women. These are people, usually women, who have acquired their skill in delivering women by working with other traditional birth attendants and from their own experience. In some countries, formal programmes have been devised for further training of these traditional birth attendants and for incorporating them within the health services. In favour of such schemes is that these attendants usually belong to the local community in which they practise, where they have gained the confidence of the families and where they are content to live and serve. Their training programme is designed to promote safer birth practices, to avoid harmful practices, to improve their technique (with particular reference to cleanliness), to recognize abnormalities which indicate the need for referral for more skilled evaluation and management, and to know their own limitations, thereby refraining from attempting to deal with problems beyond their skill. They are also supplied with simple kits which include hygienic dressings and basic equipment.

However, the education, training and skills of TBAs are not sufficient to fulfil all the requirements for management of normal pregnancies and births, and for identification and management or referral of complications. Their strong cultural and traditional beliefs may influence their practices and thereby impede the effectiveness of their training.

There is no consensus about the appropriate role for TBAs. Because of their limited skills, they should practise in close collaboration with and under the supervision of trained midwives. Their close relationship with the community could be used to advantage in promoting modern midwifery services.

First referral level for obstetric services

Analytical work has shown the crucial role of emergency obstetric care in preventing maternal deaths. The first referral level is the key anchor of community-based maternal health services. This facility is required for dealing with the complications that occur in the course of pregnancy and delivery such as obstructed labour and haemorrhage that require skilled intervention to save the life of the mother and her baby. It is estimated that at least 5% of pregnancies require some form of surgical or skilled obstetric intervention. The first referral level should be equipped to carry out the key functions including emergency obstetric care as listed in Box 12.5.

Maternal deaths occur when women with life-threatening complications do not have timely access to emergency obstetric care. The delays may occur at one or more stages:

■ delay at home in deciding to seek emergency treatment;

- delay in reaching an institution that can provide emergency obstetric care (EmOC);
- delay in providing effective EmOC at the referral institution.

POSTNATAL CARE

During the puerperium the woman recovers from the effects and injuries, if any, associated with delivery. The physiological changes that took place during pregnancy are now being reversed and her body is restored to its prepregnant state. The postnatal care services are designed to supervise this process, to detect any abnormalities and to deal with them. In particular, she should be protected against hazards such as puerperal infection to which she is liable at this stage. Postnatal care may

> ### Box 12.5: Essential obstetric care at the first referral level
>
> - Surgery (e.g. caesarean section).
> - Anaesthesia to support surgical procedures.
> - Medical treatment of complications like diabetes and hypertension.
> - Blood replacement for severe anaemia and cases of haemorrhage.
> - Manual procedures (e.g. removal of placenta, vacuum extraction, forceps delivery).
> - Monitoring and management of women at high risk.
> - Neonatal special care.
> - Family planning support, e.g. sterilization, intrauterine contraceptive devices.

be a convenient service through which to introduce family planning so as to reduce the risk of the early occurrence of another pregnancy, and also to establish breast-feeding.

SAFE MOTHERHOOD

Concern about the high mortality and morbidity associated with pregnancy has led to the development of *safe motherhood* programmes, a global effort that aims to reduce deaths and illnesses among women and infants, especially in developing countries. Specifically aimed at reducing maternal mortality, these programmes are being developed in the wider context of health services for women's reproductive health.

These programmes tackle the clinical causes of maternal deaths – haemorrhage, obstructed labour, infections, eclampsia and complications of induced abortions through improvements in maternal services with special emphasis on emergency obstetric care. However, the terminal events that cause death occur against a background of predisposing factors in the community and within the health services. Figure 12.2 illustrates the complex interaction of medical and non-medical factors that are involved in perpetuating the high maternal mortality rates occurring in the developing world. Child marriages of preteen age is associated with serious complications during pregnancy and delivery. Female genital mutilation (circumcision) is another cultural behaviour that carries serious implications for women's reproductive health. It also offers clues as

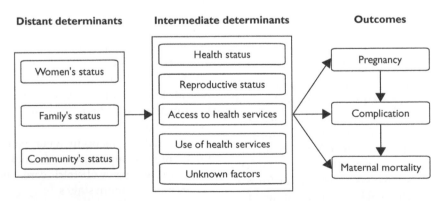

Figure 12.2: The complex interaction of factors involved in the epidemiology of maternal mortality.
Source: McCarthy & Maine 1992.

Box 12.6: A seven-point programme for safe motherhood

1. **Information**	Expand and strengthen the information base about reproductive health.
2. **Advocacy**	Disseminate relevant information about reproductive health to those who need to take action.
3. **Education**	Expand educational opportunities for girls and promote family life education for the general population.
4. **Women's status**	Improve the social, economic and legal status of women.
5. **Family planning**	Encourage women to regulate their fertility and provide access to family planning services.
6. **Health care**	Ensure that all pregnant woman receive adequate care during pregnancy and childbirth.
7. **Research**	Promote research aimed at obtaining a clearer definition of maternal health, the determinants of morbidity and mortality including operational factors, as well as the development of new technologies.

---

to the package of interventions that are required to reduce maternal mortality. WHO is promoting the concept of the 'mother–baby package' which consists of a cluster of interventions including family planning to prevent unwanted and mistimed pregnancies, basic maternity care for all pregnancies, and special care for the prevention and management of complications during pregnancy, delivery and postpartum for the mother and her newborn baby.

Essential services for safe motherhood

Services for safe motherhood should be readily available through a network of linked community health-care providers, clinics and hospitals:

- community education on safe motherhood;
- prenatal care and counseling, including the promotion of maternal nutrition;
- skilled assistance during childbirth;
- care for obstetric complications, including emergencies;
- postpartum care;
- management of abortion complications, post-abortion care and, where abortion is not against the law, safe services for the termination of pregnancy;
- family planning counseling, information and services;
- reproductive health education and services for adolescents.

Box 12.6 gives a model list of elements that would feature in a national *safe motherhood* programme.

Box 12.7: Safe motherhood – a matter of human rights and social justice

Empowerment is critical to securing safe motherhood because it enables women to:

- **articulate** their health needs and concerns;
- **access** services with confidence and without delay;
- **seek** accountability from service providers and programme managers, and from governments for their policies;
- **act** to reduce gender bias in families, communities and markets;
- **participate** more fully in social and economic development.

EMPOWERING WOMEN

The factors that place women at great disadvantage must be tackled as long-term interventions and development goals. Empowering women means enabling them to overcome social, economic and cultural factors that limit their ability to make fully informed choices, particularly in the areas affecting the most intimate aspect of their lives – their reproductive health. Women must have the means, both physical and psychological, to overcome the barriers to safe motherhood. Central to all empowerment is choice, and far too many women still have far too few choices. Box 12.7 indicates the relevance of the empowerment of women, their human rights, and social justice to the achievement of safe motherhood.

CHILD HEALTH

The past few decades have witnessed major improvements in the health of children throughout the world. The Child Survival programmes that UNICEF and WHO spearheaded have made significant contributions to the dramatic fall in child mortality rates in most developing countries (Fig. 12.3). The main interventions are usually summarized under the acronym, GOBI-FFF (growth monitoring, oral dehydration, breast-feeding, immunization, family planning, female education and supplementary feeding of pregnant women). Much remains to be done in reducing the avoidable mortality and morbidity; in developed countries, the under five mortality rate has been reduced below 10 per 1000 live births but many developing countries still record rates that are over 100 per 1000. Many of the diseases that cause severe illness and death in children in developing countries can be prevented or treated by simple affordable measures provided through simple efficient child health services. In order to be most effective, the services must reach all the children, with particular attention to the most vulnerable groups.

OBJECTIVES

The three major objectives of the child health services are to:

- *Promote the health of children* to ensure that they achieve optimal growth and development both physical and mental.

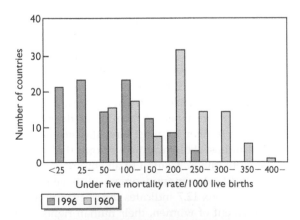

Figure 12.3: Under five mortality rates: changes from 1960 to 1996. Source: WHO (1998).

- *Protect children from major hazards* through specific measures (immunization, chemoprophylaxis, dietary supplements) and through improvement in the level of care provided by the mothers and the family.
- *Treat diseases and disorders* with particular emphasis on early diagnosis. The aim is to provide an effective remedy at an early stage before dangerous complications occur.

Promotion of health: monitoring development

The growth and development of each child should be carefully monitored. It is important that the child be seen at the clinic regularly during the first 5 years of life. The mother should be guided on matters concerning the child's diet, hygiene and other factors affecting the child's health and safety. Simple charts showing graphs of the normal growth curve can be used effectively in monitoring the child's physical development (see Fig. 9.2). Experience has shown that it is better for each mother to retain her child's growth card: it increases her involvement in monitoring the child's development. Methods and indices used in monitoring growth have been described in Chapter 9.

Protection: immunization, chemoprophylaxis, dietary supplements

Immunization of children is one of the most cost-effective public health interventions. WHO and UNICEF estimate that childhood immunization saves 3 million lives. But 30 million children do not complete the standard course of immunization. Greater coverage with immunization could save another 3 million lives (Table 12.3).

IMMUNIZATION

Each child should be immunized against the common communicable diseases for which vaccines are available. Immunization is routinely offered against tuberculosis (BCG), tetanus, whooping cough, diphtheria, poliomyelitis and measles. The choice of vaccine and the immunization schedule should be selected on the basis of local epidemiological situations, and on the most practicable routine. Box 12.8 summarizes WHO recommendations on schedules for routine vaccination and Table 12.4

gives information about individual vaccines. A new international programme, the Global Alliance for Vaccines Initiative (GAVI) is helping countries to strengthen their immunization programmes. Those countries that have achieved good coverage with standard vaccines are being supported to introduce the newer, somewhat more expensive vaccines: hepatitis B and *Haemophilus influenzae* B.

Table 12.3: Potential lives saved through infant immunization

Disease	Number of preventable annual deaths (estimated)
Hepatitis B	900 000
Measles	888 000
Tetanus (including 215 000 neonatal deaths)	410 000
Haemophilus influenzae type B (HiB)	400 000
Pertussis (whooping cough)	346 000
Yellow fever	30 000
Diphtheria	5000
Polio	720
Total	**2 979 720**

The vaccines should be handled with care to ensure that they preserve their potency. This is particularly important in the case of live vaccines that are sensitive to heat and must therefore be kept cold until administered. By the use of refrigerators at the main health centres and insulated cold boxes when the vaccine is being carried for use in the field, the continuous 'cold chain' can be preserved.

SAFETY OF VACCINATION

On the whole, immunization is highly effective, cost-effective and safe, but safety precautions must be taken to avoid risks, especially during mass campaigns. Ideally, the injection equipment should be disposable and not reused to obviate the risk of cross-infections. Because of the risk of cross-infections, the old fashioned method of reusing syringes and needles after sterilization is no longer recommended nor is the multidose jet injector gun. New technologies include:

- *auto-destruct syringes and needles* which eliminate improper reuse;
- *prefilled monodose disposable 'pouch and needle' injection devices* assure the integrity of the vaccine or drug content and also prevents reuse;

Box 12.8: National immunization schedules for infants

WHO recommends that children should be immunized as early in life as possible to protect them against vaccine-preventable diseases in their country. Because the epidemiological situation varies from country to country, the model schedule below has been adapted in some way by most countries so that it more closely meets their needs. None the less it provides a useful general guide.

The immunization schedule for infants recommended by the WHO Expanded Programme on Immunization:

Age	Vaccine	Hepatitis B vaccine* (two alternative schemes)	
		Alternative A	Alternative B
Birth	BCG, OPV-0	HB-1	
6 weeks	DPT-1, OPV-1	HB-2	HB-1
10 weeks	DPT-2, OPV-2		HB-2
14 weeks	DPT-3, OPV-3	HB-3	HB-3
9 months	Measles, yellow fever**		

OPV, oral polio vaccine; DPT, diphtheria, pertussis, tetanus triple vaccine; HB, hepatitis B vaccine; BCG, vaccine against tuberculosis.
*Schedule A is recommended in countries where perinatal transmission of HBV is frequent (e.g. South East Asia), and scheme B in countries where perinatal transmission is less frequent (e.g. sub-Saharan Africa).
**In countries where yellow fever poses a risk. Measles vaccine is usually given at 12–15 months of age in industrialized countries where the threat of the disease comes after the first year of life. Such a policy benefits from the increased vaccine efficacy after 1 year of age. The vaccine is often combined with rubella and/or mumps vaccine when it is referred to as MR or MMR vaccine. Specific inquiries about a country's immunization schedule should be referred to the national or local authorities.

Table 12.4: A guide to childhood immunizations in the tropics. After R.G. Hendrickse.

Vaccine	Recommended age of administration	Method of administration	Special problems associated with use	Other comments
Routine programme				
BCG (live, attenuated bovine strain)	Neonatal period as a routine Tuberculin-negative subjects of any age exposed to mycobacterial infections	Intradermal injection (multiple-puncture using modified Heaf Gun recommended for use by semi-skilled personnel)	Vaccine light and heat sensitive – risk of inactivation in unskilled hands	Isoniazid-resistant BCG may be used in conjunction with isoniazid chemotherapy
Triple antigen (DPT) (combined tetanus and diphtheria toxoids and pertussis vaccine)	Start at 2 months. Give 3 injections at monthly intervals. Boosters at 12–18 months and at school	Subcutaneous or intramuscular injection	Rarely encephalitis due to pertussis component	Where high risk of pertussis, can start at age of 1 month. Tetanus toxoid to all unprotected adults especially during pregnancy to prevent neonatal tetanus
Poliomyelitis: killed Salk vaccine	Start at 2 months and monthly × 3. Fourth dose at school entry	Subcutaneous or intramuscular injection	None	May be simultaneously administered with triple antigenin spearate syringe unless a combined vaccine is used. Best for small local clinics
Poliomyelitis: live Sabin vaccine	Start at 2 months and monthly × 3. Fourth dose at school entry	Oral	Cool storage required. May get poor antibody response when used on small groups in tropics	Most effective when mass vaccination campaigns undertaken (National Immunization Day)
Measles (further attenuated vaccine)	8 months	Subcutaneous injection	Refrigerated storage required	Mass campaigns being used for elimination programmes
Epidemic control				
Cholera (whole cell vaccine)	All ages – two doses	Subcutaneous or intramuscular injection		For mass immunization – one dose. No clear evidence of value in controlling epidemics
Menigococcal vaccines A, W135, C*	All ages	Subcutaneous		Depends on the particular immuno-type of the organism*
Yellow fever**	All except infants under 1 year	Subcutaneous	Encephalitis, particularly infants under 1 year	

*In countries where the predominant strain of *Neisseria meningitidis* is type C, three doses of a conjugated vaccine are immunogenic and safe in infants and are recommended for routine use, as part of EPI. Differing epidemiological conditions in various countries may require relevant alterations to these guidelines.

**This vaccine is now recommended as part of EPI in yellow fever endemic areas.

- *needle-free injection systems with disposable syringes* – this new device also eliminates risk from accidental needle prick.

Sound hygienic practices must be enforced even where the vaccines are being delivered in mass campaigns in the field. A few specific contraindications to routine immunization must be observed but generally, most children at the appropriate age should receive the routine immunization according to the national guidelines.

CHEMOPROPHYLAXIS AND DIETARY SUPPLEMENTS

In endemic areas of malaria, chemoprophylaxis is usually recommended for the highly susceptible groups including preschool children, pregnant women and visitors. Other specific prophylactic measures may be indicated as for example, the use of dietary supplements to prevent common nutritional deficiencies (see p. 264). Vitamin A deficiency causes xerophthalmia and it also has harmful effects on the immune response. It is estimated that 250 million young children have low blood levels of vitamin A but no eye signs. This subclinical deficiency has serious consequences on mortality and morbidity. It has been proved that giving supplements of vitamin A to young children who are deficient:

- significantly reduces death rates;
- particularly reduces complications and mortality in measles;
- seems to have a greater impact on diarrhoea (by reducing severity) than on respiratory diseases.

A trial in Nepal showed reduction in pregnancy-related deaths in women who received low-dose supplements of vitamin A. This observation is being tested at other sites.

Early diagnosis and treatment

Simple remedies should be made available for the treatment of the common diseases of childhood. Mothers should be encouraged to seek treatment early and where appropriate to institute simple therapy at home. They should for example learn how to clean simple cuts and abrasions, covering them with clean dressings to prevent infection. Especially in areas where they cannot gain rapid access to the clinic, mothers should learn how to prepare and administer the oral rehydration fluid in cases of diarrhoea (see p. 165 and below for a description of the integrated management of childhood illness).

INTEGRATED MANAGEMENT OF CHILDHOOD ILLNESS (IMCI)

For many sick children a simple diagnosis is often neither possible nor appropriate, for example a child presenting with cough and/or fast breathing may have pneumonia, severe anaemia, *Plasmodium falciparum* malaria or a combination of these conditions. The WHO Departments of Child and Adolescent Health and Development (CAH) and UNICEF have developed the integrated management of childhood illness (IMCI) in response to this challenge. Both agencies are actively promoting the rights of children to health and health care spelled out in the UN Convention on the Rights of the Child. The IMCI strategy is an active move to give effect to the articles concerned. It is a combination of: (i) improved management of childhood illness; (ii) improved nutrition; (iii) immunization; (iv) breast-feeding support; (v) vitamin A and micronutrient supplementation; (vi) use of insecticide impregnated nets; and (vii) compliance with treatment.

The above combination of interventions is aimed at improving practices both in the health facilities and at home and IMCI can be modified to include specific conditions that may be important in individual countries and for which effective interventions are available.

Integrated case management guidelines have been developed for use by health workers from a wide variety of backgrounds and experience.

Systems have been devised to teach patients what to do if their children fall ill – how to look after them at home, where and when to go if they are ill and the importance of following treatment advice.

Introducing IMCI into the health services is a phased process that requires adaption and co-ordination among existing health services.

SPECIAL SERVICES

Ideally, health services should reach every child within the community. This may be achieved through a combination of postnatal care, child health services, vaccination programmes and school health services (see p. 332). It is particularly important that these services identify the most vulner-able or the high-risk groups. The factors that most accurately identify the high-risk groups are best determined locally by epidemiological studies but in general high risk is associated with factors in the mother (e.g. illiteracy, poverty, past history of a child who had died) and in the child (e.g. low birth weight, haemoglobinopathy). Special attention should be given to such children, with support to the family by home visits and other measures designed to improve the level of care at home.

It may be useful to provide special services for children who have specific health problems. For example, a nutrition rehabilitation service would help to supervise the recovery of malnourished children and educate the mothers on the nutrition of their children. Services may also be provided for handicapped children, for those who are mal-adjusted or have emotional problems. The current trend is to support handicapped children with community-based services and to accommodate them as far as possible in ordinary schools; the success of such schemes depends on educating teachers, other schoolchildren and the community at large about the value of the community-based arrangements.

FAMILY PLANNING

OBJECTIVES

The objective of this service is to encourage couples to take responsible decisions about pregnancy and enable them to achieve their wishes with regard to:

- preventing unwanted pregnancies;
- securing desired pregnancies;
- spacing of pregnancies;
- limiting the size of the family.

The concept of responsible parenthood should be promoted and in the interest of the health of the family, couples should have children by choice and not by chance.

Family-planning services should be used as a tool for promoting family health and specifically for reducing maternal morbidity and mortality by preventing unwanted and high-risk pregnancies. To this end, the services should target women with serious underlying medical problems, grand multi-parae, couples who have achieved their desired family size, sexually active teenagers and any others who need or wish to avoid pregnancy. The programme should also raise community aware-ness of the need to plan families; it should pay par-ticular attention to the role of males in deciding the desired size and in choosing acceptable means of achieving the goal. Family-planning services may also provide genetic counselling (see p. 251).

Family-planning programmes are best designed in the context of promoting women's reproductive health and meeting the needs of women's health. This broader view of women's health has been developed through a series of international confer-ences. The Beijing Declaration and Platform for Action that was adopted at the Fourth World Conference on Women (4–15 September 1995) by representatives from 189 countries reflects a new international commitment to the goals of equality, development and peace for all women everywhere (Box 12.9).

ASSESSMENT OF COMMUNITY NEEDS

The family-planning programme should be based on an analysis of the needs of the community. Available data on the reproductive behaviours of the community should be carefully examined not-ing especially: birth rates in various groups, age of first pregnancy, average interval between pregnan-cies, family size, the use of contraceptive methods (both traditional and modern), knowledge of these methods and attitudes to them, the frequency of induced abortions and other indications of unwanted pregnancies.

WHO estimates that 120 million married women have unmet needs; 40–50 million women resort to abortions and that 300 million couples are not satis-fied with the methods used resulting in 8–30 million unintended pregnancies. Millions of individuals

Box 12.9: The Beijing Declaration and Platform for Action

12 critical areas of concern for women's advancement and empowerment:

1. Poverty
2. Education and training
3. Health
4. Violence
5. Armed conflict
6. Economy
7. Decision-making
8. Institutional mechanisms
9. Human rights
10. Media
11. Environment
12. The girl-child

The Platform for Action defines strategic objectives and spells out actions to be taken by governments, the international community, non-governmental organizations and the private sector.

who want and need family-planning care still do not have access to quality services that would ensure the safe and effective provision of methods based on the informed choice of the user.

CONTRACEPTION

In the context of family health, the family-planning service should make available simple, effective and safe contraceptive methods that are compatible with the family's religion and culture, and also in keeping with their needs and resources. For religious reasons, some couples cannot accept artificial methods and devices; the natural method based on the safe period should be taught to them. A variety of contraceptive devices should be available so that each couple can select the method that is most aesthetically acceptable and practicable in their circumstances. The use of condoms as a barrier contraceptive method is being advocated because of the additional benefit in preventing the transmission of HIV and other sexually transmitted diseases. Barriers to access to effective use of family-planning services, even where they exist in the community include logistic, social and behavioural factors; some medical and procedural

obstacles also impede access; and outdated policies and eligibility criteria also discourage women from using methods of their choice.

ORGANIZATION OF FAMILY HEALTH SERVICES

For reasons stated in the early part of the chapter, it is generally preferable to provide an integrated service comprising maternal, child health and family-planning services.

ACCESSIBILITY

The details of the organization would vary from place to place, but the important issue is to make sure that the services are provided in such a way that the community can make the best use of them. Rather than having a rigid format, the health personnel should seek innovative ways of promoting the coverage and the quality of care. For example, adjustments in the timing of clinics could make the service more easily accessible to the mothers: it may be particularly convenient if the services are provided in association with markets and other community activities. Special arrangements may have to be made for women who are unable to utilize the normal services. For example in Moslem communities, women in Purdah may not be able to go out to the clinics in the day time but could do so at night: evening clinics at convenient sites could solve this particular problem. The programme should pay particular attention to families that do not spontaneously use such services as the antenatal clinic; such persons may be at much greater risk than users. The goal should be to reach all families.

COMMUNITY PARTICIPATION

For the family health services, more than for any other component of the health services, the intimate involvement of the community is essential in making the best decisions. The resources of the community should be fully utilized, for example training and using voluntary health workers, and health education through women's associations.

EVALUATION

Continuous monitoring and evaluation should be built into the family health services using simple but informative indicators. Programme managers should monitor the processes (services provided, activities of the health personnel), the outputs (utilization and performance of services) and impact (changes in the health status of women and children morbidity and mortality rates).

Processes

To what extent are health centres and hospitals equipped to provide emergency obstetric care: drugs, equipment, blood transfusion, etc.? Are services available to communities for providing all the elements of the GOBI-FFF strategy? Are the staff at dispensaries and health centres trained to immunize children, manage common simple illnesses, recognize more serious conditions that require referral?

Output

The coverage of each major component of the services should be measured. For example, what proportion of pregnant women within the community is seen at least once during pregnancy? What proportion of them deliver under supervision of the health personnel? What proportion of children receive the standard vaccines, and what proportion completes the full course?

Impact

The standard rates used in health statistics should be calculated, for example perinatal mortality, infant mortality, neonatal mortality, etc. The incidence of measles, paralytic poliomyelitis, severe diarrhoea, and other important diseases of children would also provide useful indicators of the health of the child population. It is not feasible to monitor each and every condition and the inclusion of too many elements may reduce the efficiency of the system. It is much better to select a few indicators, concentrating for example on the top 10 killing diseases in childhood.

With regard to maternal health, the number of maternal deaths in each community is very low and cannot be used for monitoring the impact of maternal health services and changes over time. It is better to use process and output indicators.

Regardless of the indicators that are selected, it is important to relate the cases or events to the population at risk. It is difficult to interpret such data (e.g. number of children immunized, number of deliveries at maternity centres, cases of measles) unless they are related to the appropriate denominators.

SCHOOL HEALTH PROGRAMME

It is universally recognized that the health of schoolchildren deserves special attention. In order to derive the maximum benefit from the educational programme, the child must be healthy physically, mentally and emotionally. Children at school are exposed to a variety of hazards – physical injury, infection and emotional problems. School age is a period during which the child is undergoing rapid physical and mental development; a healthy environment is required to provide the child with the best opportunity of making the appropriate adjustments that are required during this critical period. The school provides a unique opportunity for health education: a means of establishing a firm foundation for the healthy habits of the future adult population. By safeguarding the health of the schoolchildren of today, one is ensuring the health of the adults of tomorrow. In many developing countries the need for good school health programmes is particularly critical.

Apart from the universal reasons already cited for having a special programme for schoolchildren, there is the additional factor that in many developing countries, the schoolchildren are the survivors of a high childhood mortality. Many of them still bear the sequelae of the diseases which were responsible for the deaths of the other children and most are still subject to the environmental conditions which predisposed to the high morbidity and mortality of preschool age groups. The overall objective of the school health programme is to ensure that every child is as healthy as possible so as to obtain the full benefit from his or her education.

COMPONENTS

Although the detailed organization of a school health programme varies from place to place, the following elements are usually represented:

- medical inspection;
- assessment of handicapped children;
- health education;
- safe school environment;
- nutrition.

Medical inspection

Routine, periodic medical examination is designed to detect defects that require medical attention. The medical examination also provides the opportunity of discussing with parents and teachers the health problems and needs of the children. It includes screening for defects of hearing and sight. The school examination will ascertain whether the child is fit to take part in school activities, including sports.

Assessment of handicapped children

The school health programme must include some mechanism for finding children who are physically or mentally handicapped, assessing them, supervising them and placing them in the most appropriate institution if special care is indicated. The main categories of handicapped children are:

- blind and partially sighted;
- those with a defect in hearing and/or speech;
- epileptic;
- educationally subnormal;
- maladjusted and psychotic;
- physically handicapped or delicate.

Health education

The objective of the health education programme at school is to make the children value health as a desirable asset, and to know what the individual and the community can do to maintain and promote health. At this impressionable age, the aim is to ingrain in children healthy lifestyles with regard to such issues as diet, exercise, abuse of alcohol, smoking, use of illegal drugs, and unsafe sex. The course of instruction would include basic information about the normal structure and function of the human body, the agents of disease, and the role of the environment in maintaining good health. At the appropriate age, various aspects of sex education can be incorporated into the syllabus. All fit children should participate in a well-designed programme of physical education.

Safe school environment

It is necessary to ensure that the school environment is maintained at a high standard in order to safeguard the health of the children and to provide them with a practical example of healthy living. The school environment must reinforce the theoretical lessons learnt in the classes. The school should be sited in a safe place, in an area free from excessive noise and other nuisances such as smoke or soot. The building should be well constructed so as to minimize accidents. The classrooms should be of adequate size, well lit and ventilated. Sanitary facilities for the disposal of waste should be provided, and there should be an adequate supply of safe water for drinking and washing. There should be adequate facilities for recreation.

CONTROL OF INFECTIONS

Going to school represents for many children the first opportunity to mix with children other than close relatives and immediate neighbours. Hence, schooling often represents their first contact with infections to which they are susceptible. The control of infection includes the exclusion of sick children from school and the protection of susceptible children against such infections as polio, diphtheria and typhoid by immunization. The school health service should provide a routine vaccination programme. Parents should be urged not to send sick children to school and teachers should, in the course of daily inspection of the children, note any sign of illness. The health of the schoolteachers and other school personnel should be kept under careful observation to ensure that they do not transmit infection to the children. For example, schoolteachers should be routinely screened for tuberculosis and food handlers for enteric infections.

Deworming

There is some evidence indicating infestation with intestinal helminths may affect the cognitive skills of school children in addition to causing other physical damage. Even if the degree of mental impairment attributable to helminthic infection is not as severe as suggested from some studies, it is still a good idea to deworm infested children. In cases where the prevalence is high, one should consider selective targeted mass chemotherapy using a broad-spectrum anthelminthic.

Nutrition

The school health programme should include some mechanism for the promotion of adequate diet for schoolchildren. It should be designed to ensure that each child is adequately nourished and, where specific defects are noted, to provide some means of supplementation. Some health education of parents should be included, either through group activities such as the parent–teacher associations, or individually in cases of special problems. It may be useful to have a school meal programme: this can provide a valuable demonstration of good balanced diets, but the school meal can also be specifically designed to supplement the child's home diet in such a way as to make up any major specific nutritional deficiencies. Practical instruction in nutrition can include the growing of food crops in the school garden and mother-craft and cookery classes, especially for the girls.

SPECIAL SURVEYS

Special epidemiological surveys can be conducted to investigate specific health problems. They can also be used as part of the assessment of health needs and evaluation of the school health programme.

ORGANIZATION OF SCHOOL HEALTH SERVICES

The detailed organization of the school health programme varies from one country to another. In the more developed countries, the school health services employ numerous doctors, dentists, nurses, psychologists, speech therapists and other skilled personnel. In most developing countries, such elaborate schemes are not in operation. The objective in each country should be to exploit the available resources and co-ordinate them into a national school health programme.

The following services are usually provided in school health programmes:

- medical inspection;
- screening tests for defects;
- clinics for the treatment of minor ailments; consultation; special clinics (e.g. orthopaedic, ophthalmic, ENT and child guidance);
- dental services – preventive and therapeutic.

CO-ORDINATION

The health care of the child at school requires the co-ordinated efforts of parents, teachers, school health personnel, family physicians and local health authorities. Each has an important role to perform; skilled dovetailing of these various units will provide the most effective school health programme. Since there are overlapping functions in several areas, it is important to avoid unnecessary duplication of effort especially where resources are scarce. Careful definition of roles and delineation of functions will help to prevent conflict and friction.

The provision of a safe, healthy environment is the responsibility of the school authorities. They are also responsible for health education and physical education at school. The personnel of the school health programme are responsible for the medical inspection of the children; in some places they also undertake treatment but in other countries any defect or illness is treated by the family physician. The school health personnel are also responsible for the control of communicable diseases, although again the family physician may be responsible for immunization of the children. In developing countries, medical auxiliaries who are working under the supervision of doctors perform many of these functions.

ASSESSMENT AND EVALUATION

Evaluation of the school health programme depends in the first instance on a careful definition of the objectives of the programme.

Input

There should be an assessment of the work load of the various units: the number of medical inspections, the number of cases treated at the clinics, the number of children immunized, the number of school meals served, etc.

Output

The health status of the children can be assessed from an analysis of the data gathered at the medical inspections, from sickness records and from special surveys. The data generated in the operation of the school health service should be compiled and analysed. Such information as the distribution of the heights and weights of the children, the haemoglobin level, and the frequency of dental caries can provide valuable assessment of the health of the children and the effectiveness of the school health programme.

REFERENCES AND FURTHER READING

Convention on the Rights of the Child (1989) United Nations General Assembly Resolution A/RES/44/25. United Nations, New York.

Expanded Programme on Immunization (1988) Contra-indications for vaccines used in EPI. *Weekly Epidemiological Record* 63: 279–281.

Maine D. (Ed.) (1997) Prevention of maternal mortality network. *International Journal of Gynecology and Obstetrics* 59 (Suppl 2): 1–226.

McCarthy J. (1997) The conceptual framework of the PMM network. *International Journal of Gynecology and Obstetrics* 59 (Suppl 2): S15–S22.

McCarthy J. & Maine D. (1992) A framework for analyzing the determinants of maternal mortality. *Studies in Family Planning* 23: 23–33.

Rosenfield A. & Maine D. (1985) Maternal mortality – a neglected tragedy. Where is the M in MCH? *Lancet* 2(8446): 83–85.

Universal Declaration of Human Rights (1948) United Nations General Assembly Resolution, A/RES/217 A(III). United Nations, New York.

WHO (1975) *Evaluation of Family Planning Services.* Technical Report Series No. 569. WHO, Geneva.

WHO (1976) *Statistical Indices of Family Health.* Technical Report Series No. 578. WHO, Geneva.

WHO (1978) *Induced Abortion.* Technical Report Series No. 623. WHO, Geneva.

WHO Family Health (1986) *Essential Obstetric Functions at First Referral Level to Reduce Maternal Mortality.* WHO, Geneva.

WHO (1995) Vaccination Policy. WHO/EPI/GEN/95.03. WHO, Geneva.

WHO (2000) *The World Health Report 2000. Health Systems: Improving Performance.* WHO, Geneva.

WHO/UNICEF (1996) *Revised 1990 Estimates of Maternal Mortality, a New Approach by WHO and UNICEF.* World Health Organization/United Nations Children's Fund.

WHO/UNICEF (1997) Integrated management of childhood illness. *Bulletin World Health Organization* 75 (Suppl 1).

CHAPTER THIRTEEN

ENVIRONMENTAL HEALTH

N. Roche

- Water supply
- Excreta disposal
- Waste management
- Vector control
- Shelter/housing and site planning

- Hygiene education
- Food safety and hygiene
- Protection from radiation
- Air pollution
- References and further reading

Environmental health comprises of those aspects of human health, including quality of life, that are determined by physical, chemical, biological, social and psychosocial factors in the environment. It also refers to the theory and practice of accessing, correcting, controlling and preventing those factors in the environment that can potentially affect adversely the health of present and future generations.

(Fitzpatrick and Kappos, 1999)

'Environmental Health relates to the impact the environment can have on a population. The environment refers to both the natural environment and the human created environment.

The natural environment on its own may create problems for human health as evidenced by temperature fluctuations and such natural events as forest fires, tidal waves and landslides. For example a heat wave may result in cases of heat stroke and forest fires will produce smoke resulting in respiratory problems.

The created environment also poses many risks to health. For example the slum areas of many cities are in themselves a health hazard due to poor housing and poor availability of water and sanitation.

People engaged in the sector of Environmental Health are working towards the protection of people from hazardous environments and the promotion of healthy environments.'

The definition described above is a draft definition produced by WHO at a consultation meeting held in Sofia, Bulgaria in October 1993.

The sector is very broad and covers a multitude of disciplines, both within and outside the health services. In the European context one is more likely to see reference to additional topics such as occupational health and safety, transport management, noise control and environmental impact assessment, but in relation to the tropics the main areas to cover are the following:

- water supply;
- excreta disposal;
- waste management;
- vector control;
- shelter/housing and planning;
- hygiene education;
- food safety/hygiene;
- protection from radiation;
- air quality/control of pollution.

Many of these problems are dealt with by non-health-sector professionals such as civil engineers and town planners.

WATER SUPPLY

Water is a basic human right and essential need. It has many uses including the irrigation of crops, the generation of electricity and for transport such as canals. In terms of protecting human health we are mostly concerned with the use of fresh water for domestic purposes. WHO currently estimates that over 1.1 billion people worldwide still lack access to an adequate supply of clean water.

Uses of water in the domestic setting include:

- drinking;
- personal hygiene;
- cleaning, e.g. cooking utensils;
- gardening, e.g. garden vegetables.

QUANTITY

Generally speaking a minimum of 20–40 litres per person per day is needed for drinking, personal hygiene and cleaning.

QUALITY

The water should be free from chemical and biological contamination plus be acceptable in terms of colour, taste and smell, in accordance with the WHO Guidelines on the Quality of Drinking Water (1993).

SOURCES OF FRESH WATER

- Surface water, e.g. streams, rivers, lakes and ponds.
- Ground water, e.g. wells and springs.
- Rainwater, as harvested off buildings.

Surface water

Surface water is the most easily accessible source of fresh water but also the source most prone to contamination. Human and agricultural activity nearby often contaminate surface water.

Ground water

Ground water is more likely to be of a higher quality than surface water. However, ground water can be difficult to access as complicated forms of extraction such as submersible pumps may be needed. Ground water comes from springs, shallow wells or deep wells.

SHALLOW WELLS

The water is collected from above the first impervious layer and they may be hand dug or drilled. Shallow wells may be open or fitted with a hand-pump, common examples of which are the India Mark III or Afridev. Shallow wells are often less than 10 m in depth and are potentially prone to contamination such as when a latrine is built within 30 m of the well (Plates 96 and 97).

DEEP WELLS

The water is sourced from below the first impervious layer and deep wells may be up to 100 m deep. The depth of such wells excludes the use of manual extraction systems and mechanical systems are needed. Such systems are costly to install, run and maintain.

Rainwater

In some countries it is culturally accepted practice to collect rainwater, for example Cambodia. Rainwater is a good quality source of water if surface areas on which it is collected are kept clean. Rainwater also needs to be stored safely.

PROTECTION OF SOURCES

Obviously surface water sources need a great deal more protection than ground water sources. Each source still needs protecting from contamination and in developing countries the main type of contamination to protect from is human faeces (a major source of pathogenic organisms) and animals. Excreta from small children is particularly hazardous. Protection can be achieved through the construction of physical barriers such as fences and walls and/or through hygiene promotion. Good planning is also another important means of protection by, for example, ensuring pit latrines are not constructed within 30 m of a shallow well.

STORAGE

A water supply may come from a clean source and be well protected but may still become contaminated during storage. Storage containers should be well protected from outside contamination, be used for no other purpose other than the storage of clean water and have an opening which is small and have a tight-fitting lid. Storage containers, such as water jars used in Cambodia, may also serve to promote the proliferation of disease vectors such as *Aedes agypti*, the mosquito that transmits dengue fever. Hygiene-promotion efforts are necessary to ensure storage containers are used properly.

TREATMENT

In many instances some form of treatment will be necessary. The degree of treatment will depend on the quality of the raw water sourced. Surface water sources tend to require the greatest level of treatment whereas spring water may not require any treatment at all. Treatment may be as simple as boiling in the home or a series of activities resulting in water fit for human consumption. Depending on the quality of the raw water the following are the stages of treatment that may be followed:

- flocculation and sedimentation;
- filtration;
- disinfection.

Flocculation and sedimentation

The purpose of flocculation and sedimentation is to remove as much solid matter, such as suspended particulates, from the water as possible thus aiding the stages of filtration and disinfection. Flocculation normally involves the addition of alum (aluminium sulphate), which acts as a coagulant allowing suspended particulate matter to sink and settle out of suspension. The removal of such particulates is important as their presence interferes in the disinfection process as well as giving water an unacceptable physical appearance. The aim is to reduce the turbidity to less than 5 Nephelometric Turbidity Units (NTU) which facilitates the disinfection process.

Filtration

The best known method of filtration is the passing of water through a combination of small stones and sand, often described as slow sand filtration. Filtration is aimed at not only removing remaining particulate matter but also pathogenic organisms. Filtration may also be used to remove chemical contaminants in water. In Bangladesh, for example, they have a huge problem with arsenic in the water which is currently affecting an estimated 77 million people. One of the proposed solutions is the filtration of arsenic out of ground water.

Disinfection

The most common form of disinfection is chlorination. Disinfection is the last stage in the treatment process and is aimed at killing pathogenic organisms in the water. In municipal treatment plants chlorine gas is often used whereas on a small scale other forms of chlorine are used, such as granules or tablets. One of the most common forms is granules of calcium hypochlorite containing a 70% concentration of chlorine.

Chlorine is consumed by organic matter and it is therefore important to remove as much organic matter as possible from raw water before disinfection. The stages of flocculation, sedimentation and filtration are all aimed at removing organic matter thus enabling administered chlorine to act on the pathogens that remain. When water is disinfected one aims to leave a residual of chlorine in the water to deal with additional contamination once the water leaves the point of treatment up to the point of consumption. A normal residual chlorine level is 0.2–0.5 mg/litre. This compares with the residual chlorine level found in swimming pools of 1.5–2 mg/litre.

DISTRIBUTION

Once a supply of water fit for human consumption has been achieved the next challenge is to distribute that water in an equitable manner while maintaining the quality of the water. Basically there are two options:

- individual family connections;
- public water points.

Individual water points are the ideal solution if reasonably practicable. They allow families to obtain water with a great deal of ease, thus improving their opportunities for greater hygiene. Individual water points are common in the developed world but less so in the developing world.

Public water points are most common in developing countries where individual family connections cannot be afforded. Such public water points may provide water of sufficient quality but this does not necessarily translate into the consumption and use of safe water. There are a number of important issues to consider around the provision of public water points. One of the most crucial issues is that of access. Access means that people should not have to travel too far from their home to any public water point. Access also means they should not have to queue for a long time waiting to access a tap. The Sphere Project minimum standards which apply to emergencies state that people should not have to walk more than 500 m in order to reach a water point, there should be one water point for every 250 people and the flow rate from each tap should be no less than 0.125 litres per second.

In addition to access families also need containers for the hygienic collection of water. Without such containers and others for storage the good work of providing water fit for human consumption at the point of distribution is likely to be lost. Normally two 20-litre jerrycans per family is considered sufficient.

Other issues around public water points concern the drainage of waste water, the maintenance of such water points and the protection of such from contamination or pollution.

END USE

The critical point at which water supplies need to be safe and free from pathogenic organisms is at the point of consumption. All the work in providing water in sufficient quantity and of high quality will be lost if consumers do not display hygienic practices and behaviours. This is the point where hygiene promotion/education plays a vital role. Hygiene promotion/education is discussed separately later in this chapter.

TESTING OF WATER SUPPLIES

When a new source of water supply is provided, the water from that source should be tested for physical, biological and chemical parameters. A sampling programme for periodic testing should also be established for the purpose of continuous monitoring. The frequency of testing will be largely determined by the size of population served.

The physical parameters to be looked at in determining a water supply's suitability are its colour (turbidity), smell and taste.

The key indicator of biological contamination in a water supply is the presence of *faecal coliforms*. The presence of coliforms in numbers greater than 10 coliforms/100 ml as determined in the Sphere standards indicates an unacceptable level of contamination.

There is whole range of chemical contaminants one can test for and just some of them include nitrates, phosphates, fluoride, arsenic and iron. For example the provisional guideline value set in the WHO guidelines for arsenic is 0.01 mg/litre.

All water tested should be tested with reference to the WHO Guidelines on Drinking Water Quality of 1993.

EXCRETA DISPOSAL

The main objective of the International Drinking Water and Sanitation Decade 1980–1990 was to substantially improve the standards and levels of services in drinking water supply and sanitation by the year 1990. Sanitation is taken to mean excreta disposal. As of the year 2000 an estimated 2.4 billion people still lack access to an adequate means of excreta disposal (WHO, 2000). Most urban centres in Africa and Asia have no sewage system at all including many cities with a million or more inhabitants (WHO, 1992).

Human excreta is an important source of pathogenic organisms, especially the causative agents of diarrhoeal diseases. In addition, faeces are attractive to flies who not only spread pathogenic organisms contained in the faeces but also breed in them. Therefore, the disposal of human excreta is of major public health significance. The objective of any latrine or toilet should be:

- to dispose of potentially dangerous excreta;
- to prevent the proliferation of vectors that might breed in such waste.

In the tropics there are two basic choices of excreta disposal:

- pit latrines;
- pour flush toilets.

The choice of system will depend on a number of factors including adequate site planning, availability of water, the soil type, skills present in the community, the water table, existing culture of excreta disposal within the community and the availability of material and financial resources. Whatever system is chosen there are a number of principles which should be adhered to.

PRINCIPLES OF EXCRETA DISPOSAL STRUCTURES

- They should be safe. For example it should not be possible for small children to fall into a latrine pit.
- They should be built using hygienic and easy to clean materials. For example the floor of latrines should be made from a hard and durable material such as concrete rather than compacted soil.
- They are accessible to all sections of the community including the young and the old. Note: excreta from children is particularly hazardous.
- They are designed to minimize the proliferation and harbourage of disease vectors such as flies and mosquitoes.
- They provide a degree of privacy to the users.
- They are located to avoid the potential of contaminating water sources. For example they should be a minimum of 30 m and preferably downhill from a water source.
- They avoid the need to handle fresh faeces.
- There should be no contamination of surface soil.

Pit latrines

Pit latrines are the most basic of excreta disposal systems and are further divided into two main types: (i) the simple pit latrine; and (ii) the VIP (ventilated improved pit) latrine.

SIMPLE PIT LATRINES (PLATE 98) (FIG. 13.1)

Pit latrines are characterized by their simplicity in design. Unfortunately, they are often also characterized by the presence of a foul smell and huge numbers of flies.

The simple pit latrine (Fig. 13.1) is usually dug to a depth of 2 m and is 1–1.5 m in diameter. In ideal conditions the liquid part of the waste percolates out through the surrounding soil leaving the solid

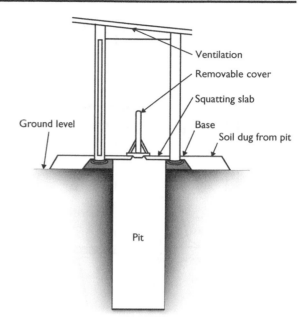

Figure 13.1: Pit latrine.

matter behind. Heavy clay soils will prevent the percolation of liquid resulting in a shorter lifespan for the latrine and more conducive conditions for the vectors of disease. Sandy soils, although providing good percolation, are prone to collapse. The pits of latrines in sandy soils therefore need to be lined to prevent collapse. The floor slab is often made from concrete or timber but in some cases is compacted soil over sticks. The floor should be raised up 150 mm above ground level to prevent the possibility of surface runoff water entering the latrine pit. The drop hole in the floor slab is sometimes provided with a cover to prevent the escape of foul smells and to prevent access/escape for disease vectors such as flies. The superstructure is usually made from local materials such as mud and wattle, bamboo and sugar palm thatch or timber and tin sheeting (Plate 98).

Common problems associated with the simple pit latrine include the presence of a foul smell and large numbers of disease vectors namely flies, mosquitoes of the *Culex* variety (in flooded latrines), which transmit filariasis, and cockroaches.

VENTILATED IMPROVED PIT (VIP) LATRINES (FIG. 13.2)

The ventilated improved pit (VIP) latrine is designed to eliminate the common problems

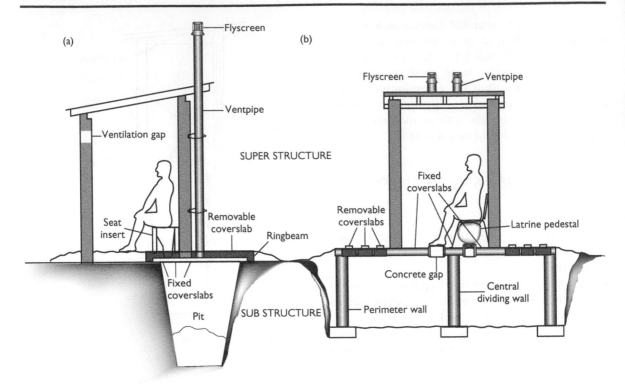

Figure 13.2: (a) Improved ventilated pit latrine; (b) improved double ventilated pit latrine.

associated with the simple pit latrine, namely foul smells and conducive conditions for the proliferation of disease vectors.

The principal difference from the simple pit latrine is the addition of a ventilation pipe, which is normally placed outside the superstructure. The vent pipe should be 110–150 mm in diameter and extend at least 0.5 m above the roof. The top of the vent pipe must be fitted with a fly-proof screen with a mesh size of 1 mm and should be made from a non-corrosive material. The superstructure must also be kept dim. The VIP latrine works due to the passing of wind over the top of the vent pipe which acts like a conventional chimney. The wind creates a draft of air up the vent pipe and down into the pit through the drop hole. The effect of this air flow is two-fold. First, the direction of air flow prevents foul smells emanating from the pit. Second, flies present or breeding in the pit are drawn up the vent pipe (they are attracted by the light at the top of the vent pipe) and become trapped by the fly-proof screen. The air flow keeps them trapped at the top of the pipe until eventually they die. In addition, female flies looking for an egg-laying site are drawn to the smell at the top

of the pipe and the fly-proof screen prevents them from gaining access to the pit.

Cairncross and Feachem (1993) quote an example of the difference between the simple pit latrine and the VIP latrine. During controlled experiments in Zimbabwe, 13 953 flies were caught during a 78-day period from an unvented pit latrine, but only 146 were caught from a vented pit latrine.

There are other types of latrines that loosely fit within the category of pit latrine. These include the twin pit latrine, bucket latrine, trench latrine and the borehole latrine. Trench latrines are often used at the beginning of an emergency where large numbers of people have become displaced.

Pour flush toilets

The alternative to the pit latrine is the pour flush latrine. The pour flush latrine also has the added advantage of preventing foul smells and removing easy access for the vectors of disease. However, pour flush latrines are dependent on an ample supply of water all year round and a population who knows how to use a pour flush latrine properly.

There are basically two types of pour flush latrine. The offset type with the pit located to the rear of the superstructure allows for easy access when it comes to the emptying of the latrine. The pour flush latrine works when a seal of water is maintained in the U-bend thus preventing smells coming out and preventing flies and mosquitoes from getting in or out.

DISPOSAL

When pit latrines or pour flush latrines become full one has a number of possible options. For pit latrines it is often possible to simply dig a new hole and build a new superstructure or move the existing superstructure over the new hole. In some countries they have a system of two pits which are used alternatively allowing the contents of one pit to be removed and used as compost/fertilizer. They are often described as compost latrines. The two-pit system allows the contents of one pit to be rendered harmless over time (often up to 6 months) before removal. In other circumstances excreta is removed by hand and disposed of into another hole which is then filled in. Pour flush latrines in particular may need a vacuum truck to pump out the waste and dispose of it in another location.

Sewerage

Although not common in the tropics, even in cities, excreta may also be disposed of by a water carriage system, also known as sewerage. Toilets connected to sewers are of the pour flush variety commonly known in the northern hemisphere as the water closet (WC). The water used in flushing (up to 9 litres per flush in the UK) is used to transport excreta through a network of sewers or pipes to a treatment plant, a collection point for additional transport, possibly out to sea or may discharge directly to a water course.

WASTE MANAGEMENT

The management of waste is another key element in the protection of public health. Different types of waste pose different problems but in general failure to manage and dispose of waste properly exposes people to increased risk of infectious disease.

Apart from excreta the other types of waste common to the tropics include:

- domestic waste, i.e. food waste;
- waste water, i.e. from bathing and other domestic washing;
- medical waste, i.e. syringes;
- the dead;
- industrial waste.

DOMESTIC WASTE

The management of domestic waste or refuse is further broken down into storage, collection, recycling and/or disposal. Domestic waste normally consists of organic material such as food waste and inorganic objects such as bottles, tins and packaging, etc.

Storage

Domestic waste accumulates continuously and the first stage in its management is storage prior to collection and disposal. Sufficient containers or bins are needed to cope with the volume of waste prior to collection. The containers need to be suitable by limiting opportunities for vectors of disease such as flies and rats to feed on and breed in the waste. Also they must be convenient to access both for the user and the collector. Organic waste may be composted directly without the need for storage and collection. Inorganic waste such as paper, tins and glass may be recycled. Often in developing countries people dispose of waste once it is produced. Good practice in this regard entails the placing of waste in a pit and dependent upon the moisture content it can either be burned or buried.

Collection

Where the collection of domestic waste is possible collections should be at regular and consistent intervals. The frequency of collection will often depend on the capacity and quality of the storage containers used. Collection workers need protective clothing and education in order to reduce the risk of infection to themselves.

Disposal

The correct disposal of waste is very important and there are a number of options available. The system of disposal needs planning from the very beginning and must consider the types of waste being produced, the volume of waste being produced and the best disposal method within the circumstances. Common disposal methods include:

LANDFILL

Landfill is probably the most common method of domestic waste disposal. Basically it consists of four steps:

- depositing waste in a planned controlled manner;
- spreading and compacting it in layers to reduce its volume;
- covering the material with a layer of earth;
- compacting the earth cover.

Landfill areas are often located on the periphery of large cities. Great care is needed in the selection of landfill sites as domestic waste can be highly polluting.

BURNING

Burning is possible where the moisture content of the waste is low. Generally, one sees burning being carried out at a localized level in the absence of adequate collection services. Burning does have a number of disadvantages in that the burning of refuse in close proximity to domestic dwellings (particularly if made of highly flammable materials such as bamboo and thatch) creates an additional fire risk in addition to producing atmospheric pollution.

COMPOSTING

Composting is best suited in situations where waste high in organic matter content is produced.

WASTE WATER

Waste water from bathing and domestic washing can also present public health problems if not dealt with properly. Waste water if not drained away can accumulate creating conditions conducive to the proliferation of disease vectors namely mosquitoes. In addition, washing water containing phosphates may also cause problems when discharged into water courses in excessive quantities.

In the absence of a sewerage system to carry waste water to a treatment plant the common solution to waste water at the individual household level is the use of a soak pit, sometimes referred to as a soakaway. The principle of the soakpit is to contain waste water and protect it from vectors (mosquitoes and flies) allowing time for percolation into the surrounding soil. The pit is filled with stones to prevent the pit from collapsing and is covered with a plastic or tin sheet prior to topsoil going on top.

MEDICAL WASTE

Medical waste also poses a special threat to health and safety. Medical waste by its very nature is potentially harmful and can be divided into two types:

- sharps;
- pathological wastes.

Sharps (syringes, needles, etc.) should be placed in sealed containers, often tin boxes and sometimes filled with disinfectant. When full these containers should be buried to a depth of at least 1 m (Davis and Lambert, 1995).

All non-metallic wastes which have been in contact with body fluids need separate collection and disposal. Disposal should be in the form of incineration.

THE DEAD

Generally, dead bodies pose minimal health risk unless they have died from a highly infectious disease such as cholera in which case they need to be disposed of as soon as possible. The form of disposal is normally dependent on the cultural practices of the population concerned. Some opt for burial (Christians and Muslims) while others opt for cremation (Buddhists and Hindus). If the method of disposal is burial, sufficient space needs to be allocated and a suitable site found which considers soil conditions and the depth of the water table. If cremation is the option sufficient fuel must also be available.

INDUSTRIAL WASTE

Industrial waste comes in many different forms and is disposed of:

- on land;
- in water;
- into the atmosphere.

The types of industry responsible for the majority of hazardous waste include the food and agricultural processing industry, metal extraction and processing, cement works, the paper industry, oil refining and the chemical industry.

Typical industrial wastes of public health significance include 'tailings' from the mining industry disposed of on land, organic waste from abattoirs discharged into water courses and the emission of sulphur dioxide into the atmosphere from a number of industries including the petrochemical industry.

The range of waste types is exhaustive and this chapter cannot deal with each one but there are a number of principles one should consider in relation to industrial waste. The principles would include:

Planning

Adequate planning can ensure that industries producing wastes of huge public health significance are not sited in close proximity to concentrations of human population or fragile environments. Sometimes planning permission needs to be denied in the interests of public health.

Design

Ideally, such industries need to design sufficient mechanisms for the safe disposal of such waste or at least to dispose of such waste within acceptable limits that are not harmful to the environment or to health. Where toxic discharges are allowed regular monitoring supported by the threat of legal action are sometimes needed to ensure discharges remain within recommended limits.

Research

The number of chemicals in use today has multiplied enormously in the latter half of the 20th century and the effects of many are not fully known. Research is continually needed to monitor the effects of industrial waste so that adjustments can be made in setting safe limits or even banning the production of certain wastes.

VECTOR CONTROL

Vector borne disease remains a substantial problem in the tropics. Malaria, which is transmitted by the *Anopheles* mosquito remains one of the top five killers in the developing world (source WHO) and alongside diarrhoea is considered a major danger for refugee or displaced populations. In addition to death malaria is also responsible for an estimated 300-500 million episodes of the disease each year, which has a huge knock on economic effect. The common vectors and their associated diseases are listed in Table 13.1.

WHAT IS A VECTOR OF DISEASE?

A vector may be any arthropod or animal which carries and transmits infectious pathogens directly or indirectly from an infected animal to a human or from an infected human to another human.

(Lacarin and Reed, 1999)

The key to vector control is to work on the following principles. One should start on the first principle and work down the list. You may be able to stop at principle number 2 but in the majority of cases a combination of actions is needed.

Table 13.1: Common vectors and their associated diseases

Vector	Associated disease
Flies	Eye infections such as conjunctivitis, and diarrhoeal diseases
Mosquitoes	Malaria, dengue fever, filariasis and yellow fever
Rats	Leptospirosis, salmonellosis
Fleas	Typhus and plague
Mites	Scabies
Lice	Epidemic typhus and relapsing fever
Ticks	Relapsing fever and spotted fever

PRINCIPLE No. 1: KNOW AS MUCH ABOUT THE VECTOR AS POSSIBLE

Know where it breeds, where it likes to rest, where it likes to feed, what it likes to feed on, what time of day it is active and what does it not like, etc. Knowledge of the vector and its habits is crucial to its control and elimination as a transmitter of disease.

PRINCIPLE No. 2: PREVENT THE VECTOR FROM BREEDING

Ideally, vector-borne disease can be prevented if the vectors don't exist in the first place. If breeding sites are eliminated then they can no longer proliferate. For example, mosquitoes breed in water and a prevention programme would fill in holes and provide good drainage, thereby preventing the formation of pools of water in which mosquitoes could breed. Other examples include the routine collection of rubbish denying flies a suitable environment for the laying of eggs.

PRINCIPLE No. 3: CONTROL/ELIMINATE THE VECTOR AT THE EARLIEST POINT IN ITS LIFE CYCLE

In most cases the total elimination of breeding sites is not possible. If not, then it is preferable to target vectors in their 'infant' stages before reaching maturity. Mosquitoes emerge from eggs as larvae where they are confined within water until reaching the adult stage. Targeting of these water sources with a larvacide such as 'Temephos', also known as Abate, can eliminate the larval stage of mosquito vectors such as those responsible for malaria and dengue fever.

PRINCIPLE No. 4: CONTROL/ELIMINATE THE VECTOR TO PREVENT DISEASE TRANSMISSION

In many circumstances and particularly during an epidemic the most suitable control measure is to target adult vectors to reduce or prevent transmission.

A number of options are available and include the use of chemical control methods including space spraying and/or residual spraying of insecticides with regard to mosquitoes or the laying of poison/ traps with regard to rodents. Other actions include the removal of potential resting sites, for example the removal of vegetation from around homes where mosquitoes may be found resting.

PRINCIPLE No. 5: PERSONAL PROTECTION

In addition to each of the other control measures mentioned in principles 2, 3 and 4 is the option of personal protection. Personal protection is best described in relation to mosquitoes. Personal protection measures against malaria include the use of chemoprophylaxis, the wearing of long sleeves and socks to reduce opportunities for mosquitoes to bite and the using of insecticide impregnated bednets while sleeping. The use of such bednets for example has been shown to reduce childhood deaths from malaria by as much as 20% (source UNICEF). In relation to leptospirosis a personal protection measure would be the use of rubber gloves if working in an area that may have been in contact with rat's urine.

SUMMARY

In summary, each of the principles described above needs to be considered in the design of any programme intending to control/eliminate vector-borne disease. In some instances treatment of cases is also considered a prevention measure. Treatment of people with malaria removes reservoirs of infection, preventing the transmission of disease from one human being to another.

SHELTER/HOUSING AND SITE PLANNING

Housing is another key component in the protection and promotion of health and carries equal priority with nutrition, water supply and sanitation and health care. Housing needs to be sited properly and constructed in such a way as to provide the physical and social needs of those housed. Housing needs to protect people from the adverse effects of the climate as well as fresh air, security and privacy to ensure dignity, health and well being (Sphere, 2000).

SITE SELECTION AND PLANNING

Site selection and planning of housing is of critical importance. In the tropics many housing developments are built without due consideration of site selection and planning. Many urban slums for example are built in locations prone to environmental health risks such as flooding, close to discharges of potentially harmful industrial waste or at risk from landslides. Many such developments are also planned without due consideration for the issues listed as follows:

- *water* (WHO recommends that 20 litres is the standard minimum per person per day);
- *security* (refugees/displaced people for example should not be placed in the firing line);
- *space* (some publications estimate that an average of 45 m² per person is needed excluding land for agricultural purposes; 45 m² covers all space to include roads, public buildings, recreation areas and markets, etc.);
- *access* (access relates to access both for the receiving of services such as food or waste collection and access to markets);
- *soil type and water table* (these will have a direct bearing on the type of excreta disposal system chosen);
- *drainage* (which is vital for the removal of storm water and preventing pools of water which might assist the breeding of mosquitoes for example);
- *availability of fuelwood* (most households in the tropics depend on biomass fuels for cooking and heating);
- *vegetative cover* (necessary to provide shade and prevent soil erosion).

HOUSING

Housing needs to take account of:

- *space per person* (the Sphere standards in relation to emergencies state that each person should have a covered area of between 3.5 and 4.5 m²);
- *suitable materials for construction* suited to the climate and culture which are environmentally friendly (such materials may need to reflect excessive heat away during the day and/or retain heat indoors at night);
- *ventilation* (enough ventilation is needed to provide a fresh throughput of air and the removal of harmful particulates produced by cooking or heating);
- *cooking facilities* (space needs to be provided for cooking facilities and if possible the use of non-flammable construction materials);
- *storage*, for items such as food (storage of food needs to protect food from vectors such as rodents and flies);
- *excreta and other forms of waste disposal* (latrine facilities need to be accessible and non-polluting of water sources);
- *access to potable water* (water also needs to be accessible preferably within 1 minute's walk, in adequate quantities and of sufficient quality).

HYGIENE EDUCATION

The promotion of hygiene is another integral component of environmental health activities and is often included as the third part of any water and sanitation programme. It is widely recognized that the promotion of hygiene (often described as software) must be included alongside the provision of clean water and excreta disposal (described as hardware) if one is to achieve an impact in the reduction of water-related diseases. 'Too often health/hygiene education is perceived as being essentially a simple matter of telling people what they ought to do to be healthy. Dangerous oversimplifications of this sort have gone hand in hand with a tendency for health education to be treated as an "instant expert" subject.' (Downie *et al.*, 1990). It is *not* an 'instant' expert subject.

Hygiene education is a specific component to health education which in turns forms a part of health promotion. Hygiene education cannot work unless the enabling factors (i.e. hardware) are in place in order for people to engage in positive behaviour change associated with the messages they receive in hygiene education.

Health promotion can be defined in the following way:

> Promoting health is more than just providing health services. It is about peace, housing, education, food, income, a sustainable environment, social justice and equity are all necessary for achievement of health. It calls for people to act as advocates for health through addressing of political, economic, social, cultural, environmental, behavioural and biological factors.
>
> (Hubley, 1993)

Health promotion covers a very broad range of issues but many of these issues are necessary if hygiene education is to achieve success as part of a wider public health programme.

Hygiene or health education is defined as:

> a process with intellectual, psychological and social dimensions relating to activities that increase the abilities of people to make informed decisions affecting their personal, family and community well being.
>
> (Hubley, 1993)

Hygiene education allows people to become better informed or aware of the influences affecting their health and, when combined with some of the other components of health promotion, enables people to make positive behaviour changes.

The types of behaviour change generally associated with hygiene education in the tropics include:

- washing your hands with soap before preparing food and after going to the toilet;
- collecting and storing water hygienically;
- boiling water if you are unsure of the water's source.

For example, hygiene education may deliver messages on the importance of washing hands after going to the toilet to prevent diarrhoeal diseases. However, such a message on its own cannot work unless there is a source of water accessible nearby and people have enough money in their pocket to pay for soap. A wider health-promotion programme will work towards ensuring a supply of clean water is available and people have opportunities to earn an income which would allow them to buy the soap.

Hygiene education can be disseminated in one of two broad ways.

FACE TO FACE CHANNELS

These are:

- person to person contact on an individual basis;
- larger numbers of people, such as a talk or focus group.

The face to face channels of communication are slower for spreading information and the use of different senders may distort the message being delivered. However face to face has a number of advantages over the mass media. These advantages include:

- one can selectively reach specific target groups;
- the communication can be tailored to fit local needs;
- direct feedback is possible at the time of message delivery through two-way dialogue;
- a greater chance of achieving behaviour change is possible through the use of face to face communication (Hubley, 1993).

MASS MEDIA

The dissemination of hygiene messages through the mass media is a common mechanism used to achieve behaviour change in addition to an information-type role. One must stress that this role is only as a supportive role to other interventions such as improving the physical and social environment. In the tropics populations are more susceptible generally to mass media interventions – due in large part to the fact that the messages are not as negative as we have received in the west and the changes sought are simple (Tones *et al.*, 1990).

The mass media can do the following:

1 Raise consciousness about health issues.
2 Help place health on the public agenda.
3 Convey simple information.
4 Change behaviour if other enabling factors are present:
   - existing motivation;
   - supportive circumstances;
   - advocating simple one-off behaviour change.

Using media is more effective if:

- it is part of an integrated campaign including elements such as one to one advice;
- the information is new and presented in an emotional context;
- the information is seen as being relevant for 'people like me'.

The media cannot:

- convey complex information;
- teach skills;
- shift people's attitudes or beliefs;
- change behaviour in the absence of enabling factors.

Generally, a well planned hygiene education programme will involve some combination of both face to face and mass media approaches utilizing the advantages inherent in both.

FOOD SAFETY AND HYGIENE

In practical terms, food safety can be defined as the absence of adverse health effects following food consumption.

'Foodborne illnesses are defined as diseases, usually either infectious or toxic in nature, caused by agents that enter the body through the ingestion of food' (WHO, 2000). The extent of the problem is difficult to estimate particularly in developing countries but given that in excess of 2 million people (mostly children) die from diarrhoea each year a great proportion of these cases can be attributed to the contamination of food as well as drinking water (WHO, 2000)

Broadly speaking food safety hazards can be classified into two categories.

BIOLOGICAL HAZARDS

Biological hazards associated with the mishandling of food at some point in the chain from harvesting, processing, storage, preparation and cooking through to consumption. The more common biological hazards include:

- *Cholera*, a major public health problem in developing countries. In addition to transmission

via water cholera can also be transmitted through contaminated food and has had severe economic consequences in parts of the world most notably in parts of South America.
- *Parasites*, which play a major role in chronic malnutrition and in turn susceptibility to other infections. Common parasitic diseases associated with food in the tropics include amoebiasis, giardia, trichinosis, liver fluke and *Taenia saginata*, also known as the beef tapeworm.
- *Other common food-borne illnesses*, which are identified in the developed world are salmonellosis, campylobacteriosis, infections due to *Escherichia coli*, such as those caused by *E. coli 0157*, and listeriosis.

OTHER HAZARDS

Other hazards include naturally occurring toxins, metals and unconventional agents.

Naturally occurring toxins include mycotoxins, such as aflatoxin and ochratoxin A, which are found in many staple foods. Aflatoxins are commonly associated with ground nuts and are linked to liver cancer. Unconventional agents such as prions are associated with cattle suffering from bovine spongiform encephalopathy (BSE) which in turn are suspected to cause new variant Creutzfeldt–Jakob disease (CJD) in humans through the consumption of meat and meat products. Metals such as lead and mercury are toxic (WHO, 2000). In more recent times there has been debate about the safety of genetically modified foods.

The responsibility for food safety rests with many different people. In the developed world there is a great deal of emphasis placed on the responsibility of government to regulate the safe production of food right through to the point of purchase/consumption. Environmental health officers (EHOs) are one group of government representatives who enforce such regulations. EHOs tend to focus on the structural, operational and personnel hygiene aspects of food premises, in addition to the taking of food samples for analysis. Thereafter, responsibility rests with the consumer influenced hopefully by public information/ education on best hygiene practice in the storage, preparation and cooking of food.

In many countries in the tropics there is an almost complete lack of regulatory control in relation to food safety and hygiene. The preventive mechanism most commonly used is hygiene education described earlier in this chapter. This gives people the opportunity to protect both their own and other people's health. The types of food hygiene messages one could give include the following:

- wash your hands before preparing food and after using the latrine;
- store foodstuffs off the floor and in areas that do not permit pests to gain access (pests include rats, flies and cockroaches);
- cook or reheat food thoroughly before consumption;
- vegetables and salads should be washed and prepared using clean water prior to consumption;
- dispose of food waste immediately and properly either by composting or burial;
- perishable foods should be stored in a cool dry place and preferably at a temperature below 4°C;
- do not store raw meat beside or above cooked meat.

These are just some of the common hygiene messages that can be delivered to individual householders or workers in the food service industry. One must stress again that such messages do not work unless 'enabling factors' are in place to allow people to adopt good hygienic practice.

PROTECTION FROM RADIATION

Matter is composed of atoms. Some atoms are unstable. As these atoms change to become stable, they give off invisible energy waves or particles called radiation.
(US Environmental Protection Agency)

Radiation is classified into ionizing and non-ionizing radiation. The most energetic form and of major public health significance is ionizing radiation. In normal circumstances 80% of our exposure to ionizing radiation comes from natural sources of which radon gas is by far the most significant. The other 20% comes from man-made sources, primarily medical X-rays.

Overexposure to ionizing radiation can have serious effects including cancers, birth deformities and mental anguish (WHO). Cancer is the most

significant health risk associated with overexposure to ionizing radiation and typically these cancers develop 10–40 years after exposure.

NATURAL RADIATION

Radon gas is by far the main source of naturally occurring ionizing radiation. Radon is a colourless, tasteless and odourless gas that comes from the decay of uranium found in nearly all soils. Radon usually moves from the ground up into dwellings where it tends to become trapped unless the house is well ventilated. Scientists believe that radon is the second leading cause of lung cancer in the United States (after smoking) (US Environmental Protection Agency). The other sources of naturally occurring ionizing radiation include other radioactive elements in the earth's crust (thorium and potassium) and radiation from outer space.

MAN-MADE RADIATION

In general, man-made radiation accounts for around 20% of an individual's exposure to ionizing radiation, primarily medical X-rays. However, certain industries and processes may expose people to high concentrations of radiation either occupationally or as the result of accidents. These activities include mining, the use of materials with high natural levels of radioactivity (such as phosphate fertilizers), nuclear power generation, weapons testing and nuclear medicine (Fitzpatrick and Bonnefoy, 1998). Most notable exposures to man-made radiation are the atomic bombs dropped on the Japanese cities of Hiroshima and Nagasaki in 1945 and more recently the nuclear accident at Chernobyl in the Ukraine.

Ionizing radiation cannot be eliminated. Natural radiation is all around us and we can only limit our degree of exposure. Perhaps most important is the control of radon gas in the indoor environment. Simple tests are available to measure radon gas and if they exceed a level of 4 picocuries per litre, the US Environmental Protection Agency standard, then corrective action should be taken. Corrective action may take the form of moving to an area where less radon gas is emitted or protecting existing homes by sealing floors and/or increasing ventilation. In industry and the medical services high standards of occupational health and safety are needed to protect and limit overexposure to ionizing radiation.

AIR POLLUTION

Air pollution is a major environmental health problem in both developed and developing countries. Increasing amounts of potentially harmful gases and particles are being emitted into the atmosphere resulting in damage to human health and the environment. Acute respiratory infection (ARI) is one of the most important causes of ill health and death in the developing world and air pollution is considered a very important risk factor in the development of ARI.

Air pollution may be divided into anthropogenic (man-made) and natural sources (e.g. dust storms and volcanic action) and pollutants are broadly classified into:

- suspended particulate matter (smoke and dusts);
- gaseous pollutants (sulphur dioxide);
- odours (hydrogen sulphide).

Air pollution has three types of sources:

- stationary sources, e.g. industry and the generation of electricity;
- mobile sources, e.g. motor vehicles;
- indoor sources, e.g. cooking fires.

STATIONARY AND MOBILE SOURCES

The primary pollutants produced by stationary and mobile sources are oxides of nitrogen, sulphur, carbon monoxide, particles and volatile organic compounds. Reactions of primary pollutants within the atmosphere generate secondary pollutants of which ozone is the best known example. The adverse health effects of these pollutants varies according to the concentration of pollutants, the weather prevailing at the time of exposure and the populations exposed. The elderly, especially those with pre-existing cardiorespiratory disorders, and the very young are most susceptible. One of the most dramatic episodes of air pollution and its effects occurred in London in 1952 where climatic conditions combined with high concentrations of smoke and sulphur dioxide resulted in 4000 extra deaths.

INDOOR SOURCES

At the individual level, indoor air pollutants are perhaps the most important for those people living in developing countries. WHO estimate that about 1.9 million people die annually due to exposure to high concentrations of suspended particulate matter in the indoor air environment. The health effects associated with poor indoor air quality are: (i) acute respiratory infections in children; and (ii) chronic obstructive pulmonary disease and lung cancer. The main source of suspended particulate matter in the indoor environment comes from the use of unprocessed solid fuels for cooking and heating. Approximately half of the world's households use unprocessed solid fuels for such purposes.

Other important indoor air pollutants include environmental tobacco smoke, biological particles, non-biological particles, volatile organic compounds, nitrogen oxides, lead, radon, carbon monoxide and asbestos. Some of these would be common in the occupational environment.

Radon is covered under Natural radiation.

SECONDARY EFFECTS OF AIR POLLUTION

In addition to the direct impact of air pollution on health there are other problems associated with the emission of pollutants into the atmosphere. Best known is the issue of global warming and associated impact plus the phenomena of acid rain.

REFERENCES AND FURTHER READING

General

Fitzpatrick M. & Kappos A. (1999) *Environmental Health Services in Thailand.* Desire, Bangkok.

Water (Late addenda see p. 352).

Adams J. (1999) *Managing Water Supply and Sanitation in Emergencies.* Oxfam, Oxford.

Sphere Project (2000) *The Sphere Project – Humanitarian Charter and Minimum Standards in Disaster Response.* Oxfam, Oxford.

White G.F., Bradley D.J. & White A.V. (1972) *Drawers of Water: Domestic Water Use in East Africa.* University of Chicago Press, Chicago.

WHO (1993) *Drinking Water Guidelines,* Vol. 1. WHO, Geneva.

Excreta

Cairncross S. & Feachem R. (1993) *Environmental Health Engineering in the Tropics: An Introductory Text,* 2nd edn. John Wiley, Chichester.

DFID (1998) *Guidance Manual on Water Supply and Sanitation Programmes.* WELL, Loughborough.

WHO Commission on Health and Environment (1992) *Our Planet, Our Health.* WHO, Geneva.

WHO (2000) *Global Water Supply and Sanitation Assessment 2000 Report.* WI IO, Geneva.

Winblad U. & Kilama W. (1992) *Sanitation Without Water.* Macmillan, London.

Waste management

Davis J. & Lambert R. (1995) *Engineering in Emergencies: A practical guide for relief workers.* RedR/Intermediate Technology, London.

Vector control

Lacarin C. & Reed B. (1999) *Emergency Vector Control Using Chemicals.* Water, Engineering and Development Centre, Loughborough.

Shelter/housing and site planning

Sphere Project (2000) *The Sphere Project – Humanitarian Charter and Minimum Standards in Disaster Response.* Oxfam, Oxford.

UNHCR (1982) *United Nations High Commissioner for Refugees Handbook for Emergencies,* UNHCR, Geneva.

Hygiene education

Downie R.S., Fyfe F. & Tannahill A. (1990) *Health Promotion: Models and Values.* Oxford University Press, Oxford.

Hubley J. (1993) *Communicating Health – An Action Guide to Health Education and Health Promotion.* TALC and Macmillan, London.

Naidoo J. & Wills J. (1994) *Health Promotion – Foundations for Practice.* Baillière Tindall, London.

Tones K., Tilford S. & Robinson Y. (1990) *Health Education Effectiveness and Efficiency.* Chapman and Hall, London.

Food safety and hygiene

WHO (2000) *Food Safety and Foodborne Illness.* Fact Sheet No. 237. WHO, Geneva.

Protection from radiation

Fitzpatrick M. & Bonnefoy X. (1998) *Environmental Health Services in Europe, Professional Profiles.* WHO, Geneva.

US Environmental Protection Agency. *www.epa.gov/radiation*

WHO. *www.who.int/peh/Radiation*

Air

UNICEF (2000) *Waterfront,* Issue 14 April 2000.

WHO (1999) *Air Quality Guidelines.* WHO, Geneva.

LATE ADDENDA

Water

Sodium dichloroisocyanate (DCCNA) is now prefered to sodium hypochlorite (Na OCE) for water disinfection *Aquatabs*®.

CHAPTER FOURTEEN

HEALTH PROMOTION AND EDUCATION

- Health education and the health services
- Community involvement
- Community participation
- Assessment of needs
- Learning from the people
- Health education methods

- Overcoming resistance to change
- Reinforcement by example
- Modern behavioural challenges
- Assessing change and progress
- Further reading

Box 14.1: Health promotion

Health promotion

Health promotion is the process of enabling people to increase control over, and to improve, their health. To reach a state of complete physical, mental and social well-being, an individual or group must be able to identify and to realize aspirations, to satisfy needs, and to change or cope with the environment. Health is, therefore, seen as a resource for everyday life, not the objective of living. Health is a positive concept emphasizing social and personal resources, as well as physical capacities. Therefore, health promotion is not just the responsibility of the health sector, but goes beyond healthy lifestyles to well-being.

The First International Conference on Health Promotion,
Ottawa, November 1986

Health promotion is a key investment

Health is a basic human right and is essential for social and economic development. Increasingly, health promotion is being recognized as an essential element of health development. It is a process of enabling people to increase control over, and to improve, their health.

The Jarkarta Declaration,
Fourth International Conference on Health Promotion,
Jakarta, July 1997

The objective of health education is to make people value health as a worthwhile asset, with a desire to live long and feel well; and with the support of health personnel, to learn what they can do as individuals, families and communities to protect and improve their own health. The more people value health, the more they will be willing to make the appropriate allocation of resources to promote and safeguard their own health. At the personal level, they will be prepared to make the effort on such matters as exercise, cleanliness in the home, diet and discipline with regard to the use of tobacco and alcohol. The community and the state will also be more prepared to allocate resources for improvement of environmental sanitation, and for other priorities within the health services.

HEALTH EDUCATION AND THE HEALTH SERVICES

Modern medicine has tended to interpret health in terms of medical interventions, and to over-emphasize the importance of medical technology. It is important to promote the concept of health as the result of the interaction of human beings and their total environment (see Chapter 1). Clinical medicine seeks to restore health through the use of drugs and surgical treatment. Public health includes medical interventions with the use of immunization and chemoprophylaxis but, more importantly, it emphasizes control of the environment and of human behaviour. Individuals, families and communities should be made to understand this concept of health, briefly summarized as: *Health, habit and habitat.*

Health education relates to all aspects of health behaviour including the use of health services and self-treatment. It is designed to help people improve their personal habits and to make the best use of the health services. Health education should feature as an integral part of the health services and all health personnel should accept responsibility for contributing to the programme. Specialists in health education are required to make accurate assessments of the needs of the population, to develop suitable materials for health education, to train other workers including voluntary health workers and to assist in evaluating local health education programmes.

Some health workers use the term 'information, education and communications' (IEC) instead of health education. Although it is more descriptive of the content, the two terms are synonymous.

COMMUNITY INVOLVEMENT

In the past, health education was practised as a one-way process with the health professional transmitting technical information and advice to individuals and to the community. This approach produced ready-made packages of ideas and plans based on the preconceived notions of the health staff. Such programmes did not always take into account traditional beliefs and practices of the local community nor did it benefit from its innate wisdom and accumulated experience.

COMMUNITY PARTICIPATION

The role of the community in the planning, organization, operation and control of health services has been repeatedly emphasized and is highlighted in the Alma Ata Declaration (see p. 304):

> *Primary health* care is essential health care ... made *universally* accessible to individuals and families in the community through their full participation and at a cost that the community and country can afford to maintain at every stage of their development in the *spirit of self-reliance and self-determination.*

The role of the community in making choices and decisions with regard to priorities and strategies should be adequately supported by health education. The degree of collaboration required to ensure success depends on the particular method of implementation. At one end of the spectrum, the sole responsibility lies with individuals and families; the role of the health personnel is to provide guidance, for example personal hygiene, nutrition, and social habits. In these cases, the individuals must learn and then do the things themselves. The individual may make a direct contribution by acting as voluntary health worker, performing a variety of simple but essential tasks. At the other end of the spectrum the tasks are such that the members of the community cannot participate directly. It is possible in such cases that specific intervention can be undertaken even if the community is indifferent or hostile, for example aerial spraying of insecticides. Even though a specific intervention can be carried out in spite of opposition from the community, this is most undesirable; it could destroy the rapport which should exist between this community and health workers. Rarely, if ever, should compulsion be used to override opposition. The range of community attitudes to a specific health measure can be classified into five levels:

- self-reliance;
- active collaboration;
- indifference;
- passive resistance;
- extreme hostility with violent rejection.

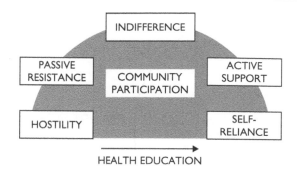

Figure 14.1: Community attitudes to health measures.

This concept is schematically illustrated in Figure 14.1. Health education is shown as the means of changing attitudes in a positive direction. The varying degrees of community participation that is required for success in different types of health programme can be illustrated using the following examples.

SELF-RELIANCE

For some health programmes the ultimate aim is complete self-reliance at the level of the individual and the family – as, for example, nutrition, (including the feeding of infants), smoking, the use of alcohol, sexual behaviour, exercise, personal hygiene and sanitation in the home. The health workers should give advice, teach, demonstrate the best methods and encourage the people in various ways, but in the final analysis the individual and the family must do these things on their own. For such activities, the minimal level to ensure success is total self-reliance within the family.

ACTIVE COLLABORATION

Indoor spraying of houses with long-acting insecticides has been extensively used in malaria control programmes. It is technically too difficult for each individual and each family to learn how to do it efficiently and safely. In this case, self-reliance is an unrealistic goal at the family level but the active collaboration of the families is essential for success. It is just possible to spray the houses if the community treats the matter with indifference, not helping and not impeding the sprayers. It would fail if a high proportion of families show passive resistance by locking up their houses during the visit of the spraying teams. For indoor spraying of houses, the desired level of community participation is active collaboration and the programme can be frustrated by passive resistance.

INDIFFERENCE

Fluoridation of municipal water supplies cannot be safely undertaken on a do-it-yourself basis and it does not call for a specific response from the individual or family. It could succeed in controlling dental caries even if a proportion of the community is indifferent on this issue. Passive resistance may, however, take the form of utilizing other sources of water and those who are hostile to the idea may actively campaign against the continuation of the service.

PASSIVE RESISTANCE

The local community could, in theory, carry out aerial spraying of insecticides for the control of arthropod vectors during an epidemic, even if there is strong opposition. It cannot be done on the basis of self-help nor does it call for active co-operation of the community.

In all cases it is important to ensure that the community is well informed about any action that is proposed, that their agreement is sought and obtained, and that their involvement in the implementation is at the optimal level. Much greater attention must be paid to the cultural context in which a health plan is implemented.

The Alma Ata Declaration (see Chapter 10), places great emphasis on the rights and responsibilities of individuals and communities in planning and implementing their health care. This concept of self-reliance has altered the role of health educators and other health personnel. The new concept of primary health care demands the involvement of the community through regular consultations. Such dialogue will help to ensure that health programmes are compatible with the social goals of the community and with their social and cultural background. In order to be effective teachers, health educators

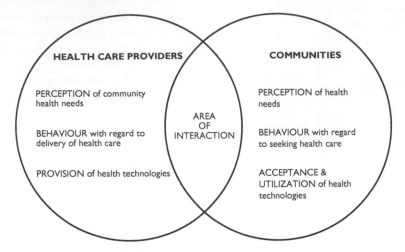

Figure 14.2: Health care as perceived by communities and health care providers (WHO, 1983).

and other health care givers must therefore also become learners, listening carefully to the views and concerns of the community and involving them in identifying health priorities and in finding feasible solutions (Fig. 14.2).

Lessons learnt from the community may help design unique solutions to local problems. For example, in tackling malnutrition in children, it would be useful to find out how the mothers of well-nourished children use locally available food-stuffs to provide a balanced diet for their children. Rather than promoting recipes that are foreign to the community, nutritional advice would be based on the use of food that is locally available and accept-able to local tastes and culture. Similarly, in dealing with the problem of diarrhoeal diseases, interest should not focus exclusively on the problem fam-ilies. By involving others, one may learn how to pre-pare and protect food under the conditions and circumstances of life of the local population.

Health education should therefore be an inter-active process between health professionals and the community, with each partner approaching the issues from a different perspective but establishing common ground where their respective views overlap (Fig. 14.2).

relevant, information is required about the current knowledge, attitudes and behaviour of the popu-lation. An educational programme can then be designed to bring about the desired changes. For example, in designing a health education pro-gramme to improve the nutrition of infants the following information should be sought:

- How many of the mothers breast-feed their babies and for how long?
- When do they introduce mixed feeding, what items do they use and how is the food prepared?
- What foods are avoided or considered unacceptable?
- What substitutes are available to provide missing nutrients and are these acceptable to the mothers?
- Which mothers are in greatest need of educa-tion on this subject as judged by the nutritional status of their infants?

Such studies aimed at identifying the needs for health education and defining the target groups are sometimes described as 'knowledge, attitude, practice' or 'KAP' studies. The broad aim is to find out what people know, what they believe, what they desire, what they expect, what they hope for and what they do in relation to their knowledge and attitudes.

ASSESSMENT OF NEEDS

The content of the health education programme should be determined by the needs of the target groups. In order to ensure that the material is

LEARNING FROM THE PEOPLE

Health workers who have acquired appropri-ate skills can gather useful information from communities through interview and social surveys. More complex studies benefit from the knowledge and skills of professional sociologists, anthropologists and political scientists. These experts employ a variety of methods for eliciting valuable information that would improve understanding of community opinions and ideas, and can be used to strengthen the design of appropriate health messages. Social scientists employ both quantitative and qualitative methods for data gathering. Quantitative studies use structured questionnaires eliciting answers to a set of standard questions. The answers can be coded and analysed numerically; the instruments can be completed by the respondent or by an interviewer. Qualitative methods also use interviews but instead of precoded responses, the answers are more open-ended. The interview may be semi-structured in that it includes a set of preset questions but the interviewer can add supplementary probing questions. Skilled interviewers can also obtain useful information from unstructured interviews in which respondents are asked to comment on selected topics with follow-up questions determined by the direction of the discussion.

Mailed questionnaires can be used to obtain information. An anonymous questionnaire may be useful for dealing with sensitive issues. Low response rate and the bias created by the group of respondents may skew the results.

FOCUS GROUPS

Instead of interviewing one person at a time, investigators sometimes use focus group discussions in which 8–10 persons take part in a group discussion. The participants are selected from similar age, sex, and social background so as to encourage free debate. A moderator guides the discussions, asks questions and helps the group to have a natural and free conversation. The questions asked help to focus the discussion on one or two topics of interest to the organizer. The aim is to elicit the feelings, attitudes and opinions of people about the topic of interest. The focus group method is used in health programmes to:

- explore a topic about which little is known;
- discover community attitude to a service, project or plan;
- fine tune a project from suggestions offered by participants;

- identify why the community is not responding to an initiative, e.g. change of behaviour, use of a service, etc.;
- evaluate a project from the point of view of the community and of the staff.

HEALTH EDUCATION METHODS

A variety of methods, both formal and informal, are used in health education. Some are personal, that is, involving a health worker in direct contact with an individual or a group. Others are impersonal, in which the communication does not involve such contact, for example the use of posters, leaflets, and the mass media (newspapers, radio, television, internet). Each method has its advantages and limitations.

PERSONAL

The personal methods, either in an interview on a one to one basis or in a group discussion, have the advantage that the content can be specifically tailored to match the needs of the individuals present. There is also the opportunity for discussion where obscure points can be clarified, objections raised and doubts expressed. Through such interactive exchange, the health worker can learn more about local beliefs and habits. It provides the opportunity for reviewing alternative approaches to the solution of specific problems and thereby the community and the individuals can determine how best to put the new lessons that they have learnt into practice in their own circumstances.

Communication skills

Whether talking to individual patients or groups of people, health workers must strive to be effective communicators. They must learn how to explain technical information in simple language that is easily understood. They must learn the skill of capturing and retaining the attention of their audiences. They must learn to deliver clear, interesting messages using humour where appropriate to highlight important issues. Where possible, they should enliven their presentations with vivid visual and sound materials.

IMPERSONAL METHODS

However, with the personal approach, each health worker can reach relatively few persons. The impersonal methods, especially the use of the mass media, have the advantage of reaching large numbers of people who may not have direct contact with health workers. The messages can be repeated over and over again, serving as reminder and reinforcement. In some communities, material read in the newspapers or heard on the radio carries more authority than information that is obtained from local sources.

Without the opportunity for questions and discussions, however, such messages may be misunderstood; constant repetition may dull their impact; and individuals may have difficulty in relating the messages to their own circumstances. By pretesting health education materials on a small scale before they are widely distributed one may overcome some of these limitations. On the findings from the pretest, one can modify the material and thereby make the message clearer.

COMBINED APPROACH

It is sometimes possible to combine the advantages of both methods. For example, wall charts, radio and television programmes and similar impersonal methods could be used as the focus for small group discussions. Alternatively, after a subject has been discussed, gifted members of the community could be encouraged to produce wall charts and other teaching materials for others in the community.

INNOVATIVE APPROACHES

Some health workers have experimented with innovative approaches to health education including music and drama as means of projecting health messages. Film star, sporting heroes, charismatic leaders and politicians are used to launch and sustain specific projects. Learning from commerce, some health workers have adapted marketing techniques for promoting health. Box 14.2 briefly summarizes this social marketing approach.

Box 14.2: Social marketing

Social marketing is the application of marketing principles and techniques to achieve social goals. The process usually involves four elements:

- Clearly defined, measurable goals, e.g. to promote the use of bed nets or condoms.
- Research to define community needs and perspectives: to find out what people want and need, and what they are prepared to buy.
- Design and optimization of product design based on research findings: packaging the product in a way that is attractive and usable.
- Effective communication of expected benefits (advertisement): promoting the product to the target audience.

OVERCOMING RESISTANCE TO CHANGE

Health workers are sometimes upset and can feel frustrated when they find that people do not immediately accept their advice. They seem surprised that people do not immediately change their behaviour once new information is given to them. Especially in matters affecting personal behaviour and on emotional issues like pregnancy and childcare, people are reluctant to have their ideas changed or even challenged. Although it is not always easy to change people's ideas one should explore strategies that have worked well in some cases.

PRESENT THE MATERIAL IN A NEW FORM WHICH IS MORE ACCEPTABLE TO THE PEOPLE

For example, if for religious reasons, the community does not eat meat, the health workers should devise a nutritionally balanced diet based on vegetables and, if acceptable, milk.

ASSOCIATE THE NEW IDEA WITH DESIRED GOALS

This is the approach favoured by commercial advertisers who link the use of their products with outcomes which are highly valued by the community. The general format of such advertisements is 'Use A (our product) to get B (what you want)'. The same approach can be effectively used in health education, provided false claims are not made.

REINFORCE THE SOCIAL NETWORK

By providing the same information to a wide circle of families and friends, one can reinforce the message that the individual receives. For example, the whole community should be educated about danger signs during pregnancy and childbirth. (see Chapter 12). This will reinforce the messages given to individual pregnant women and would facilitate decision-making during crises.

DRAW ATTENTION TO SUCCESSFUL EXAMPLES

Individuals, families and communities may provide useful examples for others in adopting a new idea. A useful strategy for introducing a new idea is to offer it first to groups who are most likely to accept it and put it into practice. They can then serve as useful examples for others. One device is the health show where prizes are awarded to individuals, families and communities who excel with regard to some particular health issue, for example the community with the highest immunization rate among children, the cleanest streets, etc.

WORK THROUGH OPINION LEADERS

In each community there are leaders whose views have a great influence within their society. Some of them are formal leaders holding recognized posts as political or religious leaders. Others hold important positions in local organizations such as women's clubs. However, there are other influential persons, the informal leaders, who do not hold such positions but who nevertheless have considerable influence on the community. Both groups should be identified and persuaded to adopt the new ideas and also to influence others to do so.

IDENTIFY AND PERSUADE INNOVATORS

Whereas some members of the community tend to be rigid in their views, there are others who tend to be more receptive to new ideas. It is worthwhile identifying such innovators, encouraging them and using them as instruments of change within their communities. On the whole, children tend to be more receptive than adults are, especially the elderly. Priority should be given to the health education of children, especially school children who in the process of their general education would be prepared to accept and test new ideas. At home they can influence their parents.

BE PATIENT AND AVOID CONFRONTATION

Head-on collision and confrontation could damage relationships between the health workers and the community. Even though the health workers are very anxious that the new ideas be accepted in the interest of the health of the population, they must be patient, retaining cordial relationships with the individuals and families in the hope of winning them over eventually. Table 14.1 outlines a simple framework for approaching traditional practices and beliefs.

Table 14.1: Official attitude to traditional practices and treatments

Health effect of the traditional practice or treatment	Examples	Recommendation
Beneficial	Prolonged breast-feeding	Reinforce and encourage
Harmful	Female genital mutilation	Discourage
Neutral	Traditional rituals	Leave to the discretion of individuals
Not known	Many traditional medicines	Research to determine effect

Table 14.2: Examples of modern risky lifestyles

Lifestyle	Comment
Sedentary habits	Risk factor for cardiovascular diseases and type II diabetes
Smoking, use of tobacco products	Rising epidemic of lung cancer and other diseases associated with the use of tobacco
Spirits and excessive use of other alcoholic drinks	Liver disease and other personal health problems and road traffic accidents associated with alcohol abuse
Substance abuse – marijuana, cocaine, etc;	Global epidemic of substance abuse including designer drugs like ectasy
Sex – multiple partners, unsafe sexual habits	The pandemic of HIV/AIDS is a compelling need for promoting safer sexual behaviour
Sugars, sweets and other refined foods	Modern processed foods tend to comprise highly refined carbohydrates with minimal roughage, with excess of fat, salt and/or sugars – risk factors for various chronic diseases
Stress	Faulty work habits; lack of leisure pursuits

REINFORCEMENT BY EXAMPLE

Health personnel should reinforce the formal teaching in health education by their own example. The members of the community observe the behaviour of the health workers and compare it with what they have learnt from lectures, interviews, posters and other forms of health education. They note the standard of personal hygiene of the health workers and of environmental sanitation at health centres, clinics and other health institutions; they observe social habits with regard to smoking and the use of alcohol; they compare the lessons that they have learnt about balanced diets with the food provided for patients in hospitals; and in many other ways they seek to reassure themselves about the value of the health education that is offered to them. If they consistently observe gross discrepancies between what is taught to them and what their teachers do, they are liable to become cynical and reject health education as a farce. It is therefore important that every contact with the health personnel and the health institutions should be a continuous exercise in health education.

MODERN BEHAVIOURAL CHALLENGES

Ignorance in health matters is not restricted to the illiterate people but it goes through all sections of society. In the past, health education in developing countries concentrated largely on basic hygiene and other measures for the prevention of classical communicable diseases. Now, populations in developing countries are adopting modern lifestyles that carry significant health risks (Table 14.2).

ASSESSING CHANGE AND PROGRESS

Assessment of the success of health education should relate to the objectives of the programme:

- increased awareness of relevant health issues;
- knowledge that is based on credible information;
- behavioural response.

Health workers should build into health education programmes indicators that would enable them to assess the changes that occur over time. Is there increased awareness of the particular problem? Are people in possession of correct information that would guide their decisions? Have they made appropriate response in the light of the new knowledge?

FURTHER READING

Anderson R. & Kickbusch I. (1990) *Health promotion: a resource book.* WHO Regional Office for Europe, Copenhagen.

Badura B. & Kickbusch I. (1990) *Health promotion research: towards a new social epidemiology*. WHO Regional Office for Europe, Copenhagen.

Dhillon B.H.S. & Philip L. (1994) *Health promotion and community action for health in developing countries*. WHO, Geneva.

Hubley J. (1993) *Communicating Health: An Action Guide to Health Education and Health Promotion*. Macmillan, London.

Maibach E. & Parrott R.L. (Eds) (1995) *Designing Health Messages: Approaches from Communication Theory and Public Health Practice*. Sage, Thousand Oaks, CA.

WHO (1983) *New Approaches to Health Education: Report of An Expert Committee*. Technical Report Series No. 690. WHO, Geneva.

WHO (1997) *Promoting Health Through Schools: Report of a WHO Expert Committee on Comprehensive School Health Education and Promotion*. Technical Report Series No. 870. WHO, Geneva.

Wurzbach M.E. (1997) *Community Health Education and Promotion: A Guide to Program Design and Evaluation*, 2nd edn. Aspen, New York.

ADDENDUM ADDED AT REPRINT

AVIAN FLU

Avian flu is acquired by infection with the H5N1 avian flu virus. Outbreaks of H5N1 disease have been reported among poultry in China, Kazakhstan, Cambodia, Indonesia, Japan, Lao People's Democratic Republic, Malaysia, Thailand, Vietnam and, more recently, Romania, Russia and Turkey (Asian part), and several countries in Europe. Mongolia has reported outbreaks of H5N1 in wild migratory birds, while the virus was found among migrating swans in Croatia. So far all known human cases, as well as all deaths, have occurred in Asia.

Transmission

The common mode of transmission is by direct contact with infected birds, e.g. slaughtering, defeathering, gutting and preparation of chicken and duck. Eating infected poultry is another mode of transmission. **No human to human transmission has been reported**.

Control

Culling is the most effective measure, complimented by vaccination. Greater public awareness of the problem is required.

WHO has advised governments, if they can afford it, to stockpile oseltamovir (Tamiflu), to stop a human pandemic, or possibly mitigate its impact, in the event that H5N1 mutates and human to human transmission is established. A global action plan to control avian flu in animals and the threat of a human avian flu pandemic has been outlined under the auspices of WHO.

CHAPTER FIFTEEN

INTERNATIONAL HEALTH CO-OPERATION

- Globalization and health
- Definition
- Mechanisms of international health co-operation
- The World Health Organization
- Other United Nations agencies
- The World Bank
- Bilateral aid agencies

- Non-governmental organizations
- Private foundations
- Other national organizations
- Public–private partnerships in international health
- International health regulations
- Further reading

GLOBALIZATION AND HEALTH

This is the age of globalization. Regional international treaties are bringing nations into union, multinational companies are merging to form larger and larger conglomerates whose branches spread all over the world; every year, millions of people travel from country to country for business and leisure, whilst war or famine displace others from their homes; rapid electronic communications transmit information around the world within seconds; and satellite communications bring events in real time from distant lands into living rooms. These trends have converted the world to what has been described as a global village with profound effects on the health of populations in every part of the world. Even in the most remote communities, these global trends affect human health and welfare. The effects of globalization on the health sector, both the opportunities and the risks, have stimulated greater interest in international co-operation for health.

DEFINITION

A simple definition of international health: '*A health activity involving persons, communities and/or institutions in two or more countries*'.

Interest in international health has its origins in the early ventures of international trade and travel and it antedates recent global events. Its history and evolution can be summarized in three simple phrases:

- born in fear;
- nurtured by compassion;
- sustained by the realization of mutual benefit.

FEAR

International health was born of fear. In earlier times, fear of the spread of epidemic diseases was the most prominent stimulus for international health action. For example, because of the fear of

Box 15.1: History of WHO and international co-operation in public health

1830	Cholera overruns Europe.
1851	First International Sanitary Conference is held in Paris to produce an international sanitary convention, but fails.
1892	International Sanitary Convention, restricted to cholera, is adopted.
1897	Another international convention dealing with preventive measures against plague is adopted.
1902	International Sanitary Bureau, later renamed Pan American Sanitary Bureau, and then Pan American Sanitary Organization, is set up in Washington DC. This is the forerunner of today's Pan American Health Organization (PAHO), which also serves as WHO's regional office for the Americas.
1907	L'Office International d'Hygiène Publique (OIHP) is established in Paris, with a permanent secretariat and a permanent committee of senior public health officials of Member Governments.
1919	League of Nations is created and is charged, among other tasks, with taking steps in matters of international concern for the prevention and control of disease. The Health Organization of the League of Nations is set up in Geneva, in parallel with the OIHP.
1926	International Sanitary Convention is revised to include provisions against smallpox and typhus.
1935	International Sanitary Convention for aerial navigation comes into force.
1938	Last International Sanitary Conference held in Paris. Conseil Sanitaire, Maritime et Quarantinaire at Alexandria is handed over to Egypt (the WHO Regional Office for the Eastern Mediterranean is its lineal descendant).
1945	United Nations Conference on International Organization in San Francisco unanimously approves a proposal by Brazil and China to establish a new, autonomous, international health organization.
1946	International Health Conference in New York approves the Constitution of the World Health Organization (WHO).
1947	WHO Interim Commission organizes assistance to Egypt to combat cholera epidemic.
1948	WHO Constitution comes into force on 7 April (now marked as World Health Day each year), when the 26th of the 61 Member States who signed it ratified its signature. Later, the First World Health Assembly is held in Geneva with delegations from 53 Governments that by then were Members.

the introduction of plague by ships coming from foreign lands, Italy required such vessels to remain anchored offshore for 40 days before docking to be sure that the crew and passengers were not infected with the plague. The Italian word *quaranta*, meaning 40, thus became the origin of the familiar term quarantine.

COMPASSION

Beyond fear, another strong motive for international health action is compassion. Medical missions, religious and humanitarian agencies, non-governmental organizations, and private voluntary organizations respond to health crises not only in their own communities but also in distant lands. With the rapid communications by satellite television and the internet, medical disasters are brought to the attention of people in their own homes and they respond by supporting international health

action. In situations of conflicts and natural disasters including epidemics, various agencies provide emergency relief and some of them stay on to strengthen routine health care.

MUTUAL BENEFIT

Fear and compassion are powerful motivations for international health but they have their limitations. Fear often generates illogical responses and after some time, its effect wanes. Similarly, compassion provides strong motivation in the spirit of solidarity with the poor and the afflicted, but it is difficult to sustain these strong emotions indefinitely; and as the feelings subside, donor fatigue may occur.

The third motivation for international health is the realization of mutual benefit. There is now a broader appreciation of international health as providing mutual benefits for all the participants, both developed and developing countries, both rich and poor, and both giver and recipient of aid. Rather than a donor–recipient relationship, the modern concept of international health is of co-operation and partnership based on mutuality and reciprocity. Partnership implies joint investment of effort towards the achievement of a common goal and an equitable sharing of the products. International co-operation based on the realization of mutual benefit is likely to be more enduring and sustainable than actions based solely on fear and/or compassion.

Collaborative programmes for disease control and health research illustrate the mutual benefit derived from international health.

Disease control

The eradication of smallpox is a good example of the mutual benefit resulting from international health action. The United States and other developed countries had long eliminated this infection from their countries but they faced the constant threat of the reintroduction of the infection from other countries. They were, therefore, obliged to establish and maintain mechanisms for protecting their populations from imported smallpox. These precautions were complex and costly. When smallpox was finally eradicated, they were able to dismantle the protective mechanisms. It is estimated that since smallpox was eradicated, the United States government has saved the equivalent of its annual contributions to WHO every 6 weeks! Now that poliomyelitis has been eliminated from the western hemisphere, there is a strong drive to protect this gain by achieving global eradication of the infection.

Health research

The last century has demonstrated the value of health research as a vital tool for health development. Although health research is mainly organized through national institutions, there is a growing appreciation of the value of international collaboration. WHO has organized major health research programmes on human reproduction and tropical diseases. These international networks have produced useful products that are being successfully applied in health programmes.

Reverse benefits

Research carried out by scientists in the north has greatly benefited people living in developing countries. Less well known and often overlooked are the occasions when the flow of benefit has been in the opposite direction; cases in which developed countries benefited from research done in developing countries. In the field of health-care delivery, the north has adopted some innovative ideas that were first tested out in the south. For example, studies that were done in India showed that supervised ambulatory care of tuberculosis gives as good results as the traditional institutional care in sanatoria. This finding reshaped the tuberculosis control programmes of developed countries. Similarly, experiments in the use of paramedical personnel in health-care delivery, innovative community-based programmes in mental health and similar initiatives in the south have informed and influenced the north.

MECHANISMS OF INTERNATIONAL HEALTH CO-OPERATION

Mechanisms for international health co-operation include bilateral agreements between nations including financial and technical support, exchange of scientific information and various forms of assistance. Co-operation may be multilateral, involving the governments of many nations on a regional or global scale.

INTERNATIONAL AGENCIES PROMOTING HEALTH

Agencies may be divided into the following categories:

- *multilateral governmental agencies*, e.g. WHO, UNICEF, UNFPA and other UN agencies, The World Bank, regional groups of countries, e.g. the European Union;
- *bilateral government aid programmes*, e.g. UK Department for International Development (DFID), Swedish International Development Agency (SIDA), United States Agency for International Development (USAID);

- *non-governmental organizations*, e.g. the International Committee of the Red Cross, League of Red Cross and Red Crescent Associations, private foundations, charities.

THE WORLD HEALTH ORGANIZATION

Within the United Nations (UN) System, the World Health Organization (WHO) has the constitutional responsibility for co-ordinating international co-operation for health and it plays a leading role in this area in collaboration with other UN agencies as well as non-governmental organizations. Founded in 1947, WHO now has 191 member states. Its headquarters are located in Geneva, Switzerland and it has six regional offices:

- *African Regional Offices* (AFRO) Harare, Zimbabwe;[1]
- *Regional Office for the Americas* (AMR0) Washington, DC, USA;
- *Eastern Mediterranean Regional Office* (EMRO) Cairo, Egypt;
- *European Regional Office* (EURO) Copenhagen, Denmark;
- *South East Asia Regional Office* (SEARO) New Delhi, India;
- *West Pacific Regional Office* (WPRO) Manila, Philippines.

In many countries, there is a resident WHO representative, who is responsible for WHO's activities in the country, and who supports the government in the planning and management of national health programmes.

STRENGTHENING OF HEALTH SERVICES

WHO co-operates with member states in the strengthening and reorientation of their health services, with particular reference to the primary health care services. The foundation of current policy about health care is based on the Alma Ata Declaration that

---

Box 15.2: WHO's objectives and functions

The objective of WHO is the attainment by all peoples of the highest possible level of health. Health, as defined in the WHO Constitution, is *'a state of complete physical, mental and social well-being and not merely the absence of disease or infirmity'*. In support of its main objective, the organization has a wide range of functions, including the following:

- to act as the directing and co-ordinating authority on international health work;
- to promote technical co-operation;
- to assist governments, upon request, in strengthening health services;
- to furnish appropriate technical assistance and, in emergencies, necessary aid, upon the request or acceptance of governments;
- to stimulate and advance work on the prevention and control of epidemic, endemic and other diseases;
- to promote, in co-operation with other specialized agencies where necessary, the improvement of nutrition, housing, sanitation, recreation, economic or working conditions and other aspects of environmental hygiene;
- to promote and co-ordinate biomedical and health services research;
- to promote improved standards of teaching and training in the health, medical and related professions;
- to establish and stimulate the establishment of international standards for biological, pharmaceutical and similar products, and to standardize diagnostic procedures;
- to foster activities in the field of mental health, especially those activities affecting the harmony of human relations.

WHO also proposes conventions, agreements, regulations and makes recommendations about international nomenclature of diseases, causes of death and public health practices. It develops, establishes and promotes international standards concerning foods and biological, pharmaceutical and similar substances.

---

[1] Temporarily evacuated from Congo, Brazzaville.

was adopted in 1978. WHO continues to promote the goal of 'Health for All', by which it means that resources for health should be evenly distributed and that essential health care be accessible to everyone.

TECHNICAL SERVICES

WHO's technical services are briefly illustrated in Box 15.3.

TECHNICAL INFORMATION

The Organization publishes a number of technical documents – printed material as well as a very active website on the internet (http://www.who.int/) from which documents can be downloaded:

- *Technical Report Series* – summarizing views of expert committees and other scientific groups on specific subjects;

Box 15.3: WHO's technical services on major communicable and non-communicable diseases

Preventing and controlling specific health problems:

- vaccine-preventable diseases;
- tropical diseases;
- malaria;
- tuberculosis;
- diarrhoeal diseases;
- acute respiratory infections;
- integrated management of childhood illness;
- HIV/AIDS;
- sexually transmitted diseases;
- new and re-emerging infectious diseases;
- heart disease;
- mental health.

Special programmes that have been organized to promote action in some high-priority areas:

- human reproduction programme (HRP);
- tropical diseases research (TDR);
- integrated management of childhood infections (IMCI);
- global programme for vaccination (GPV) (expanded programme of immunization – EPI);
- special programme on AIDS (GPA);
- roll back malaria (RBM);
- STOP TB initiative.

- *World Health Bulletin* – publishing scientific papers, either original articles or scientific reviews;
- *World Health Report* (WHR) – annual publication usually focusing on a specific issue or problem, e.g. WHR 2000 *Health Systems*: *Improving Performance*. WHR 2001 *Mental Health*: *New Understanding, New Hope*.
- *Weekly Epidemiological Records* – this contains epidemiological information about the occurrence of communicable diseases.

OTHER UNITED NATIONS AGENCIES

Apart from WHO, other UN agencies play a significant role in health. WHO collaborates with these other agencies:

- *United Nations Children's Fund* (UNICEF) is concerned with matters affecting the welfare of children (see below). It co-sponsored the Alma Ata conference;
- *Food and Agricultural Organization* (FAO) collaborates in the area of nutrition and also African trypanosomiasis and other infections which affect both humans and farm animals;
- *International Labour Organization* (ILO) deals with matters affecting the health of workers (see p. 243).
- *United Nations Environmental Programme* (UNEP) is concerned with matters affecting the environment (see Chapter 13);
- *United Nations Development Programme* (UNDP) co-ordinates UN activities in the area of development.

UNICEF

The United Nations Children's Emergency Fund was established after the Second World War. Now renamed the United Nations Children Fund, UNICEF defines its mandate and mission as being an advocate for children's rights and helping to meet their needs. UNICEF 'is guided by the Convention on the Rights of the Child and strives to establish children's rights as enduring ethical principles and international standards of behaviour towards children'.

UNICEF now works in 161 countries, areas and territories on solutions to the problems plaguing poor children and their families and on ways to realize their rights. It is financed very largely by voluntary contributions from governments, private foundations and public donations.

Aims

It attempts to mobilize all groups in societies to be concerned about improving the survival of children through the widespread dissemination of technologies that can save children's lives and improve their well-being. UNICEF's approach implies that technology can and will bring about great changes in the likelihood of children reaching adolescence even when social and economic conditions appear to be unsatisfactory. UNICEF has also campaigned for increased attention to child health and well-being in countries that are economically deprived and are undergoing structural adjustment.

Programmes

Its activities are as varied as the challenges it faces, encouraging the care and stimulation that offer the best possible start in life, helping prevent childhood illness and death, making pregnancy and childbirth safe, combating discrimination and co-operating with communities to ensure that girls as well as boys attend school.

As the main prop of its child survival programme, UNICEF has been particularly concerned with the delivery of a package of interventions: GOBI-FFF: growth monitoring, oral rehydration, breast feeding, immunization, family planning,

Box 15.4: Examples of UNICEF health-related programmes developed and implemented with partners

- The Global Alliance for Vaccines and Immunization (GAVI).
- Eradication of poliomyelitis.
- The vitamin A global initiative.
- Controlling malaria, a major child killer.
- Education for All.
- Reducing global poverty.

female literacy and supplementary feeding, particularly for pregnant women.

THE WORLD BANK

The World Bank is involved in lending funds for development. Activities such as the creation of man-made lakes and large-scale irrigation schemes carry major implications for health. The World Bank is therefore involved in the assessment of the health aspects of development projects which it sponsors. More recently, the World Bank is playing an increasingly active role in organization and reform of the health sector. Its publication, *Investing in Health: World Development Report 1993*, provided useful guidance for the reform of health services to improve efficiency, cost-effectiveness and equity.

PROGRAMMES

Themes in the Bank's present health sector work include: (i) strengthening of management systems; (ii) health policy; (iii) for Africa south of the Sahara developing peripheral health care systems; and (iv) training of health sector staff and establishing appropriate strategies for health sector financing. The Bank is also concentrating on specific health problem areas which it believes are not being examined and tackled in a systematic fashion, including maternal mortality, malaria, nutrition and non-communicable chronic diseases. Through its Population, Health and Nutrition department, it works with WHO and other partners, health research and other initiatives.

POVERTY AND DEBT RELIEF

International organizations are much concerned about the impact of poverty and macro-economic policies on health. For example, under pressure from the international finance agencies, some developing countries undertook structural adjustment programmes (SAP) and markedly reduced public investment in health and other social sectors. UNICEF and other agencies drew attention to negative impact of SAP on the health of children; they proposed modification of the programme to protect essential health functions – 'structural adjustment with a human face'.

The burden of debt on the poorest countries has also invited attention in recent years. Currently, the 52 poorest countries of which 37 are in Africa, owe a total of $376 billion. These countries pay the same amount in debt service as they spend on health and education combined. It has been estimated that if funds were diverted back into health and education from debt repayment, the lives of 7 million children a year could be saved.

In response to the concerns about the impact of macro-economic policies, WHO set up a Commission on Macroeconomics and Health (CMH); it produced a series of studies on how concrete health interventions can lead to economic growth and reduce inequity in developing countries. It recommended a set of measures designed to maximize the poverty reduction and economic development benefits of health sector investment (Boxes 15.5 and 15.6).

BILATERAL AID AGENCIES

Much of the foreign aid provided to developing countries is made available through bilateral

---

Box 15.5: Report of the Commission on Macroeconomics and Health: Investing in Health for Economic Development

Key findings on the linkages of health and development

1 Health is a priority goal in its own right, as well as a central input into economic development and poverty reduction. The importance of investing in health has been greatly underestimated, not only by analysts but also by developing-country governments and the international donor community.
2 A few health conditions are responsible for a high proportion of the health deficit: HIV/AIDS, malaria, TB, childhood infectious diseases (many of which are preventable by vaccination), maternal and perinatal conditions, tobacco-related illnesses, and micronutrient deficiencies. Effective interventions exist to prevent and treat these conditions. Around 8 million deaths per year from these conditions could be averted by the end of the decade in a well-focused programme.
3 The HIV/AIDS pandemic is a distinct and unparalleled catastrophe in its human dimension and its implications for economic development. It therefore requires special consideration. Tried and tested interventions within the health sector are available to address most of the causes of the health deficit, including HIV/AIDS.
4 Investments in reproductive health, including family planning and access to contraceptives, are crucial accompaniments of investments in disease control. The combination of disease control and reproductive health is likely to translate into reduced fertility, greater investments in the health and education of each child, and reduced population growth.
5 The level of health spending in the low-income countries is insufficient to address the health challenges they face. We estimate that minimum financing needs to be around $30 to $40 per person per year to cover essential interventions, including those needed to fight the AIDS pandemic, with much of that sum requiring budgetary rather than private-sector financing. Actual health spending is considerably lower. The least developed countries average approximately $13 per person per year in total health expenditures, of which budgetary outlays are just $7. The other low-income countries average approximately $24 per capita per year, of which budgetary outlays are $13.
6 Poor countries can increase the domestic resources that they mobilize for the health sector and use those resources more efficiently. Even with more efficient allocation and greater resource mobilization, the levels of funding necessary to cover essential services are far beyond the financial means of many low-income countries, as well as a few middle-income countries with high prevalence of HIV/AIDS.
7 Donor finance will be needed to close the financing gap, in conjunction with best efforts by the recipient countries themselves. ... This funding should be additional to other donor financing, since increased aid is also needed in other related areas such as education, water, and sanitation.

Box 15.6: Report of the Commission on Macroeconomics and Health: Investing in Health for Economic Development

Highlights of major recommendations

An Action Agenda for Investing in Health for Economic Development:

1   Each low- and middle-income country should establish a temporary National Commission on Macro-economics and Health (NCMH), or its equivalent, to formulate a long-term programme for scaling up essential health interventions ... The WHO and the World Bank should assist national Commissions to establish epidemiological baselines, operational targets, and a framework for long-term donor financing.

2   The financing strategy should envisage an increase of domestic budgetary resources for health of 1% of GNP by 2007 and 2% of GNP by 2015. ...

3   The international donor community should commit adequate grant resources for low-income countries to ensure universal coverage of essential interventions as well as scaled-up R&D and other public goods.

4   The international community should establish two new funding mechanisms, with the following approximate scale of annual outlays by 2007: The Global Fund to Fight AIDS, Tuberculosis, and Malaria (GFATM), $8 billion; and the Global Health Research Fund (GHRF), $1.5 billion. Additional R&D outlays of $1.5 billion per year should be channelled through existing institutions such as TDR, IVR, and HRP at WHO, as well as the Global Forum for Health Research and various public–private partnerships that are currently aiming toward new drug and vaccine development. Country programmes should also direct at least 5% of outlays to operational research.

5   The supply of other Global Public Goods (GPGs) should be bolstered through additional financing of relevant international agencies such as the World Health Organization and World Bank by $1 billion per year as of 2007 and $2 billion per year as of 2015. These GPGs include disease surveillance at the international level, data collection and analysis of global health trends (such as burden of disease), analysis and dissemination of international best practices in disease control and health systems, and technical assistance and training.

6   To support private-sector incentives for late-stage drug development, existing 'orphan drug legislation' in the high-income countries should be modified to cover diseases of the poor, such as the tropical vector-borne diseases. In addition, the GFATM and other donor purchasing entities should establish pre-commitments to purchase new targeted products at commercially viable prices.

7   The international pharmaceutical industry, in co-operation with low-income countries and the WHO, should ensure access of the low-income countries to essential medicines through commitments to provide essential medicines at the lowest viable commercial price in the low-income countries, and to license the production of essential medicines to generics producers as warranted by cost and/or supply conditions....

8   The World Trade Organization member governments should ensure sufficient safeguards for the developing countries, and in particular the right of countries that do not produce the relevant pharmaceutical products to invoke compulsory licensing for imports from third-country generics suppliers.

9   The International Monetary Fund and World Bank should work with recipient countries to incorporate the scaling up of health and other poverty-reduction programmes into a viable macroeconomic framework.

government to government programmes involving industrialized countries as donors and developing countries as recipients. This pattern of aid is usually an important element of donor governments' overseas policies and is administered by an agency that is part of the Ministry of Foreign Affairs or equivalent within the donor government. Examples of such agencies include USAID, Britain's DFID, Norway's NORAD, Denmark's DANIDA, Canada's CIDA and Japan's JICA. Bilateral donors frequently join up

with multilateral organizations (in multi-bi projects) especially when large schemes are being envisaged.

Usually about 5% of a bilateral agency's budget is made available for health sector work. Most bilateral agencies' health policies now make direct reference to encouraging the development of primary health care. However, in practice programmes have to be negotiated between the donor and recipient countries and the number of different commercial, political and economic factors may determine the eventual shape of a health sector aid programme.

DONOR STIPULATIONS

Bilateral agencies may require that this aid is used to purchase goods manufactured within the donor country. Donor programmes are frequently oriented towards the provision of capital costs and not recurrent costs; this can be a serious problem if the donor supplies high technology goods or buildings which the recipient country needs to maintain once donor support ceases. There is always a tendency for donor assistance to be directed by priorities determined from within the donor country. Aid may not be responsive to the recipient country's needs or concerns.

RECENT IMPROVEMENTS IN INTERNATIONAL AID POLICIES

Co-ordination

In the last few years bilateral agencies have been reassessing health sector aid policies, especially how they can co-operate with each other and link their health programmes with general development activities aimed at the alleviation of poverty. Generally, these external agencies operate independently of each other but there have been some attempts at co-ordination and collaboration. UNICEF and WHO have established mechanisms of collaboration including such formal mechanism as the Task Force for Child Survival. WHO also sometimes executes health programmes on behalf of other external agencies. A more ambitious attempt at interagency collaboration is the UNAIDS programme; six UN agencies jointly manage this programme for the global control of HIV/AIDS epidemic.

Bilateral aid programmes vary considerably in their content, their duration and their interaction with other external agencies. Some of them narrowly focus on the specific interest of the donor countries, for example family planning. There is, however, a new move to achieve more effective co-ordination of external aid through the mechanism of sector-wide expenditure planning. The idea is to develop in each country a programme based on national priorities and funded from national resources supplemented by donor aid. All participating donors subscribe to the national plan and contribute their donation to a common fund without earmarking to specific projects.

NON-GOVERNMENTAL ORGANIZATIONS

A number of non-governmental organizations are actively involved in international health and development. These include multinational groups like the Christian Medical Commission (which is a medical body of the World Council of Churches), the League of Red Cross Societies and the Save the Children Alliance.

THE INTERNATIONAL RED CROSS

The International Council of the Red Cross and the League of Red Cross Societies (Crescent) play an important part in providing relief in cases of natural disasters.

THE GLOBAL FORUM FOR HEALTH RESEARCH

The Global Forum for Health Research is an international foundation managed by a Foundation Council, representing a broad range of partners, for example representatives from governments, multilateral and bilateral aid agencies, international and national foundations and NGOs, women's organizations, research institutions and universities, pharmaceutical companies and the media.

Spending on health research by both the public and private sectors amounts to about US $56 billion per year (1992 estimate). However, less than 10% of this is devoted to diseases or conditions that account for 90% of the global disease burden. The central objective of the Global Forum for Health Research is to help correct the 10/90 gap and focus research efforts on the health problems of the poor by improving the allocation of research funds and by facilitating collaboration among partners in both the public and private sectors.

PRIVATE FOUNDATIONS

Most of these foundations work within national boundaries, but some have substantial international activities, for example Rockefeller Foundation, Wellcome Trust, Ford Foundation, Melinda and Bill Gates Foundation, and Sasakawa Foundation.

OTHER NATIONAL ORGANIZATIONS

Some large organizations based in developed countries are concerned with disaster relief. These rely on public donations and often have a high profile though the overall scale of their overseas programmes is relatively small. Some are missionary organizations, others secular. Some are primarily concerned with disaster relief, others with long-term development. World Vision, Christian Aid, Medecins sans Frontieres, Oxfam and Save the Children Fund are all well-known examples of such organizations. Some of these organizations are concerned with specific diseases or disabilities, such as the World Commonwealth Society for the Blind or the European Leprosy Association.

PUBLIC–PRIVATE PARTNERSHIPS IN INTERNATIONAL HEALTH

In recent years, there has been a trend towards increasing collaboration between the public sector and private industry. This relationship is reflected in collaborative ventures in international health involving research and development as well as programmes for increasing access to medicines in developing countries. For example, the tropical diseases research programme that is jointly co-sponsored by the World Bank United Nations Development Programme and the World Health Organization co-operates closely with pharmaceutical companies in research and development of new drugs and diagnostics for parasitic and infectious diseases. Several major programmes involving large donations of drugs from private companies have also involved collaboration between the private and public sectors. For example, Merck & Co.'s donation of 30–40 million doses of ivermectin a year for the control of onchocerciasis is currently the main strategy for the elimination of onchocerciasis as a blinding disease. Similarly, Pfizer is donating the broad-spectrum antibiotic, azithromycin, in support of collaborative programmes for the elimination of trachoma.

INTERNATIONAL HEALTH REGULATIONS

One of the early functions of the health programme of the League of Nations was to establish sanitary regulations dealing with various problems but most prominently the control of infectious diseases that were regarded as international threats. The international health regulations are intended to ensure the maximum security against the international spread of disease with the minimum interference of world traffic. Rapid travel by jet aeroplane has increased the risk of international transmission of infectious disease. Not only can sick travellers transmit infections but arthropod vectors can also be rapidly moved from one end of the world to the other. For example, mosquitoes can survive over long distances in aeroplanes and 'airport malaria' has occurred in countries where the disease is not normally transmitted, for example Britain, France, Belgium.

The World Health Assembly adopted the current International Health Regulations (IHR) in 1971, replacing the International Sanitary Regulations, which had been in force since 1951. They were first introduced to help monitor and control four serious diseases, which had significant potential to spread between countries. The goals of the IHR are to:

- detect, reduce or eliminate sources from which infection spreads;
- improve sanitation in and around ports and airports;
- prevent dissemination of vectors.

The IHR require mandatory declaration of cholera, plague and yellow fever (smallpox was removed in 1981). They do not cover several diseases of international importance including ebola and other haemorrhagic fevers. International Health Regulations (IHR) are currently being revised in accordance with a resolution adopted by the World Health Assembly in 1995. The on-going revision process aims to develop IHR which will effectively adapt to emerging trends in the epidemiology of communicable diseases as well as international trade in the 21st century.

These regulations have been modified over time:

- smallpox has been removed from the list of diseases subject to IHR and therefore an international certificate of vaccination should no longer be required from any traveller;
- the only certificate that is now required, from a limited number of international travellers, is that for yellow fever vaccination;
- the requirement of cholera vaccination certificates, or indeed any other vaccination certificates, is in excess of the terms of the International Health Regulations.

NATIONAL PORT HEALTH PROGRAMMES

Most countries have a Quarantine and Epidemiology Branch at the Ministry of Health which deals with:

- port health;
- airport health;
- quarantine stations or hospitals;
- vaccination.

The aim of such a division is to guard against the import and export of diseases, thus keeping the indigenous population reservoir as small as possible and honestly notifying WHO of the latest situation in the country, irrespective of the local consequences. Regulations need to be supported by the epidemiological surveillance of disease: the study of a disease as a dynamic process involving the ecology of the infectious agent, the host, the reservoirs, the vectors and the role of the environment.

Seaports

When a ship is infected (e.g. with a case of plague) the following action has to be taken:

- isolation of case;
- revaccination of those passengers and crew without valid certificates;
- isolation of close contacts (incubation period of 14 days);
- surveillance of other contacts (14 days);
- disinfection of patient's cabin, etc. (not whole ship);
- international notification.

At quarantine stations and hospitals compulsory revaccination takes place, as well as group isolation and medical surveillance. Sanitary examination of ships, especially water, toilets, kitchen and food storage compartments should be carried out and the deratization certificate examined. When a ship flies the 'Q' flag, no one is permitted to board or leave the ship before the Port Health Officer.

With most travellers now using air rather than sea and with the advent of container ships carrying relatively small numbers of crew members, port health is now a good deal less important than in the past. The smuggling of narcotics and arms now pose a greater threat.

Airports

The increase in the volume as well as speed of travel means that travellers infected in one country may still feel quite well when they arrive in another, if they are in the early stages of their illness. In these circumstances, the surveillance and the precautions taken at airports of arrival are often ineffective. None the less, airport health services are rapidly being developed all over the world. They may perform the following functions:

PASSENGERS AND STAFF

- Vaccination and inoculation of passengers and crews when necessary.
- Vaccination and inoculation of all airport personnel who come in contact with aircraft from infected ports.
- Examination of suspected passengers.
- Placing of passengers under surveillance when necessary.

AIRCRAFT

- Inspection of aircraft coming from yellow fever infected areas for the presence of *Aedes* mosquitoes and to carry out disinsectation, if necessary (knock down spraying to kill anopheles).
- Sending of specimens of toilet wastes from planes for bacteriological examination to ascertain whether adequate disinfection is being carried out.

- Periodic sampling of food and potable water supplied to the aircraft to ascertain whether these are fit for human consumption and that they have not been contaminated by bacteria or chemical substances.

AIRPORTS

- Inspection to ensure that the airport precincts are kept in a satisfactory state including the airport restaurant and flight kitchen.
- Supervision of the control of *Aedes* and other mosquitoes within the control zone of the airport perimeter.
- Maintenance and running of the casualty clearing station in case of air disaster.
- Provision of outpatient treatment facilities for cases of minor illnesses (for passengers and airport staff).

FURTHER READING

Global Forum for Health Research (1999) *The 10/90 Report On Health Research.* Global Forum for Health Research, Geneva.

Newell K.W. (1985) Global strategies – developing a unified strategy. In: Holland W.W., Detels R. and Knox G. (Eds) *Oxford Textbook of Public Health.* Oxford University Press, Oxford, pp. 261–271.

Patten C. (1988) Britain's role and responsibility for health in the tropics. *Transactions of the Royal Society of Tropical Medicine and Hygiene* 82: 660–664.

UNICEF (1999) *The State of the World's Children 1998.* Published for UNICEF by the Oxford University Press (annual publication).

WHO (1997) *International Travel and Health – Vaccination Requirements and Health Advice.* WHO, Geneva.

WHO (2001) *Macroeconomics and health: investing in health for economic development.* Report of the Commission on Macroeconomics and Health, December 2001.

World Bank (1993) *World Development Report 1993: Investing in Health.* Oxford University Press, New York.

World Bank (1994) *Better Health in Africa: Experience and Lessons Learnt.* World Bank, Washington, DC.

WEBSITE ADDRESSES OF SELECTED ORGANIZATIONS ACTIVE IN INTERNATIONAL HEALTH

Major intergovernmental agencies

World Health Organization (WHO)
http://www.who.int/

World Bank
http://www.worldbank.org/

United Nations Children's Fund (UNICEF)
http://www.unicef.org/

United Nations Population Fund (UNFPA)
http://www.unfpa.org/

United Nations Development Programme (UNDP)
http://www.undp.org/

Examples of other international agencies and programmes

Task Force for Child Survival and Development
http://www.taskforce.org/

International Trachoma Initiative
http://www.trachoma.org/

Global Forum for Health Research
http://www.globalforumhealth.org/

INDEX

Abbreviations: GI, gastrointestinal.

Printed and bound by CPI Group (UK) Ltd, Croydon, CR0 4YY

23/10/2024

01778255-0002